BACKPACKING WASHINGTON

From the book . . .

OLYMPIC COAST: NORTH (TRIP 1)

The wild Olympic coast is a national treasure. . . . You will see crashing waves, scenic off-shore rocks, dense inland forests, and abundant wildlife.

ENCHANTED VALLEY–LACROSSE BASIN LOOP (TRIP 4)

Amid glorious mountain scenery, the trip samples every major environment in the range, from lush rainforests to glaciers. There is also plenty of wildlife—including marmots, deer, elk, and black bears—to enjoy. The route runs alongside a strikingly beautiful stream and climaxes in the most sublime alpine basin in the entire range.

CHELAN SUMMIT TRAIL (TRIP 12)

Protected by the moisture-loving ranges to the west, these drier mountains feature open forests and beautiful meadows that provide endless vistas of distant peaks. . . . In the last few days of September and the first week of October, [Lyall "alpine" larches] put on arguably the best fall-color display in the state.

DOWNEY CREEK TO CUB LAKE (TRIP 14)

Itswoot Lake and its soul-stirring blue depths are complemented by a waterfall with a jagged skyline of mountains behind it and hungry trout beneath its surface. If the berries are ripe and the weather is good, this area is as close to paradise as most backpackers can get.

GLACIER PEAK LOOP (TRIP 15)

Taking in all of this remarkable landscape requires a long and rugged adventure. . . . But if you are up for the challenge, this could be the trip of a lifetime.

MOUNT RAINIER: WONDERLAND TRAIL LOOP (TRIP 19)

The route provides a generous sampling of all the attractions in the Cascade Range, including meadows choked with wildflowers, abundant and varied wildlife, old-growth forests, huge glaciers, impressive waterfalls, and scenic lakes.

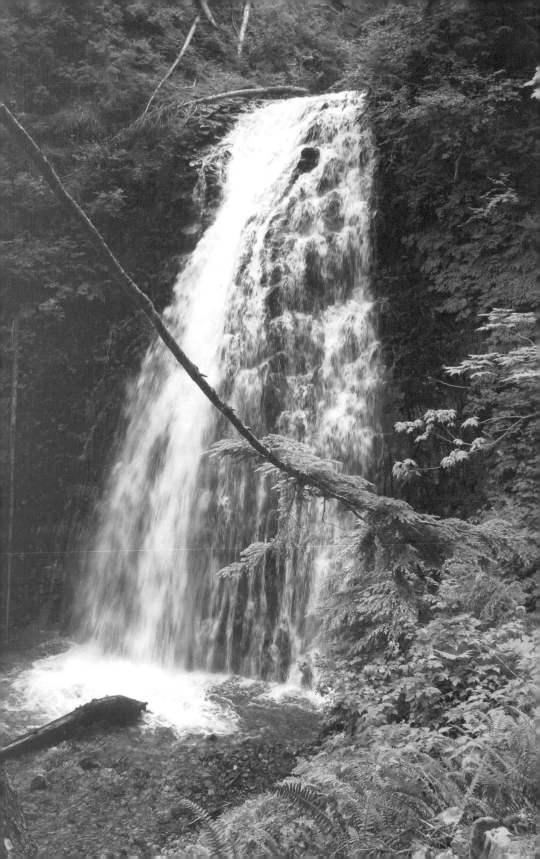

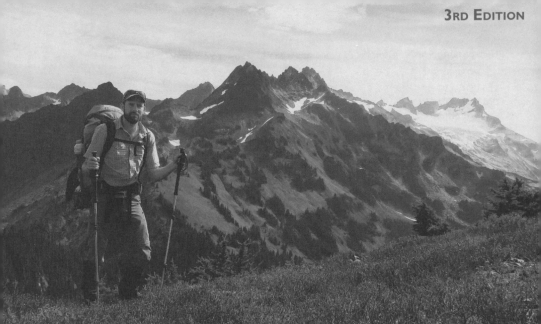

BACKPACKING
WASHINGTON

From Volcanic Peaks to Rainforest Valleys

DOUGLAS LORAIN
and
MARK WETHERINGTON

 WILDERNESS PRESS . . . **on the trail since 1967**

Backpacking Washington: From Volcanic Peaks to Rainforest Valleys

1st EDITION 2000
2nd EDITION 2007
3rd EDITION 2020
   3rd printing 2021

Library of Congress Cataloging-in-Publication Data

Names: Lorain, Douglas, 1962- author.
Title: Backpacking Washington : from volcanic peaks to rainforest valleys / Douglas Lorain and Mark
    Wetherington.
Description: Third Edition. | Birmingham, Alabama : Wilderness Press, [2020] | "2nd EDITION 2007"—
    T.p. verso. | "Distributed by Publishers Group West"—T.p. verso. | Includes index.
Identifiers: LCCN 2019016591| ISBN 9780899978567 (paperback) | ISBN 9780899978574 (ebook)
Subjects: LCSH: Backpacking—Washington (State)—Guidebooks. | Hiking—Washington (State)—Guidebooks.
    | Day hiking—Washington (State)—Guidebooks. | Walking—Washington (State)—Guidebooks.
    | Camping—Washington (State)—Guidebooks. | Mountaineering—Washington (State)—Guidebooks.
    | Rock climbing—Washington (State)—Guidebooks. | Trails—Washington (State)—Guidebooks. |
    Outdoor recreation—Washington (State)—Guidebooks. | Washington (State)—Guidebooks.
Classification: LCC GV199.42.W2 L67 2020 | DDC 796.509797—dc23
LC record available at https://lccn.loc.gov/2019016591

Manufactured in the United States of America

Published by: **WILDERNESS PRESS**
   An imprint of AdventureKEEN
   2204 First Avenue S., Ste. 102
   Birmingham, AL 35233
   800-443-7227; FAX 205-326-1012

Visit wildernesspress.com for a complete listing of our books and for ordering information. Contact us at our website, at facebook.com/wildernesspress1967, or at twitter.com/wilderness1967 with questions or comments. To find out more about who we are and what we're doing, visit blog.wildernesspress.com.

Distributed by Publishers Group West

Front cover photos: top: Trip 14, Downey Creek to Cub Lake (page 126); photographed by Mark Wetherington. *Bottom, left to right:* Trip 14, Downey Creek to Cub Lake (page 126); photographed by Mark Wetherington. Trip 23, Loowit Trail Loop (page 221); photographed by Mark Wetherington. Louis Creek Falls (Trip 15, page 132); photographed by Douglas Lorain.
Back cover photo: Trip 5, Northeastern Olympics Loop (page 52); photographed by Mark Wetherington.
Frontispiece: Martha Falls (Trip 19, page 177); photographed by Douglas Lorain.

Safety Notice: Although Wilderness Press and the authors have made every attempt to ensure that the information in this book is accurate at press time, they are not responsible for any loss, damage, injury, or inconvenience that may occur to anyone while using this book. You are responsible for your own safety and health while in the wilderness. The fact that a trail is described in this book does not mean that it will be safe for you. Be aware that trail conditions can change from day to day. Always check local conditions and know your own limitations.

CONTENTS

Map Legend

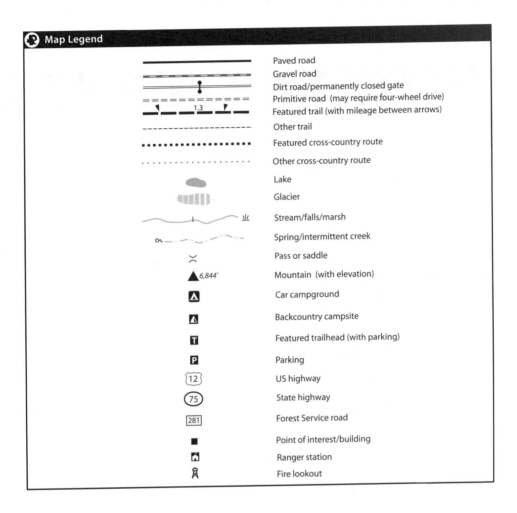

	Paved road
	Gravel road
	Dirt road/permanently closed gate
	Primitive road (may require four-wheel drive)
1.3	Featured trail (with mileage between arrows)
	Other trail
	Featured cross-country route
	Other cross-country route
	Lake
	Glacier
	Stream/falls/marsh
	Spring/intermittent creek
	Pass or saddle
▲ 6,844'	Mountain (with elevation)
	Car campground
	Backcountry campsite
T	Featured trailhead (with parking)
P	Parking
12	US highway
75	State highway
281	Forest Service road
■	Point of interest/building
	Ranger station
	Fire lookout

FEATURED TRIPS SUMMARY TABLE

	TRIP NUMBER & NAME (grouped by typically best month)
MAY	
1	Olympic Coast: North (p. 16)
24	Yakima Skyline Trail (p. 228)
JUNE	
22	Mount Margaret Backcountry Loop (p. 212)
23	Loowit Trail Loop (p. 221)
26	Wenaha-Tucannon Loop (p. 241)
JULY	
4	Enchanted Valley–LaCrosse Basin Loop (p. 43)
5	Northeastern Olympics Loop (p. 52)
6	Dungeness–Marmot Pass Loop (p. 60)
10	Buckskin Ridge–Ptarmigan Peak Loop (p. 94)
13	Entiat River Loop (p. 119)
14	Downey Creek to Cub Lake (p. 126)
20	Goat Rocks Circuit (p. 193)
25	Salmo-Priest Loop (p. 234)
AUGUST	
3	High Divide–Hoh River Traverse (p. 35)
7	Northern North Cascades Loop (p. 67)
8	Southern North Cascades Loop (p. 74)
9	Western Pasayten–Ross Lake Loop (p. 83)
15	Glacier Peak Loop (p. 132)
16	Chiwaukum–Ladies Pass Loop (p. 146)
17	Alpine Lakes Traverse (p. 154)
18	Northern Mount Rainier Loop (p. 168)
19	Mount Rainier: Wonderland Trail Loop (p. 177)
21	Mount Adams Highline Trail Loop (p. 200)
SEPTEMBER	
11	Eastern Pasayten Loop (p. 104)
12	Chelan Summit Trail (p. 111)
OCTOBER	
2	Olympic Coast: South (p. 28)

RATINGS (1–10)			LENGTH IN:		ELEVATION GAIN	SHUTTLE MILEAGE
SCENERY	**SOLITUDE**	**DIFFICULTY**	**DAYS**	**MILES**		
9	4	9	4–7	33	1,100'	68
6	3	4	2–3	27	6,800'	n/a
9	3	9	3–5	28	6,300'	n/a
9	4	9	3	34	4,700'	n/a
7	8	8	4–7	46	8,450'	n/a
10	4	7	5–7	59	10,350'	n/a
9	5	7	4–5	46	12,400'	n/a
8	6	6	3–6	30	6,600'	4
8	9	10	4–6	52	13,300'	n/a
9	5	6	4–7	43	10,900'	n/a
10	8	10	3–4	24	5,600'	n/a
10	5	6	3–5	37	6,050'	18
7	8	5	3–4	37	5,800'	n/a
10	1	7	4–6	38	5,350'	73
9	4	8	3–5	48	10,550'	n/a
9	5	6	5–10	66	14,200'	8
8	5	8	7–11	80	17,600'	n/a
10	5	8	9–12	110	23,700'	3.6
8	4	6	4–6	38	10,000'	4
8	4	6	5–9	66	12,050'	135
8	3	5	3–5	36	9,300'	n/a
10	2	8	8–13	91	25,150'	n/a
10	5	9	4–5	33	6,700'	n/a
8	8	7	6–7	54	9,100'	n/a
9	6	6	3–5	42	9,200'	29
10	5	8	2–4	18	1,700'	38

PREFACE

Guidebook authors face a dilemma. Without dedicated supporters the wilderness would never be protected in the first place. The best and most enthusiastic advocates are those who have actually visited the land, often with the help of a guidebook. On the other hand, too many boots can be destructive. It is the responsibility of every visitor to tread lightly on the land and to speak out strongly for its preservation.

To their credit, almost every agency official who reviewed this material stressed the need for hikers to leave no trace of their visit. The authors believe the time has come for us to go beyond the well-known Leave No Trace principles. It must be our goal to leave behind a landscape that not only shows no trace of our presence but is actually in *better* shape than *before* we arrived. Here are some guidelines:

- Obviously, be scrupulous to leave no litter of your own. Even better, remove any litter left by others (blessedly little these days).

- Do some minor trail maintenance as you hike. Kick rocks off the trail, remove limbs and debris, and drain water from the path to reduce mud and erosion. Report major trail-maintenance problems, such as large blowdowns or washouts, to the land managers so they can concentrate their limited dollars where those are most needed.

- Always camp in a designated site or at a place that either is compacted from years of previous use or can easily accommodate a tent without being damaged—sand, a gravel bar, or a densely wooded area is best.

- Never camp on fragile meadow vegetation or immediately beside a lake or stream. If you see a camp established in an inappropriate place, be proactive: place a few limbs or rocks over the area to discourage further use, scatter horse apples, and remove fire-scarred rocks. Report those who ignore the rules to rangers (or offer to help the offenders move to a better location).

- Never feed wildlife, and encourage others to refrain.

- Choose not to build campfires, especially in alpine areas where trees grow extremely slowly and wood is scarce. You simply don't need a fire to have a good time, and it's damaging to the land. When you discover a fire ring in an otherwise pristine area, scatter the rocks and cover the fire pit to discourage further use.

- Leave the following at home: soap (even biodegradable soap pollutes); if at all possible, pets (even well-mannered pets are instinctively seen as predators by wildlife); anything loud; and any outdated attitudes you may have about going out to "conquer" the wilderness.

A WORD ABOUT MOTORCYCLES

Many U.S. Forest Service trails also allow motorcycles, which disrupt the quietness hikers expect on a path. Motorcycle tires also hasten trail erosion, making the paths more difficult for hikers. For frustrated hikers, here are some things you should do:

- Hike the trails and see what's at stake.
- Contact your elected representatives urging wilderness status for these lands, or at least restrictions on wheels by local district rangers.
- Hike before trail maintenance is completed; logs lying over the trail effectively keep out motorcycles.

A WORD ABOUT THE THIRD EDITION

Thanks to the enthusiastic response of outdoors lovers such as yourself, *Backpacking Washington* now goes proudly into its third edition, bigger and better than ever. Fans of the first two editions will notice that most of their favorite trips have been retained (they were just too good to omit). A few trips were removed to make room for several exceptional new backpacking outings; one trip, the Larch Pass: Hidden Lakes Loop, had to be removed because a huge fire in 2017 blackened the entire area, making it unattractive and virtually unhikable. Another trip, the Kettle Crest Trail, was once one of the finest backpacking trips in eastern Washington, but recent fires have reduced its overall quality to such a degree (and even made it unsafe with all the hazard trees at the logical locations for camping in the northern section) that it is no longer suitable to be recommended in this book.

In addition, several of the older trips have been rewritten and reworked to include outstanding new side trips or to reflect what the authors feel is a superior way to take the hike. Due to reader requests, this edition also includes a few especially rugged trips that require some off-trail travel, giving experienced and adventurous backpackers additional options for challenge and solitude. Finally, we have updated and improved the maps for all trips.

Like the original trips, this book's new adventures frequently visit parts of the Evergreen State that many readers are probably unfamiliar with. Some of these trips have never been fully described in any guidebook before. The solitude these trips provide is a nice bonus, but it's the scenery that you will likely remember the most. All of the new hikes offer enough spectacular sights to make even the most experienced outdoors lover stand in awe and wish they had scheduled more vacation time in the backcountry.

We invite all readers to use this third edition as your guide to years of great adventures in the wildlands of Washington. We hope you enjoy touring these trails as much as we did. Please feel free to contact Wilderness Press with your suggestions and updates, so this book can continue to be the best and most accurate backpacking guide for the Evergreen State.

ACKNOWLEDGMENTS

The help of many people made this book possible. First of all, we would like to thank the countless wilderness rangers and fellow hikers who provided trip companionship and recommendations. Special thanks go to the following people:

For her love, support, time, and other reasons too numerous to list, Doug owes a huge and unpayable debt to his wife, Becky Lovejoy.

Doug's friend and occasional hiking partner, Dave Elsbernd, deserves a shout-out.

Doug would also like to thank his coauthor on this third edition, Mark Wetherington. Without Mark's enthusiasm, determination, and, most of all, his much younger and stronger legs, it would not have been possible to do all the necessary fieldwork to get this third book accomplished.

Mark would like to offer his appreciation to his parents for their support of his hiking and writing endeavors; to the friends (especially Justin Montgomery and John Murphy) who have joined him in the backcountry over the years; to the staff and volunteers at the Bitterroot Public Library in Hamilton, Montana, for their support and warm welcomes when returning from fieldwork trips; to Tia Beavert (program manager, Tribal Forestry, Yakama Nation Department of Natural Resources) for information about access to Yakama Nation lands on the east side of Mount Adams; and to all the trail crew workers and those involved in outdoor education across the country. Last but not least, Mark must offer his sincerest thanks to the original author and coauthor for this edition, Doug Lorain, for his endless patience, guidance, and humor throughout this project.

These hikes are on the ancestral lands of indigenous tribes who occupied it before being forcibly removed. We would like to acknowledge their occupation and stewardship of the land—past, present, and future. Please take a moment to consider the displacement, violence, and injustice that is part of the history of the lands upon which we now hike.

While the contributions and assistance of the persons listed above were invaluable, all of the text, maps, and photographs herein are the work and sole responsibility of the authors. Any and all omissions, errors, and just plain stupid mistakes are strictly our own.

INTRODUCTION

Although people on the East Coast may find this hard to believe, by Western standards, Washington is a small state. It's smaller, in fact, than any other state west of the Great Plains except Hawaii. Within these boundaries, however, are some of the most spectacular wildlands in the country and many of the continent's finest hiking trails. Washington has more wild beaches, dense rainforests, glacial ice, and outstanding mountain scenery than any other state outside of Alaska. Despite such a wealth of world-class landscapes, with a few notable exceptions, the trails in Washington are often less famous and frequently less crowded than those in other parts of the United States.

In addition to spectacular vistas, the mountains in Washington have another big advantage over those in most other parts of the American West: the northern latitudes and extremely heavy winter snowpack keep timberline down to relatively low elevations. Nearly all hiking is below 7,000 feet, so hikers can enjoy sublime alpine scenery without having to gasp for oxygen as they would in the high altitudes of California's Sierra Nevada, Wyoming's Wind River Range, or the Colorado Rockies. For the typical hiker who lives at low elevation and heads to the mountains only once or twice a year, this means less time wasted getting acclimated and more time enjoying the trip.

There are many ways to see and appreciate the beauty of Washington. Many parts of the state can be seen just as easily by day hikes, rafting trips, and bicycle tours—even from your car. The focus of *this* book, however, is on the best ways for backpackers to see the state. Most of the state's best scenery is far from roads and can be truly appreciated only by backpackers. After many years and thousands of trail miles, the authors have chosen what they believe to be Washington's very best backpacking trips. The focus is on *longer* trips— from three days to two weeks. Most of these are beyond a simple weekend outing, but they make terrific vacations and give you enough time to fully appreciate the landscape. Best of all, you'll have the chance to really get to know and love the country.

HOW TO USE THIS GUIDE

Each featured trip begins with an information box that provides a quick overview of the hike's vital statistics and important features. This allows you to rapidly narrow down your options based on your preferences, your abilities, how many days you have available, and the time of year. Also, see the Featured Trips Summary Table on pages viii–ix.

Scenery This is the authors' subjective opinion of the trip's overall scenic quality, on a scale of 1 (an eyesore) to 10 (absolutely gorgeous). This rating reflects the authors' personal biases in favor of qualities like abundant wildflowers, photogenic views, and clear streams. If your tastes run more toward lush forests or good fishing, then your own rating may be quite different. Also keep in mind that the rating is a *relative* one. *All* the featured trips are beautiful, and if they were located almost anywhere else in North America, they would justifiably draw crowds of admirers.

Solitude Because solitude is one of the things that backpackers are seeking, it helps to know roughly how much company you can expect. This rating is also on a 1 (bring stilts to see over the crowds) to 10 (just you and the mountain goats) scale. Of course, even on a trip rated 9 or 10, there's always an outside chance that you could end up plagued by a pack of wild Cub Scouts.

Difficulty This is yet another subjective judgment by the authors. The rating is intended to warn you away from the most difficult outings if you are not in shape to try them. The scale is *only relative to other backpacking trips*. Most Americans would find even the easiest backpacking trip to be a very strenuous undertaking. So this scale of 1 (barely leave the La-Z-Boy) to 10 (the Ironman Triathlon) is only for people already accustomed to backpacking.

Miles This is the total mileage of the recommended trip in its most basic form (with no side trips). The authors, however, have never seen the point of a bare-bones, Point A–to–Point B kind of trip. After all, if you're going to go, you may as well explore a bit. Thus, for most trips a second mileage number is listed in parentheses that includes distances for recommended side trips. These side trips are also shown on the maps and included in the "Possible Itinerary" section. (*Note:* Some exact mileages were not available. The mileage shown may be only an approximation, based on extrapolation from maps or the authors' own on-site calculations.)

Elevation Gain For many hikers, how far *up* they go is even more important than the distance. This item shows the trip's *total* elevation gain, including all ups and downs, not simply the net gain. As with the mileage section, a second number in parentheses also includes the elevation gain in recommended side trips.

Days This is a *rough* figure for how long it will take the average backpacker to do the trip. It's based on the authors' preference for traveling about 10 miles per day. Also considered were the spacing of available campsites and the trip's difficulty. Hard-core hikers may cover as many as 25 miles a day, while others saunter along at 4 or 5 miles per day, a good pace for hikers with children. Most trips can be done in more or fewer days, depending on your preferences and abilities.

Shuttle Mileage When appropriate, this is the shortest one-way driving distance between the beginning and the ending trailheads. Be sure to schedule enough time at both ends of your trip to complete the necessary car shuttle.

Map Every trip includes a map that is as up-to-date and accurate as possible. As every hiker knows, however, you will also need a good contour map of the area. This entry identifies the best available map(s) for the described trip. All references to United States Geological Survey (USGS) maps are for the 7.5-minute series.

Usually Open This entry tells you when a trip is usually snow-free enough for hiking (which can vary considerably from year to year).

Best This note lists the particular time(s) of year when the authors feel the trip is at its very best (when the flowers peak, the fall colors are at their best, or the mosquitoes have died down, and so on). Unfortunately, the best season may also be the most crowded, so you may prefer to visit when conditions aren't as good, but you'll enjoy more solitude.

Permits Regulations are rapidly changing in the Washington backcountry. All national parks and many wilderness areas require backpackers to obtain and carry permits, several of which require a fee. Managers are also restricting the number of hikers allowed into traditionally crowded locations, and some places require advance reservations. Generally, it's best to obtain backcountry permits from the nearest U.S. Forest Service or National Park Service ranger station. It's always advisable to call ahead and ask about current restrictions and the need for reservations because the regulations are constantly changing.

Rules This section lists any restrictions on fires, camping, or the number of people in your party, as well as other regulations for the area.

Contact This is the phone number and the website (though trail information is very rarely updated on U.S. Forest Service websites) for the local land agency responsible for the area. Be sure to check on road and trail conditions, as well as any new restrictions or permit requirements, before your trip.

SPECIAL ATTRACTIONS

This section focuses on attributes of this particular trip that are rare or outstanding. For example, almost every trip has views, but some have views that are *especially* noteworthy. The same is true of areas with a particularly good chance of seeing wildlife, excellent fall colors, and so on.

CHALLENGES

This is the flip side to the "Special Attractions" section. It lists the trip's special or especially troublesome problems. Expect to read warnings about areas with particularly abundant mosquitoes, poor road access, lots of bears, or limited water.

HOW TO GET THERE

This section includes driving directions to the trailhead(s), as well as GPS coordinates.

NOTES, TIPS, AND WARNINGS

Throughout the text are numerous helpful hints and ideas. These all come from the authors' experiences. A pessimist once said that experience is something you never have until just *after* you need it. By relying on the hard-won experience of others, these prominently labeled Notes, Tips, and Warnings should make your trips safer and more enjoyable.

POSSIBLE ITINERARY

This is given at the *end* of each trip. To be used as a planning tool, it includes daily mileages and total elevation gains, as well as recommended side trips. Your own itinerary is likely to be different. Although the authors have hiked all the book's trips, many were not done exactly as written here. If we were to rehike a trip, we would follow the improved itinerary shown here.

VARIATIONS

Shown at the end of a hike's description, this gives general information on ways you could significantly alter the described trip by using different routes to shorten or lengthen a trip, use alternate exit or entry points, return by a different loop route, and the like.

BEST SHORTER ALTERNATIVE

Because many readers may not have the time or desire to tackle a longer backpacking trip, most featured trips include a section at the end that details the best way to get a sampling of the area with day hikes or shorter backpacking adventures. These options often miss the best areas that are farther from the roads, but this will at least give time-strapped hikers the opportunity to see some of the wonders that each described area has to offer.

SAFETY NOTICE

The trips in this book are long and often difficult, and some go through remote wilderness terrain. In the event of an emergency, supplies and medical facilities may be several days away. Anyone who attempts these hikes must be experienced in wilderness travel, carry proper equipment, and be in good physical condition. While backpacking is not inherently dangerous, the sport does involve risk. Because trail conditions, weather, and hikers' abilities all vary considerably, the authors and the publisher cannot assume responsibility for the safety of anyone who takes these hikes. Use plenty of common sense and a realistic appraisal of your abilities so you can enjoy these trips safely.

References to water in the text attest only to its availability, not its purity. You should treat all backcountry water before drinking it.

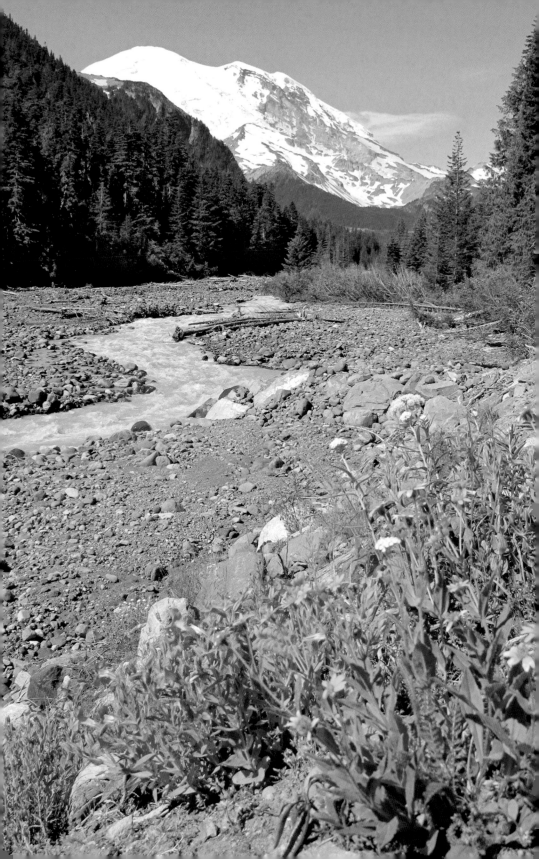

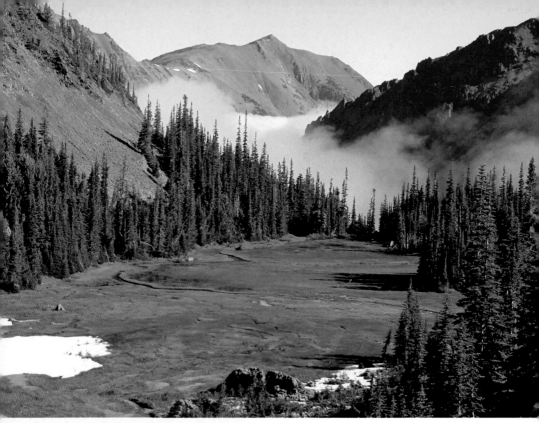

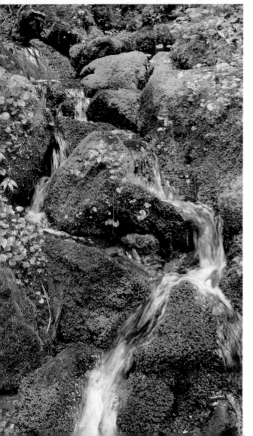

Previous page: *Mount Rainier over White River (Trip 19)*
photographed by Douglas Lorain

Above: *Baldy looms over a meadow above Royal Lake (Trip 6).*
photographed by Douglas Lorain

Left: *Tiny Creek below Mowich Lake (Trip 19)*
photographed by Douglas Lorain

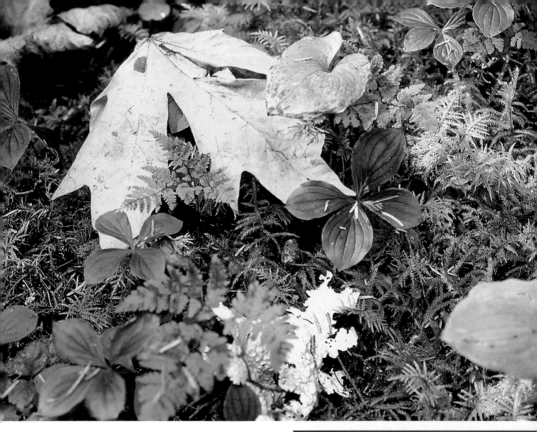

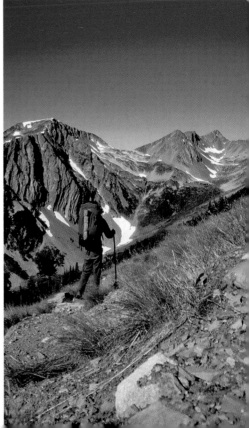

Above: *Fall color scene along the
Hoh River Trail (Trip 3)*
photographed by Douglas Lorain

Right: *Taking in the view from above
Big Face Basin (Trip 9)*
photographed by Douglas Lorain

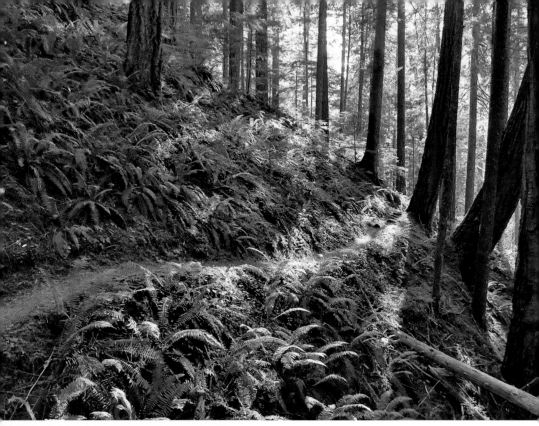

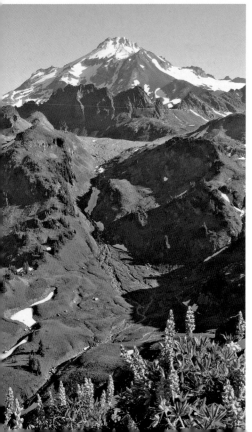

Above: *Downey Creek Trail (Trip 14)*
photographed by Mark Wetherington

Left: *Glacier Peak from a ridge east of White Mountain (Trip 15)*
photographed by Douglas Lorain

Opposite page, top: *"Devils Pipe Organ" basalt formation below South Puyallup Camp (Trip 19)*
photographed by Douglas Lorain

Opposite page, bottom left: *Tiger lilies (Trip 25)*
photographed by Mark Wetherington

Opposite page, bottom right: *Salmon in Chilliwack River (Trip 7)*
photographed by Mark Wetherington

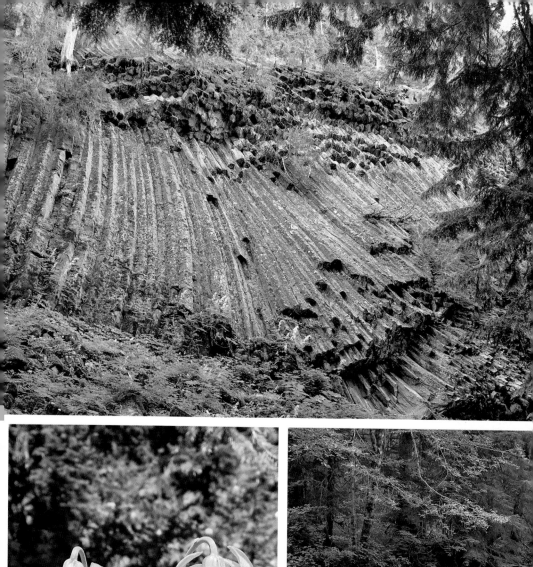

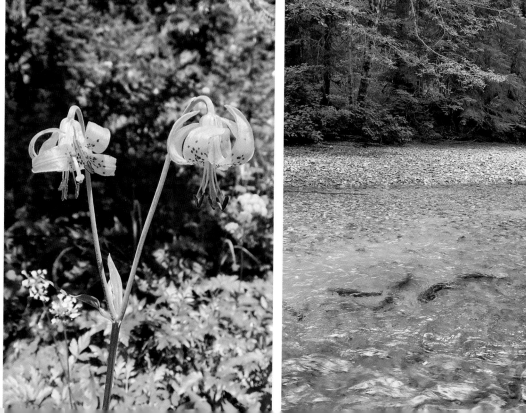

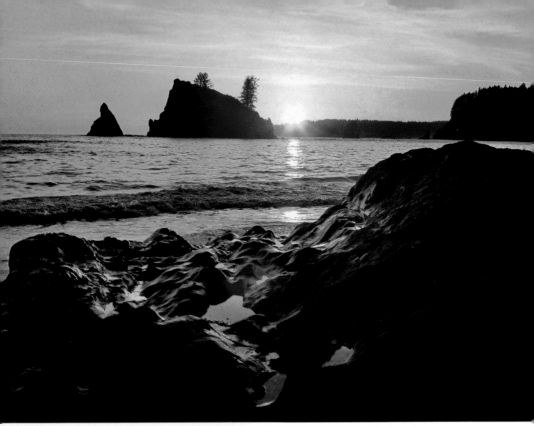

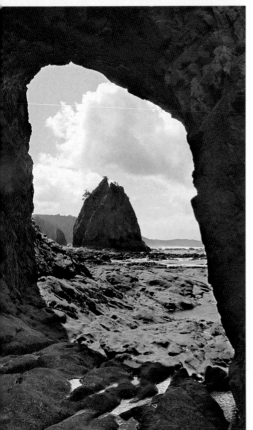

Above: *Sunset near Scott Creek (Trip 2)*
photographed by Douglas Lorain

Left: *Looking through the arch at Hole-in-the-Wall (Trip 1)*
photographed by Douglas Lorain

Opposite page: *Sea stars in a cove north of Shi Shi Beach (Trip 1)*
photographed by Douglas Lorain

Next page: *North Fork Bridge Creek (Trip 8)*
photographed by Douglas Lorain

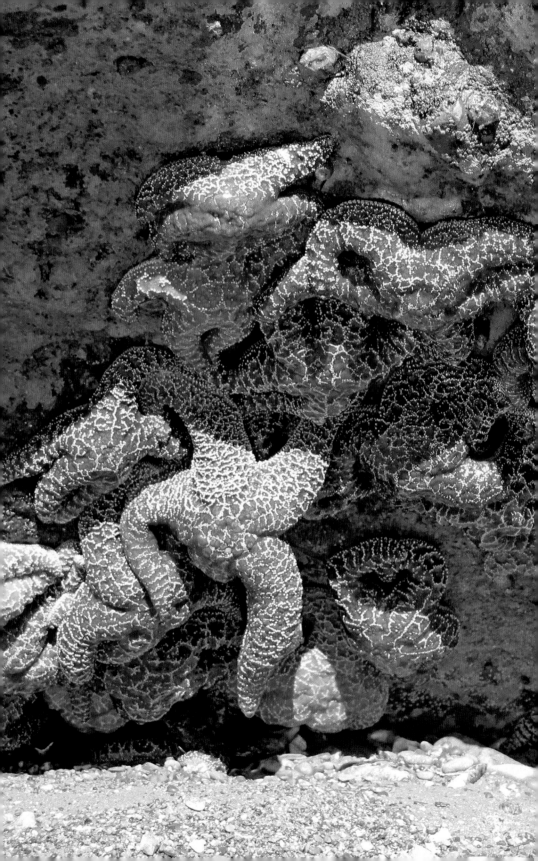

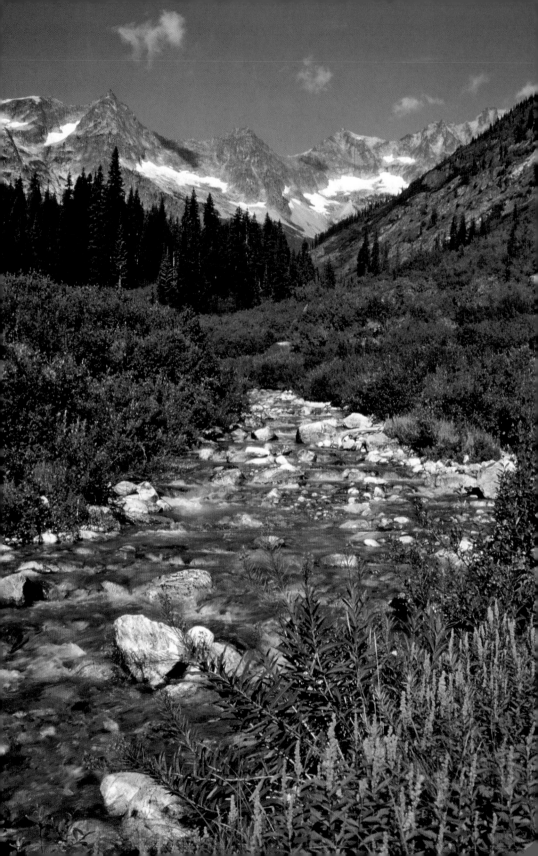

GENERAL TIPS ON BACKPACKING IN WASHINGTON

This book is not a how-to guide for backpackers. Anyone contemplating an extended backpacking vacation will (or at least should) already know about equipment, the Leave No Trace ethic, conditioning, food, selecting a campsite, first aid, and all other aspects of this sport. A myriad of excellent books cover these subjects. It is appropriate, however, to discuss some tips and ideas that are specific to Washington and the Pacific Northwest.

- Most national forests in Washington require a trailhead parking pass. In general, a windshield sticker is required for cars parked within 0.25 mile of most developed trailheads. In 2019 daily permits cost $5, and an annual pass, good in all the forests of Washington and Oregon, was $30 (actually a pretty good deal). The fees are used for trail maintenance, wilderness rangers' pay, and trailhead improvements. Olympic and Mount Rainier National Parks have separate entry fees.

- The winter's snowpack has a significant effect not only on when a trail opens, but also on peak wildflower times, stream flows, and how long seasonal water sources will be available. You can check the snowpack around April 1, and make a note about how it compares to normal. This information is available through the local media or by going to www.wcc.nrcs.usda.gov. If the snowpack is significantly above or below average, adjust the trip's seasonal recommendation accordingly.

- When driving on Washington's forest roads, keep a wary eye out for log trucks. These scary behemoths often barrel along with little regard for those annoying speed bumps known as passenger cars.

- The Northwest's frequent winter storms create annual problems for trail crews. Early-season hikers should expect to crawl over deadfall and search for routes around slides and flooded riverside trails. Depending on current funding and the trail's popularity, maintenance may not be completed until several weeks after a trail is snow free and officially open. Unfortunately, this means that trail maintenance is often done well after the best time to visit. On the positive side, trails are usually less crowded before the maintenance has been completed.

- The weather in Washington's Cascade and Olympic Mountains will come as something of a nasty shock to hikers from other parts of the country. It can rain here for days on end, and in some years summer never truly arrives. Good raingear, gaiters, a weatherproof shelter, a rain cover for your pack, and a flexible schedule to allow for tent-bound layover days are all essential. The situation is somewhat better in the southern Cascades and markedly better east of the Cascade Divide, but even there you must always carry raingear no matter how short the trip.

  In this wet climate, down sleeping bags are *not* recommended. If that is all you own, however, be sure to take extra precautions to keep the bag dry. Many veteran hikers in these mountains pack their sleeping bags in two garbage bags in addition to using a pack cover.

- Another annoyance to hikers in the Washington Cascades and Olympics is rarely mentioned in guidebooks. The thick vegetation and abundant insect population make this an ideal habitat for spiders. The first person to hike a trail in the morning will spend considerable time (and a lifetime's vocabulary of swear words) wiping away spiderwebs from their face, hair, clothing, and pack. Waving a walking stick in front of you helps, as does alternating the lead with your hiking partner, but if you're an early riser who likes to hit the trail before anyone else, then spiderwebs are a problem you're just going to have to put up with.

- For environmentally conscious backpackers, one good solution to the old problem of how to dispose of toilet paper is to find a natural alternative. Two excellent options are the large, soft leaves of thimbleberry at lower elevations, and the light green (old man's beard or *Usnea*) lichen that hangs from trees at higher elevations. They're not exactly Charmin soft, but they get the job done.

- General deer-hunting season in Washington runs from the second or third weekend of October to the end of the month or early November. Also, every year September 15–25, Washington holds a high buck season in the Lake Chelan National Recreation Area and the Alpine Lakes, Glacier Peak, and Pasayten Wildernesses. For safety, anyone planning to travel in the forests during these periods (particularly those doing any cross-country travel) should carry *and wear* a bright red or orange cap, vest, pack, or other conspicuous article of clothing.

- Along the same line as the above, elk hunting season is generally held in late October or, more often, early November. The exact season varies in different parts of the state.

- Mushrooms are a Northwest backcountry delicacy. Although the damp climate makes it possible to find mushrooms in any season, late August–November is usually best. Where and when the mushrooms can be found varies with elevation, precipitation, and other factors.

  WARNING: Mushroom collecting has become a big and very competitive business. A few people have even been murdered in recent years in disputes over prize locations. Secondly, make absolutely sure that you know your fungi. Several poisonous species grow in our forests, and you don't want to make a mistake.

WILD AREAS OF WASHINGTON

What follows is a general overview of the principal remaining wild areas in the state of Washington. All of these have at least one backpacking trip in this book. Whether you prefer wild beaches, virgin forests, high mountains, or lonesome ridges, there's a choice of outstanding trips for you.

OLYMPIC COAST

The United States is blessed with thousands of miles of shoreline. Outside of Alaska, however, almost every inch of this coastline is closely paralleled by roads. One of the few exceptions is the wild coast of the Olympic Peninsula. Protected in a narrow strip of Olympic National Park, this incredibly beautiful coastline includes the longest stretch of roadless shoreline in the contiguous United States. Backpackers from all over the country come here to enjoy the coastal hiking experience of a lifetime.

The scenery is a spectacular mix of craggy headlands, strips of sand, offshore rocks, cobblestone beaches, tidepools, and rainforests. Sunsets along the coast are absolutely glorious. Finally, wildlife—including bald eagles, sea otters, deer, raccoons, an amazing array of tidepool life, seabirds galore, and whales—is abundant. The amount of life is positively overwhelming.

With all of these attractions, visitors must also be aware of the difficulties of hiking here. First and foremost, of course, is the weather. To call it unpredictable is too kind because the weather is actually *very* predictable—it's *bad!* Rain and wind are the norm, and in summer, when rain is less frequent, fog often hugs the immediate coast and blocks the view. To enjoy this area you need either exceptional luck or the proper frame of mind.

The second major challenge is tides. You should always carry a tide table and a map that indicates which headlands require a low tide to get around. Be prepared to wait—sometimes for hours—for the tide to cooperate with your hiking schedule. Also remember to camp well above the tide line.

Looking at the map, a hiker might assume that because routes here closely follow the ocean, this will be easy walking with little or no elevation gain. *Wrong!* Much of the going is actually quite rugged, including miles of slippery rocks, scrambles over headlands (often using rickety ladders), treacherous stream crossings, and muddy inland trails.

The final consideration is the National Park Service's permit and reservation system. Permits are required for the entire coast. There is a fee, but for most of the coast, permits can be easily obtained at any trailhead. In the popular Cape Alava/Ozette area, however, the National Park Service requires reservations. With the notoriously lousy weather, it would be nice if you could watch the weather forecast and plan to go on short notice when there is an expected break in the rain. The need to get reservations weeks or even months in advance, however, makes this plan impossible.

OLYMPIC MOUNTAINS

Inland from the coast rise hills covered with thick greenery and lots of clear-cuts. Beyond these foothills are the jagged peaks of the Olympic Mountains. This spectacular area of uplifted rock includes numerous glaciers, deep stream canyons, wildflower-covered alpine meadows, and all the other beauties of mountains in the Pacific Northwest. They also have an extensive network of trails, providing countless opportunities for the backpacker.

Hopkins Lake (see Trip 9, page 83)
photographed by Douglas Lorain

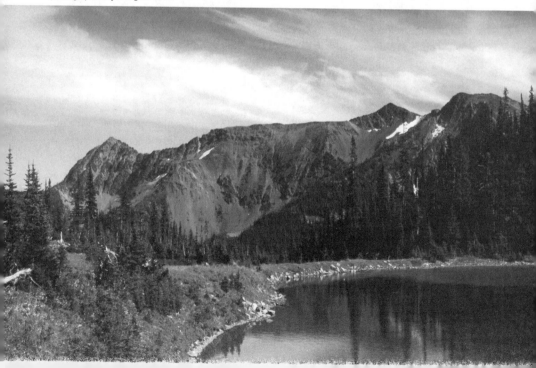

Cut off from other North American mountains by Puget Sound and surrounding lowlands, the Olympics have developed a unique mix of flora and fauna. Several common mountain species like grizzly bears and mountain goats never reached this range, although goats were later introduced. Other animals, such as the local marmots and chipmunks, have evolved to become separate species from their nearby relatives. Several species of plants are found here and nowhere else.

While the trails are a joy, hikers must come prepared for rain. It is *possible* to hike for a week or more without getting wet, but equally possible (in fact, more likely) to encounter a week or more of nonstop rain even in the summer "dry" season. The western Olympics get as much as 14 *feet* of rain annually. This moisture results in incredibly lush temperate rainforests that support the highest concentration of biological material (biomass) of any ecosystem on Earth. The eastern Olympics are in the rainshadow of peaks to the west, so while they're not exactly arid, they are generally drier and less humid.

NORTH CASCADES

The North Cascades contain some of the wildest country left in the contiguous 48 states. Roads are few and trails reach only a small part of the many wonders. Much of this region is strictly the domain of the dedicated bushwhacker and mountaineer.

The incredibly rugged nature of this landscape shaped its history and explains its appeal. It was the difficult terrain that kept roads out of this country long enough for much of it to be preserved in 1968 as North Cascades National Park. This complex includes not only the park but also the Ross Lake and Lake Chelan National Recreation Areas. The steep, glacier-carved valleys and high ridges preserved here are truly awe-inspiring. There is, in fact, so much splendor that it's difficult to take it all in.

As for difficulties, the North Cascades share the same problem with flies as the Glacier Peak region (see later section). Black bears are quite common, and there are even a handful of grizzlies prowling around, so store all of your food properly. Finally, while the North Cascades are not as notoriously soggy as the Olympic Mountains, you must still come prepared for rain.

PASAYTEN WILDERNESS

In the eastern rainshadow of the North Cascades, this huge wilderness looks very different from the heavily glaciated peaks to the west. There is less precipitation here—a real blessing for those who tire of getting wet all the time—and the peaks are less heavily eroded. Although there are only a few spectacular peaks, the wilderness features scenic attributes that are outstanding in their own right. Endless miles of high, rolling meadows and thousands of acres of wildflowers are among the top attractions. In season, this wilderness supports some of the finest flower displays in Washington. The flower season runs early July–early August, with the peak display working its way from east to west as the summer progresses.

Solitude is another big attraction. Greater distances from major cities help to keep the trail population low. Also, the sheer enormity of this wilderness spreads out visitors and gives long-distance backpackers plenty of room for wandering. This is prime country for devotees of long loop trips because the trails connect to form loops ranging from 50 to 100 miles or more.

In addition to the flower season, an equally spectacular time to visit is late September and early October when the Lyall alpine larch trees turn gold. Solitude at that time is also nearly guaranteed, with the excellent possibility of hiking for several days without seeing another human being.

WARNINGS: While free of both people and bugs, autumn visits risk a shortage of water, the possibility of snow, and the near certainty of freezing nights.

One other thing to keep in mind is that recent years have seen several huge forest fires sweep through the Pasayten Wilderness. Trails now frequently travel through miles of blackened timber and suffer from a plague of blowdown. Call ahead about the latest conditions.

GLACIER PEAK AREA

Aptly named Glacier Peak and its surrounding lesser summits fill a huge area of spectacular wild country between Stevens Pass and North Cascades National Park. With a plethora of glaciers, rugged peaks, and flowery meadows, this delightful region shares much in common with the more famous North Cascades. One important and welcome difference for backpackers, however, is the greater number and variety of trails that crisscross this area. Unlike the true North Cascades, most of the highlights here can be reached by trail, and doing so is a joy.

Although the area is not as crowded as the Alpine Lakes, and less well known nationally than North Cascades National Park, local backpackers still come here in large numbers. The sheer size of this wilderness, however, means that only a few places are truly crowded.

While people are not abundant, there is never a shortage of bugs. Mosquitoes are a nuisance, but flies are the biggest problem. These nasty creatures buzz around, bite, and generally make a decidedly negative impression. In midsummer there are *billions* of them, and their preferred habitats are warm, sunny areas and the bodies of sweaty backpackers. Climbing a hot, south-facing slope at fly time is enough to make the most dedicated backpackers question their sanity. When it rains the flies miraculously disappear.

All that said, the Glacier Peak region is much more of a backpacker's dream than nightmare. Memories of incredible vistas, snow-covered peaks, and wildflower-filled meadows quickly overwhelm those of rain and flies. The best advice is to savor the delights and learn to live with the minor downsides.

ALPINE LAKES

Serving as a spectacular transition area between the icy crags of the North Cascades and the gentler southern Cascades, the Alpine Lakes Wilderness is an impressive area of forested canyons, ice-sculpted peaks, and countless lakes. Its close proximity to the Puget Sound megalopolis makes this wilderness extremely popular. On weekends, solitude is practically impossible to find here, and even midweek trails are busy. As a result, the U.S. Forest Service has been forced to impose a range of restrictions, reservation requirements, and quotas.

Despite all the regulations, the Alpine Lakes are well worth the headaches. Hundreds of miles of trails lead to beauties too numerous to list. A few of the more impressive areas are described in this book, but adventurers will find plenty of opportunities for further exploration. Even a casual look at a map of the wilderness will suggest enough trips to keep a hiker busy for years.

The famous Enchantments are a string of strikingly beautiful lakes in a high granite basin in the eastern part of the Alpine Lakes Wilderness. They are generally acknowledged to be the supreme scenic experience in the region and perhaps the entire state. This wide fame has led to a host of cumbersome restrictions on visitor numbers, group size, and campsite selection, but the biggest obstacle is the need to get reservations long in advance of your visit. There is a lottery system, but the demand is so enormous that snagging a permit for any time during the summer and fall hiking season is a less-than-10% proposition. Good luck—you'll need it. Primarily for that reason, the Enchantments have been excluded from this book.

MOUNT RAINIER

As the undisputed king of the Cascade Range, Mount Rainier dominates its surroundings like few other mountains. Serving as a landmark for much of the state, this bulky mass of rock and ice is among the nation's greatest scenic wonders. In fact, one of the world's first national parks was established here to protect this treasure. The massive peak is surrounded by a stunning array of attractions, including world-famous wildflower gardens, grand viewpoints, ancient forests, abundant wildlife, and an unusually high concentration of waterfalls. Though many highlights are visible from roads, the best way to get to know this icy giant is to hike the trails.

There are miles of fine paths, but for long-distance backpackers the around-the-mountain Wonderland Trail is a must. In its long, rugged course, the trail samples all of the park's many attractions. Significant restrictions on when and where you can camp make careful planning and reserving a permit a must, but these hassles are minor in comparison to the joys.

When planning your trip, you should know that, in addition to rain from Pacific storms, Mount Rainier is so high that it actually creates its own weather. Many summer days find clouds and rain (or snow) on the mountain while the surrounding hills are bathed in sunshine.

SOUTHERN CASCADES

Only a few generations ago the southern Washington Cascades were an endless rolling ocean of trees. Several snow-covered islands rose above this sea, providing scenic variety and spectacular landmarks. Over the years, people have riddled this once great expanse of trees with clear-cuts and logging roads. On May 18, 1980, another, more sudden change occurred when one of those "islands" (Mount St. Helens) blew itself to pieces and created a massive natural clear-cut. Almost 40 years later the blast zone is recovering, but devastation is still prevalent.

Most of the hiking in the southern Cascades centers on the great volcanic peaks of Mount Adams, Mount St. Helens, and the eroded remains of an ancient volcano called the Goat Rocks. The alpine landscape is truly outstanding, and of course, the volcanic devastation at Mount St. Helens, while not "pretty," is fascinating and spectacular in its own right.

Much of the eastern slopes of the southern Cascades is owned by the Yakama Nation and is generally off-limits to the public. East of Mount Rainier, however, lies the delightful William O. Douglas Wilderness, which has scenic ridges, pretty lakes, lots of wildflowers, and beautiful fall colors. All in all, it's a wonderful place for hiking.

COLUMBIA BASIN

While the Columbia Basin lacks the mountain majesty of other areas of Washington, it more than makes up for this in its sheer expansiveness and fascinating natural history. This arid landscape of south-central Washington, with its sweeping plateaus and steep canyons, feels almost otherworldly compared to the more familiar Cascade and Olympic Mountains. Repeated prehistoric glacial floods and the volcanic character of the under-lying geology result in scenery that is impressive both in the vastness and in the details. Basalt columns, desert wildflowers, and stunning Palouse Falls in the heart of the chan-neled scablands of this region are highlights every nature lover should put on his or her must-see list. In spring, when the wildflowers are blooming, the temperatures are mild, and the aroma of sagebrush fills the air, it's a hiker's paradise. In summer heat with a relentless sun beating down, miles to the next reliable water source, and rattlesnakes slith-ering across the trail, it might seem more like a nightmare.

The Columbia Basin lacks the large roadless areas that are necessary for an extended wilderness experience, and much of the region is privately owned, which significantly limits access. Additionally, the trail infrastructure is generally lacking when compared to other public lands in Washington. However, the Umtanum Ridge area and the Yakima Sky-line Trail provide backpackers with enough trail mileage and public land, not to mention panoramic views and enchanting high-desert scenery, to make for a worthy destination.

NORTHEASTERN WASHINGTON MOUNTAINS

Northeastern Washington is dominated by an attractive expanse of rolling hills and for-ested mountains. Several mountain ranges, most prominently the Selkirk and Kettle River Ranges, extend south into the United States from the rugged interior of British Columbia. Following these Canadian ranges is an interesting assortment of wildlife that is rare or absent in other Washington mountains. You may be fortunate enough to see a wolf, lynx, moose, or even a grizzly bear.

In the rainshadow of the North Cascades, these mountains are drier and less eroded than those to the west, so the scenery is more subdued. Instead of icy crags, you'll enjoy view-packed ridges, open forests, and attractive meadows. Another bonus of hiking here is the lack of crowds. The greater distance from major cities makes for fewer people and less competition for campsites.

Although most of these mountains are riddled with logging scars, the wild areas that remain provide many scenic destinations for those afoot. This pleasant corner of the state is well worth the extra drive and time to get to know its charms.

BLUE MOUNTAINS

By and large, southeastern Washington is a wasteland for backpackers. Wheat farms, vineyards, rolling hills, and the Snake River's canyon country dominate the region. Most of the land is privately owned and off-limits to hiking. Poking across the border from Oregon, however, is the northern extension of the Blue Mountains, where the prospects for backpacking are much brighter. These little-known mountains feature high, forested tablelands; ridges; the best canyon scenery in the state; and abundant wildlife, especially elk and bighorn sheep. The elk draw crowds of hunters in the fall, but at other times the rugged trails here are rarely traveled.

There are also, of course, a few drawbacks to hiking here. With such a significant difference in elevation between the ridges and the canyons, connecting trails are often steep and rocky. The elevation change also creates a problem with seasonal timing. In April and May, when the canyon bottoms are most attractive, the ridges remain snow covered and most trailheads are unreachable. Later in the summer the ridges are open but the canyons are often uncomfortably hot. Fall would be a good choice, but then you must contend with hunters. Early June is usually your best compromise, although by then many of the canyon's flowers will have faded and some snow patches will remain on the higher ridges. The area has been hit by huge forest fires in recent years, so you'll encounter many miles of blackened snags. You should also expect to encounter significant deadfall, especially early in the season. Finally, rattlesnakes are fairly common at lower elevations, so watch your step.

Opposite page: *Mount Rainier and Packwood Lake from the Lily Basin Trail (see Trip 20, page 193)*
photographed by Douglas Lorain

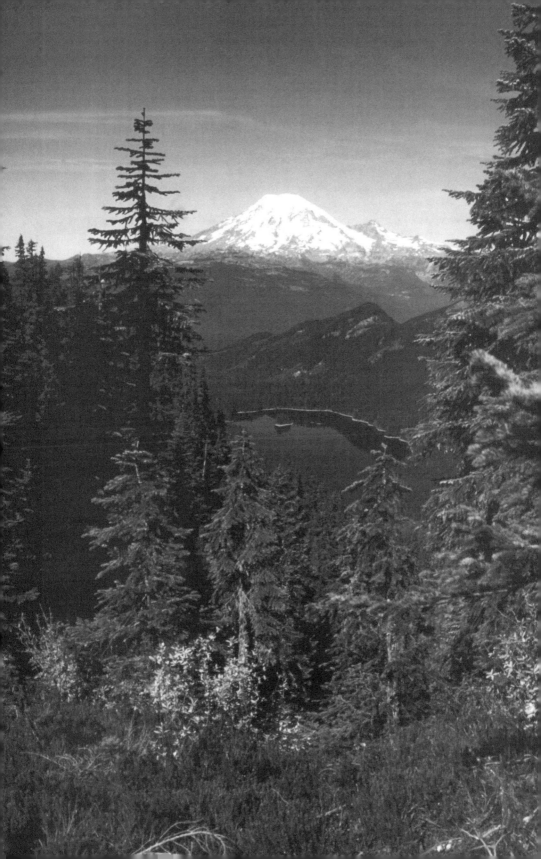

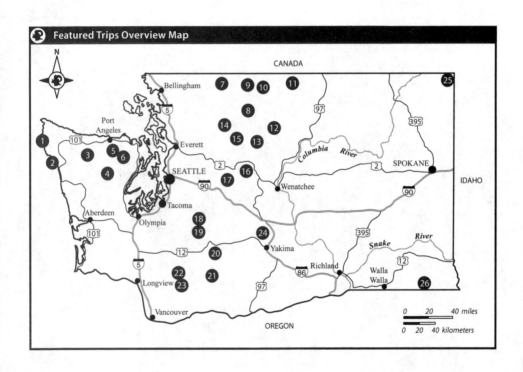

Featured Trips Overview Map

N

CANADA

Bellingham ⑦ ⑨ ⑩ ⑪ ㉕

⑤

⑧

Port
Angeles ⑭ ⑫

① ⑮ ⑬

② ③ ⑤ ⑥ Everett Columbia River SPOKANE

④ SEATTLE ⑯ Wenatchee IDAHO
⑰

Aberdeen Tacoma

Olympia ⑱
⑲

⑳ Snake River

⑫ Yakima ㉔

㉒ ㉑ Richland Walla
Longview ㉓ Walla ㉖

Vancouver

OREGON

0   20   40 miles

0   20   40 kilometers

Opposite page: *Entiat Meadows*
(see Trip 13, page 119)
photographed by Douglas Lorain

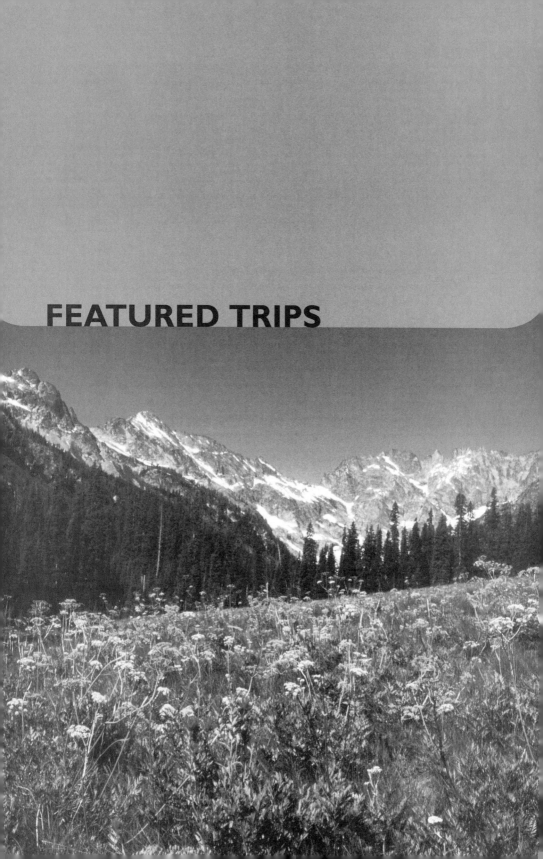

FEATURED TRIPS

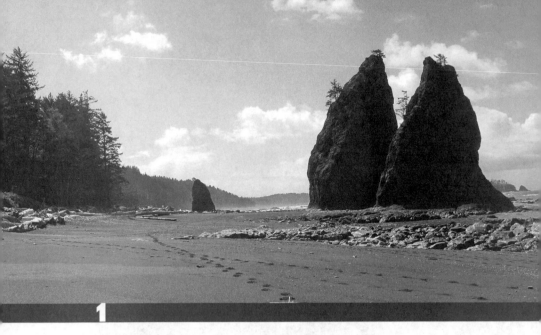

OLYMPIC COAST: NORTH

RATINGS: Scenery 9 **Solitude** 4 **Difficulty** 9

MILES: 33 (33)

ELEVATION GAIN: 1,100' (1,140')

DAYS: 4–7 (4–7)

SHUTTLE MILEAGE: 68

MAP: Custom Correct *North Olympic Coast*

USUALLY OPEN: Year-round

BEST: May/September–October

PERMIT: Required. As of 2019, the nonrefundable cost of a permit is $6 with an additional charge of $8 per adult in your party per night in the park. Alternatively, for $55 you can purchase an annual Olympic National Park Wilderness Pass, which covers all nightly fees for one person for the entire year. Hikers under the age of 16 are free.

Permits are limited for certain campsites on the suggested itinerary for this trip, and reservations are strongly recommended. Visit nps.gov/olym /planyourvisit/wilderness-reservations.htm for up-to-date information about quotas and reservations. Reservations are accepted starting 6 months in advance of your planned trip, either in person at one of the park's wilderness information centers or online via recreation.gov. Check the park's website for the latest procedures and requirements.

Above: *Looking south down Rialto Beach from Hole-in-the-Wall*

photographed by Douglas Lorain

From Ellen Creek in the south to just below Yellow Banks, and on Shi Shi Beach north of Point of the Arches, permits are not limited and no reservation is needed (just pick up a permit at the nearest ranger station). From Yellow Banks to Point of the Arches, however, you are required to have a permit that *must be reserved in advance*. No first-come, first-served permits are given out unless the quota for an area has not been filled, which almost never happens.

RULES: Secure all food and other odorous items in hard-sided containers, such as bear canisters, to keep out raccoons; maximum group size of 12 people; designated camps must be used at Sand Point; dogs are not allowed; fires are prohibited from Yellow Banks north to Wedding Rocks.

CONTACT: Olympic National Park, 360-565-3100, nps.gov/olym

SPECIAL ATTRACTIONS

Sublime coastal scenery, abundant wildlife

CHALLENGES

Often foggy and/or rainy weather; tide concerns; extraordinarily rugged hiking and/or bushwhacking over steep and brushy headlands or on slippery rocks south of Point of Arches; muddy inland trails; long car shuttle; food-stealing raccoons

HOW TO GET THERE

From Forks, drive 1 mile north on US 101 to a junction with La Push Road (also known as WA 110).

To reach the recommended starting point, turn left (west), drive 7.9 miles, then go right (west) on Mora Road. Proceed 5 miles to the road-end trailhead at Rialto Beach Picnic Area.

To reach either of the two possible ending points, you continue north on US 101 from the La Push Road junction and drive 10.5 miles to the tiny community of Sappho. Turn left (north) onto WA 113, following signs to Northwest Coast and Ozette Lake, drive 10.2 miles, and then go straight at a junction, now on WA 112. Proceed 11 miles to a well-signed junction with the Hoko-Ozette Road.

If you are making this a shorter trip by finishing at Ozette Lake, then turn left (south) and drive 21.8 miles to the spacious gravel parking lot at road's end, just past the seasonally staffed Ozette Ranger Station.

Those planning on doing the longer trek to Shi Shi Beach should continue on WA 112 from the Hoko-Ozette junction. Follow this scenic highway 15.4 miles to the town of Neah Bay and Washburn's General Store on your left. Stop here to purchase a tribal recreation use permit, which allows you to hike on Makah Reservation land. As of 2019, the price was a very reasonable $10 for an annual pass. From here you continue on the main road for 0.9 mile, make two 90° turns (first left on Fort Street, then right on Third Avenue), and come to a junction. Go left (southwest) on Cape Flattery Road, drive 2.4 miles, then turn left (southeast) onto Hobuck Road, following signs to

continued on page 21

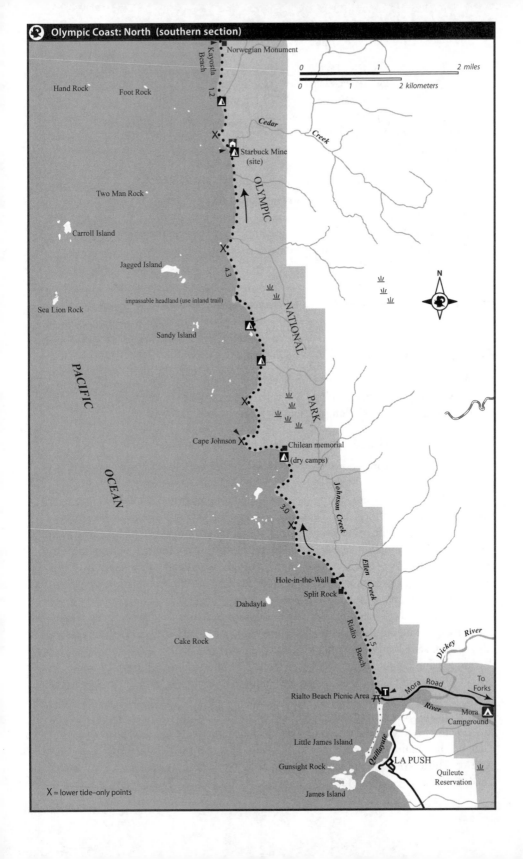

Norwegian Monument

Kayostla Beach

1.2

Hand Rock   Foot Rock

Cedar   Creek

X

Starbuck Mine
(site)

OLYMPIC

Two Man Rock

Carroll Island

X

Jagged Island   4.3

Sea Lion Rock

impassable headland (use inland trail)

NATIONAL

Sandy Island

PACIFIC

X

Cape Johnson X

Chilean memorial

(dry camps)

PARK

OCEAN

3.0

X

Johnson Creek

Ellen Creek

Hole-in-the-Wall

Dahdayla   Split Rock

Rialto Beach

1.5

Cake Rock

Dickey   River

To
Forks

Rialto Beach Picnic Area   T   Mora   Road

River   Mora
Campground

Little James Island

Quillayute

LA PUSH

Gunsight Rock

Quileute
Reservation

James Island

X = lower tide–only points

0   1   2 miles

0   1   2 kilometers

N

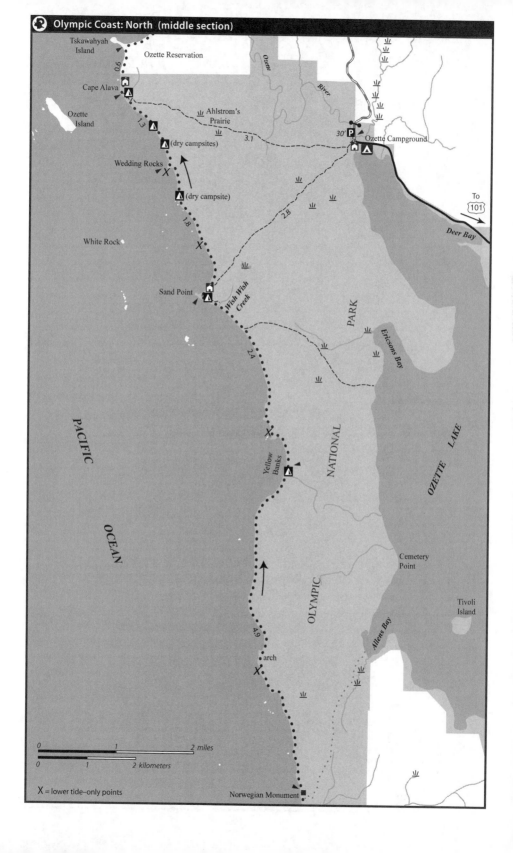

Tskawahyah
Island

Ozette Reservation

Ozette
River

.90

Cape Alava

Ozette
Island

Ahlstrom's
Prairie

1.3

3.1

30'

P

Ozette Campground

(dry campsites)

Wedding Rocks X

To
101

(dry campsite)

2.8

Deer Bay

1.8

White Rock

X

Sand Point

Wish Wish Creek

PARK

Ericsons Bay

PACIFIC

2.4

OZETTE LAKE

X

Yellow
Banks

NATIONAL

Cemetery
Point

OCEAN

Tivoli
Island

OLYMPIC

Allens Bay

4.9

arch

X

0   1   2 miles
0   1   2 kilometers

X = lower tide–only points

Norwegian Monument

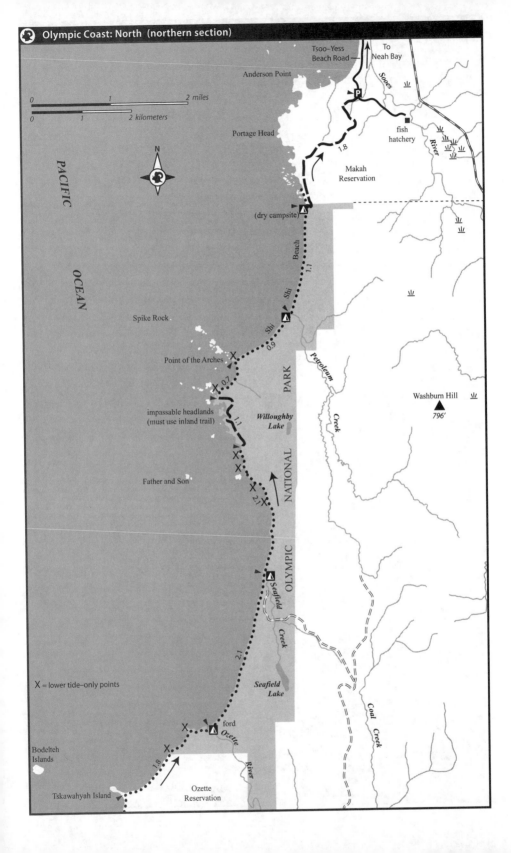

To
Neah Bay

Tsoo–Yess
Beach Road

Anderson Point

Staaes

P

Portage Head

fish
hatchery

River

PACIFIC

N

1.8

Makah
Reservation

(dry campsite)

OCEAN

Beach

1.7

Shi

Spike Rock

Shi

0.9

Point of the Arches

Petroleum

Washburn Hill
796'

0.7

*Willoughby
Lake*

PARK

impassable headlands
(must use inland trail)

1.1

Creek

Father and Son

NATIONAL

2.1

OLYMPIC

Seafield

Seafield
Creek

X = lower tide–only points

2.1

*Seafield
Lake*

Coal Creek

Bodelteh
Islands

ford
Ozette

X

X

1.8

River

Tskawahyah Island

Ozette
Reservation

0
1
2 miles

0
1
2 kilometers

continued from page 17

the Fish Hatchery. This road immediately takes you over a bridge spanning the Waatch River. After just 0.1 mile you keep straight at a four-way junction, and go 1.8 miles to another junction. Go straight on Tsoo–Yess Beach Road, which makes an immediate sharp left, and stay on the main paved road for another 2 miles. Turn left (southeast) onto Fish Hatchery Road, and go 0.2 mile to a gravel trailhead parking area on the right.

> **WARNING:** This trailhead has experienced periodic problems with car break-ins. It is safer to arrange a shuttle than to leave a car parked here for several days. Without that, your best bet is to park at a private home 0.6 mile short of the trailhead and pay a parking fee to the homeowner.

GPS TRAILHEAD COORDINATES:
Southern (Rialto Beach): N47° 55.285' W124° 38.285'
Central alternate ending (Ozette Lake): N48° 09.282' W124° 40.136'
Northern ending (Shi Shi Beach): N48° 17.616' W124° 39.890'

INTRODUCTION

The wild Olympic Coast is a national treasure. With most of our country's shoreline altered by roads, cities, and mobs of tourists, it's a blessing to have this stretch of wilderness beach to remind us of what we've lost. The dramatic coast is broken by roads on either side of the Quillayute River, but north and south of this obstacle stretches the most spectacular wild shoreline in the continental United States.

Both the northern and the southern sections of the Olympic Coast have popular and highly rewarding hiking routes, and hikers with adequate time and energy are encouraged to do both sections. On either trip you will see crashing waves, scenic offshore rocks, dense inland forests, and abundant wildlife. The northern section is longer but, except for the extremely rough far northern section just before you reach the Point of Arches, is generally less rugged. Previous editions of this guide recommended that hikers exit at Ozette Lake and skip that particularly rugged far northern section. Although that stretch is still very rough and should only be attempted by experienced and determined hikers, increased use in recent years has made it somewhat more hikable. In addition, by adding Point of Arches and Shi Shi Beach to your itinerary, you'll enjoy some of the finest coastal scenery in the world. So if you're up for the considerable challenge, it's well worth the extra time and effort. Less athletic hikers can exit at Ozette Lake and still have a great trip.

Obviously the beach can be hiked in either direction. Your choice will probably be dictated by when you can get a permit and by the weather, because it's always nicer to hike with the wind at your back. The trip is described here from south to north.

DESCRIPTION

The trail heads north from the parking lot, traveling near the edge of the forest as it wanders past the popular Rialto Beach Picnic Area. After just 100 yards the forest ends at the edge of the wide sandy expanse of Rialto Beach. The "sand" here is really a deep layer of loose gray pebbles, which makes the hiking rather tiring. Your efforts are handsomely rewarded, however, with pretty views looking south-southwest to large James Island, north to distant Cape Johnson, and west to the waves and seemingly endless expanse of the Pacific Ocean. Take time to explore the many jagged rocks and tidepool areas immediately along the shore. Just inland from the beach are hundreds of dead snags—the former trees killed by salt spray—where you are likely to see bald eagles perched and taking in the scene.

You should expect this initial section to be very crowded because this easily accessible and scenic beach is understandably popular. Once you wade across Ellen Creek at 0.8 mile, however, the crowds rapidly diminish and eventually peter out to just a handful of hardy backpackers. Dogs are not permitted on the beach beyond Ellen Creek, but on the plus side, backpackers are allowed to camp anywhere north of the stream.

About 0.6 mile north of Ellen Creek, you pass Split Rock, a very photogenic pair of sharply pointed rock pinnacles rising directly out of the sand.

Only 0.1 mile beyond Split Rock is another major highlight: Hole-in-the-Wall. This enormous arch protrudes well out onto the sand and can only be rounded at extremely low tide. However, you have two other options. At medium tides you can hike out across a shelf of mussel-covered rocks and walk through the huge hole in the arch to the other side. At high tide, you can bypass the arch entirely by taking a steep scramble trail that climbs over the inland side of the formation. All routes take you to a lovely little cove just north of Hole-in-the-Wall, which is well worth taking the time to explore for both its scenery and abundant tidepools.

Now the hiking becomes more challenging, as you must negotiate sandy areas, large boulders, tidepools, and jumbles of slippery rocks. Your progress will be relatively slow, but hiking this wilderness shoreline is all about the scenery and the wildlife, not setting a fast pace. Dozens of offshore pinnacles and hulking rocks offer excellent photo opportunities.

As you pass the first major rocky headland north of Hole-in-the-Wall, look for a boot-hardened path on the inland side that makes for easier and safer travel than scrambling over the slippery rocks. At high tide this rocky spot may be temporarily impassable until the water recedes. Past this point you travel on a narrow pebbly beach, from which you can look north to the large jutting headland of Cape Johnson. The beach itself is tucked neatly between a line of tangled driftwood and Sitka spruce forest on your right and a shelf of seaweed-covered rocks on your left. Thus, while walking on the pebbles can be tiring, it is clearly a better option than either fighting through the driftwood or taking a fall on the slippery rocks.

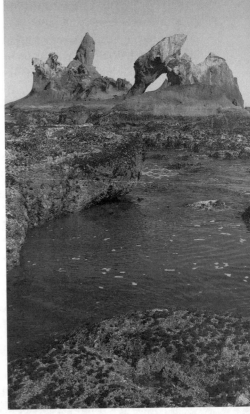

An arch in the cove north of Shi Shi Beach
photographed by Douglas Lorain

You follow this sweeping beach to the north end of a little cove where there are two possible (but usually dry) campsites a little more than 2.2 miles from Hole-in-the-Wall. A small memorial just inland from the camps commemorates the crash of a Chilean ship near this spot in November 1920.

Continuing northward, you make a rugged scramble around the tall cliffs of Cape Johnson, which requires a medium to low tide. You then round a seaweed-choked cove to a second lower-tide-only point with numerous slippery rocks. Past this point, things get easier as you stroll northward on an attractive pebbly beach. The principal obstacles along the way are numerous logs across the narrow sand, which are created by waves undercutting trees and eventually causing the trees to topple. This is a hazard you will encounter at several places along this trip, so you'll need to become accustomed to crawling around, over, or under these arboreal obstacles. A more welcome feature of this beach is a pair of small but usually reliable creeks that offer fresh water and the first really good places to camp on your journey.

At the north end of this beach you're faced with the impassable cliffs of a small, bulbous-shaped headland. Look for a signed inland trail that crosses the narrow neck of this headland and accesses the next beach to the north. This strip of sand is a joy because it consists of nice hard-packed sand that offers easy hiking. In addition, you'll enjoy continuously fine scenery looking west to the offshore rocks and islands around descriptively named Jagged Island. The beach has one low rocky area that requires a medium tide to get around (an inland bypass trail is available), but for the most part it's a simple stroll on hard sand. At the north end of the beach lies Cedar Creek, where you'll find excellent campsites on both sides of the crossing and a seasonal ranger tent. Like many coastal streams, Cedar Creek's water is the color of dark tea, but it is perfectly drinkable once filtered. Nearby are the rusting remains of the old Starbuck Mine.

NOTE: River otters live in Cedar Creek, so don't be surprised if a pair of these playful animals entertains you in the evening.

A little beyond Cedar Creek, you round another low-tide-only headland. Look for a wooden sand ladder leading to an inland trail that offers a way around, as well as a nice viewpoint from the top. North of this point stretches lovely Kayostla Beach, which features a couple of particularly scenic rocks that rise out of its hard-packed sand. At the southern end of this beach, a nice campsite lies next to a small creek, your last reliable water for several miles. About 0.5 mile north of this creek, you'll pass an easy-to-miss obelisk memorial to a Norwegian ship that wrecked on this beach in 1902. The maps show an old trail leading inland from this point to Allens Bay on Ozette Lake, but finding this unmarked route is difficult.

As you continue north on Kayostla Beach, the slopes on your right get higher and rockier, and the strip of sand eventually peters out, leaving you to scramble carefully over slippery rocks for the next 3 miles. Your progress will be slow, but the wildlife, both coastal and offshore (look for whales), is abundant. You round one lower-tide-required headland and come to an interesting rock arch on your right. From here it's slow going on a rocky shelf that takes you past a series of shallow coves and small headlands before you round a final headland and come to a pleasant little creek, where you'll find nice campsites.

The beach stretching north from this creek, called Yellow Banks, is a particularly scenic spot to rest or spend the night. At low tide several jagged rocks are exposed and tidepool life is everywhere. From here north, all the way to Point of the Arches, backpackers must have a reserved permit to camp. In addition, campfires are prohibited for the next 4.2 miles to Wedding Rocks.

At the north end of Yellow Banks is a rocky headland that requires a medium to low tide to get around. If the tide is up, you'll have to wait, as there is no overland trail.

From here it's easy walking on a lovely, sandy beach that takes you northwest toward the grass-covered bump at the tip of Sand Point. This beach is usually fairly crowded because day hikers and weekend backpackers can easily access this area from Ozette Lake. About 0.2 mile before reaching Sand Point, small but reliable Wish Wish Creek crosses the beach. To reach the excellent campsites at Sand Point, crawl over the driftwood just past Wish Wish Creek to the inland trail that travels through the trees paralleling the shore. If you camp at Sand Point, you are required to use one of the designated campsites. A seasonal ranger station is located nearby.

Hikers who have left a car at Ozette Lake and who plan to cut their trip short can take the inland trail heading northeast from Sand Point. In 2.8 miles this mostly boardwalk route travels through dense forest to the trailhead. Even if you plan to end your trip at Ozette Lake, however, it's better to make your trip a bit longer by continuing along the beach for another 3.1 miles to Cape Alava before heading east to your car. With this itinerary you'll see as much of the beautiful coastal scenery as possible before you have to reluctantly return to civilization.

Continuing north with the coastal route, you follow a narrow beach often blocked by fallen logs, which takes you 0.8 mile to a lower-tide-only point peppered with scenic little rock pinnacles. The number of pinnacles and tidepools continues to increase as you keep going north, often over slippery rocks or pebbly sand, to round another small headland, where a large pinnacle sports a tiny sea arch. Directly across from this scenic spot is a waterless campsite.

About 0.4 mile north of this camp is Wedding Rocks, where an outcrop of dark boulders sticks out from the shore. At low tide you can explore these boulders to discover an assortment of Makah petroglyphs. With patience and a lot of searching, you should find carvings that depict fish, whales, dogs, and other animals, and even one of a sailing ship. If the tide is high, you will be forced to take the short inland scramble trail around the Wedding Rocks.

Starting about 0.2 mile beyond Wedding Rocks, you'll pass a series of small campsites that offer excellent scenery but usually no water. Slippery rocks will slow your progress, but you're used to that by now. Adding to the scenery is large and forest-covered Ozette Island, which sits about a mile offshore. At really low tide an enormous rocky shelf full of tidepools extends almost all the way out to this island. Exploring this area is highly rewarding, but beware of sharp rocks and slippery seaweed. In addition, check your tide table, because you *do not* want to get so caught up in your explorations that you forget about the returning tide, which can easily trap unwary tidepool lovers. Even when the tide is up, however, the Cape Alava area is a haven for wildlife on both land and sea. On the water, look for various species of whales, sea lions, sea otters, and several types of birds, including ravens, black oystercatchers, and bald eagles. On the inland side, raccoons and black-tailed deer are both abundant.

Shortly before reaching the rounded tip of Cape Alava, you hop over a small creek and come to a spot where you can make a short detour up the grassy hillside to an inland trail. Numerous excellent campsites are in the vicinity, and a seasonal ranger station sits at the north end of the cape.

If you are ending your coastal hiking at Cape Alava, you can follow a 3.1-mile trail from here that goes briefly up to a forested plateau and then heads east to Ozette Lake. The path is a pleasant up-and-down walk with many boardwalk sections to avoid the mud, and it visits a large marshy meadow called Ahlstrom's Prairie along the way. This shorter alternative to the longer recommended trip is highly rewarding and fairly popular. It misses the remarkable scenery around Point of the Arches, but you won't have to deal with the difficult hiking required to reach that point.

Experienced and particularly athletic backpackers who are up for the full coastal experience should continue north from Cape Alava, walking on a nice sandy beach and past the rusting remains of an old shipwreck that can be seen at very low tide. Along the way you enter the tiny Ozette Reservation. You are not allowed to explore inland on reservation lands, but hikers can travel on the beach without restriction. At about 0.6 mile from the cape, you cross the narrow peninsula of sand that connects the shore with small Tskawa-hyah Island. Hikers are asked to avoid this island, which is considered sacred by the American Indians.

Your northward journey is now mostly on rocks and seaweed as you round a medium-tide point, where you leave the Ozette Reservation, and a second lower-tide point shortly thereafter. North of this point is a beach and the crossing of the Ozette River. During the winter months and/or after a heavy rain, fording this stream can be challenging. Things are much easier at low tide, when the water spreads out on the sand. With the lower river levels in the summer months, this crossing should not be a problem. There are nice camps here, including one up in the trees just after the crossing.

The next couple of miles are easy hiking, as most of the way is on pebbly sand until you reach tiny Seafield Creek. A short scramble trail on the north side of this creek leads to a forested bench with nice campsites.

North of Seafield Creek is easy travel for a little over 1 mile on beach and loose cobbles, and then it's either bouldering (at high tide) or tidepool-hopping (at low tide) around a rocky headland. Shortly beyond this is a second cliff-lined headland. This is the start of the toughest part of this trip, so be prepared to expend considerable energy over the next couple of miles.

To tackle this first obstacle you can either round the little headland at low tide or use a very steep rope to pull yourself up a cliff and then scramble down to the next pocket beach.

TIP: From the top of these cliffs, you can often observe sea otters lounging in the nearby pools and feeding on sea urchins and other critters.

After the pocket beach, another rope ladder leads you almost 200 feet up a cliff to an extended inland trail. Unfortunately, it can be very hard to find this rope, and you may have to make a ridiculously steep bushwhack up the slope instead. This route is necessitated by a series of cliffs and headlands that can only be very carefully rounded at extreme low tide. The best plan is to time your trip for a minus tide in the middle of the day. The inland trail (sometimes more of a muddy cross-country route) keeps you out of the surf but takes you into a tangle of mud and roots that makes for sloppy and slow going. Fortunately, the inland trail lasts for only about 0.7 mile before you steeply drop to another pocket beach, climb over a ladder to a bigger beach, and then scramble over yet another headland. The pattern is tiring, but at least you are rewarded with outstanding coastal scenery with lots of pinnacles and rocks and great views from the high points.

Finally back at water level, you round a medium-tide headland and happily stroll along a narrow, curving beach, which in 0.5 mile reaches spectacular Point of the Arches.

Try to time your visit to reach Point of the Arches at the lowest tide possible. This will allow you to safely round the headland here, but more important, it will give you the treasured opportunity to explore this scenic wonderland at its best. And the exploring simply couldn't be any better. A fantasyland of sea arches, towering rocky islands topped with shrubs and trees, dozens of scenic pinnacles, and countless great tidepools surrounds you. This is one of the finest collections of sea arches and pinnacles in the world, so enjoy. The opportunities for photographers are unlimited.

On the north side of Point of the Arches stretches magnificent Shi Shi Beach. Despite its remoteness, the long strip of sand earns accolades with its impressive waves, lots of scenic offshore rocks, and some of the best tidepooling anywhere. The beach is fairly popular with both day hikers and overnighters, however, so don't expect to be lonesome.

The walk on this idyllic beach begins with 0.9 mile of hard-packed sand to Petroleum Creek, which, despite its name, is not the least bit oily and whose waters are perfectly drinkable with the usual filtering. Fine campsites are found on the sand on both sides of the easy wade across this stream.

Beyond Petroleum Creek, the remainder of the beach walk is just as scenic but a bit more tiring due to the loose sand. Still, it sure beats all the slippery rocks you've negotiated over the last few days, so no complaining. After 1.1 miles, and shortly before the beach ends at a minor rocky headland, look for a path on your right that goes into the forest to some nicely sheltered campsites. Unfortunately, there is usually no fresh water in this vicinity.

From this campsite you'll notice an obvious trail heading up the steep and forested hillside. This is your exit route for the trip.

A sea arch at Point of the Arches
photographed by Douglas Lorain

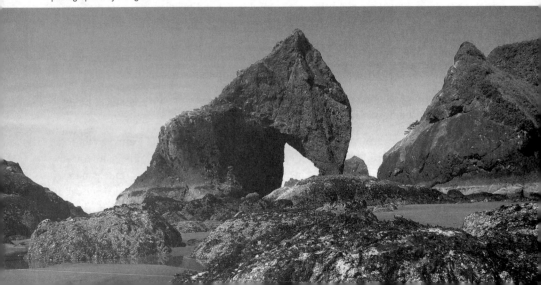

SIDE TRIP TO COVE NORTH OF SHI SHI BEACH: Before leaving the beach, set aside 20 minutes for one last coastal highlight. To reach it, explore north for about 0.1 mile to the end of Shi Shi Beach, then scramble over a little headland. On the other side is a spectacular little cove with one of the most amazing collections of tidepools you will ever see. In addition, this cove is stuffed full of incredibly scenic pinnacles and several dramatic arches that make for some of the best photo opportunities of this trip.

Having gathered enough coastal memories to last a lifetime, take the steep inland trail from the campsite and ascend a series of short switchbacks that gain about 150 feet to the forested plateau above. Here, there is a sign for the park boundary (to the north lies the Makah Reservation) and a permit registration box for those entering the park by this route.

The trail now heads north, and although nearly level, it is a mess of deep black holes of gooey mud. Some of the mud can be bypassed, but you should plan on more mud-slinging than a typical political campaign, and everyone in your party will probably get just as dirty as the politicians. On the plus side, a few short side trails go left to partially obstructed clifftop viewpoints overlooking the ocean. After about 1 mile of muddy travel, things improve dramatically when you pick up a newly designed trail that wends its way through forest and shrubbery, crosses a couple of plank bridges, and includes several gravel or boardwalk areas to avoid the mud. There are some minor ups and downs along the way but not much overall change in elevation. The trail ends about 1.8 miles from Shi Shi Beach at the northern trailhead.

VARIATION

As mentioned previously, you can shorten this trip, and make it much less rugged, by ending your hike at Ozette Lake instead of Shi Shi Beach.

POSSIBLE ITINERARY

	CAMP	MILES	ELEVATION GAIN
Day 1	Cedar Creek	8.8	50'
Day 2	Sand Point	8.5	50'
Day 3	Seafield Creek	7.6	50'
Day 4	Petroleum Creek	4.8	500'
Day 5	Out	2.9	450'
	Side trip to cove above Shi Shi Beach	0.3	40'

BEST SHORTER ALTERNATIVES

Day hikes from either end of this traverse, to Hole-in-the-Wall from the south or Point of the Arches from the north, are highly rewarding. The very popular Ozette Triangle in the middle of this route (starting at Ozette Lake and visiting Sand Point and Cape Alava, with the connecting beach route in between) is a reasonable overnight sampler, although getting the required reserved permits can be difficult.

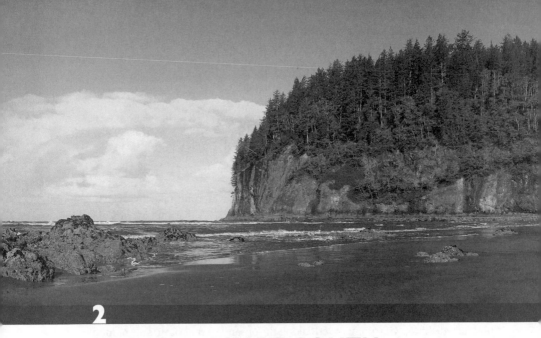

2

OLYMPIC COAST: SOUTH

RATINGS: Scenery 10   **Solitude** 5   **Difficulty** 8
MILES: 18
ELEVATION GAIN: 1,700'
DAYS: 2–4
SHUTTLE MILEAGE: 38
MAP: Custom Correct *South Olympic Coast*
USUALLY OPEN: Year-round
BEST: April–November
PERMIT: Required. As of 2019, the nonrefundable cost of a permit is $6 with an additional charge of $8 per adult in your party per night in the park. Alternatively, for $55 you can purchase an annual Olympic National Park Wilderness Pass, which covers all nightly fees for one person for the entire year. Hikers under the age of 16 are free. Permits are unlimited, and reservations are not needed for this area.
RULES: Maximum group size of 12 people; bear canisters required—to thwart the raccoons (free rentals available)
CONTACT: Olympic National Park, 360-565-3100, nps.gov/olym

SPECIAL ATTRACTIONS •

Wildlife, great coastal scenery

Above: *Jefferson Cove*
photographed by Douglas Lorain

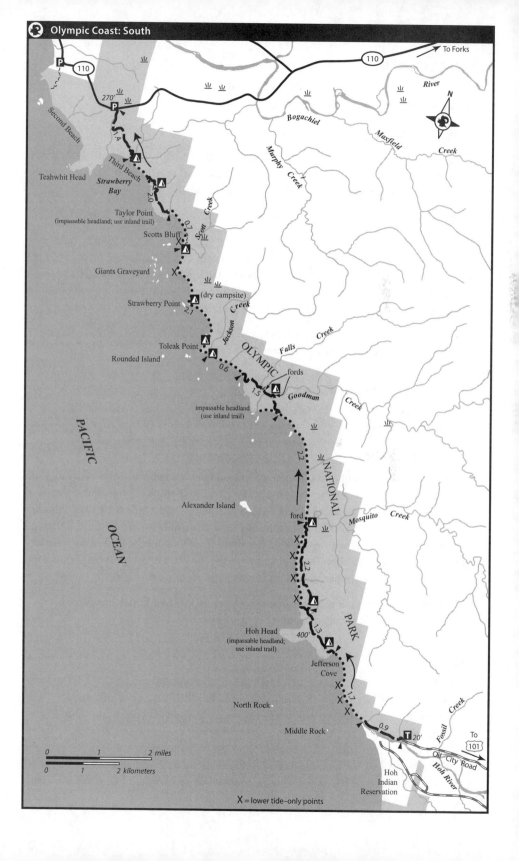

P
110
To Forks

110

River

Bogachiel

Maxfield

Creek

N

270'
P

Second Beach

1.4

Third Beach

Teahwhit Head

Strawberry Bay

2.0

Murphy Creek

Scott Creek

Taylor Point
(impassable headland; use inland trail)

0.7

Scotts Bluff

Giants Graveyard

(dry campsite)

Strawberry Point

2.1

Jackson Creek

Falls *Creek*

OLYMPIC

Toleak Point

Rounded Island

0.6

fords

1.5

Goodman Creek

impassable headland
(use inland trail)

2.2

NATIONAL

PACIFIC

Alexander Island

ford

Mosquito Creek

OCEAN

X

X

2.2

X

PARK

X

Hoh Head
(impassable headland;
use inland trail)

400'

1.3

Jefferson Cove

North Rock

X

1.7

X

X

Middle Rock

0.9

T 20'

Fossil Creek

To
101

Oil City Road

Hoh River

0   1   2 miles

0   1   2 kilometers

Hoh
Indian
Reservation

X = lower tide–only points

CHALLENGES

Difficult stream crossings, muddy inland trails, very rugged scrambles over boulders and headlands, tide problems, poor weather

HOW TO GET THERE

To reach the south trailhead from Forks, drive south on US 101 for 14 miles, then turn right (west) on Oil City Road (signed Cottonwood Recreation Area) and follow this paved and then gravel road for 10 miles to the road-end trailhead.

WARNING: The last 0.4 mile of this road is narrow and plagued with potholes. Take it slow.

To reach the north trailhead from Forks, drive north on US 101 for 1.5 miles, and turn left (west) onto La Push Road (also known as WA 110). After 3.1 miles, veer left at a junction, and 4.8 miles later go straight at a second junction. The Third Beach Trailhead is on the left side of the road, 3.8 miles from the last junction.

WARNING: Signs at this trailhead properly alert hikers to leave no valuables in their cars. Theft has been a consistent problem here.

GPS TRAILHEAD COORDINATES:
Southern (Oil City): N47° 44.960' W124° 24.517'
Northern (Third Beach): N47° 53.428' W124° 35.955'

INTRODUCTION

The hike along the southern Olympic coast is shorter but generally more difficult than all but the very challenging far northern part of Trip 1, Olympic Coast: North. The wild terrain here is more rugged, and hikers must deal with greater tide problems, muddier inland paths, and two potentially dangerous stream crossings. For experienced hikers, all of this adds to the trip's appeal, but this is a poor choice for inexperienced backpackers or those hiking with children. As compensation for the extra effort, the southern coastal strip has somewhat fewer people and no advance reservations are required.

TIP: You'll need a good pair of waterproof boots for this hike to get you through the muddy inland sections with dry feet.

DESCRIPTION

Starting from the south, the trail initially follows a shelf above the gravel bars and glacial waters of Hoh River. The vegetation here contains a lush mixture of Sitka spruce, western hemlock, and deciduous trees, with various ferns, skunk cabbage, and salmonberry crowding the forest floor. After 0.7 mile the trail leaves the forest and disappears. From here you crawl over driftwood logs and follow gravel bars beside the Hoh River to the Pacific Ocean at the river's mouth. There is a house on the Hoh Indian Reservation across the stream. Sharp-eyed hikers will be able to spot the lighthouse on Destruction Island about 3.5 miles southwest.

Your route turns north and crosses an attractive beach of sand and small stones, with lots of driftwood above the tide line. Here, as elsewhere along this hike, you should watch for bald eagles overhead, often being harassed by the ever-present gulls and crows. The trip's first major obstacle, an extended area of rough and slippery boulders at the base of a series of small headlands and cliffs, occurs less than 1 mile north of the Hoh River. The direct distance through this obstacle is only 0.5 mile, but you'll actually cover about twice that and gain quite a bit of elevation as you pick your way up, over, and around the boulders. This area requires medium to low tide to cross and is easier at very low tide.

WARNING: It's rare that hikers manage to get through here without slipping at least once. Watch your step so you don't turn an ankle.

North of these rocks, the route crosses the sands of tiny but very scenic Jefferson Cove to the sheer cliffs of massive Hoh Head, which cannot be rounded at beach level. At the end of the beach, a well-marked sand ladder climbs very steeply up the side of this headland. This ladder, like all the others along this route, simply hangs from the cliffs above and is made of solid wooden rungs between two parallel metal cables. A rope hangs down the middle for hikers to pull themselves up. The arrangement is functional but quite strenuous for typical hikers with 40 or so extra pounds on their backs. For safety, only one hiker at a time should ascend each section of the ladder.

TIP: If you carry a walking stick, you should have a convenient place to strap the stick to the outside of your pack. You will need both of your hands free to help pull yourself up the ladders.

You climb two ladders, and then steeply ascend a rocky path to a third ladder, followed by more steep trail. The total elevation gain to the top of Hoh Head is only about 400 feet, but it will seem like a lot more. About two-thirds of the way up, you'll pass a nice, flat campsite right beside the trail. The closest water, however, is from a tiny creek back on the beach, not an attractive alternative given the steepness of the trail. In addition to the steep trail, another problem you will surely notice is the mud. The trail has several muddy segments that make footing both messy and dangerous.

Once you're atop Hoh Head, the trail becomes much easier, as it makes an almost level tour through a lush forest of Sitka spruce and western hemlock. In May you'll be treated to the white blossoms of oxalis, an abundant ground cover plant with shamrock-shaped leaves. After extended rainy periods (pretty much *always* on the Olympic coast) you can expect large sections of this forest path to be muddy quagmires. To reduce your impact on the land, simply slog right through the mud rather than widening the trail by trampling vegetation along the fragile edges of muddy areas.

After just 0.4 mile of level path atop Hoh Head, the trail loses elevation as it begins a series of short, steep ups and downs. Views are limited by the trees, but three small creek crossings along the way help to break up the monotony. After about 0.5 mile of ups and downs, you come to a signed junction and a choice of routes. To the left a sign points to the EXTREME LOW TIDE ROUTE. Under this a helpful hiker has scratched in BELIEVE IT. These words speak for themselves.

If the tides are favorable, the trail down to the beach makes a wickedly steep descent, often over slippery mud. Near the bottom, a couple of soggy ropes have been installed to help daredevil backpackers. Once on the beach the route begins with a deceptively easy ramble along a narrow stretch of sand and pebbles. Next you round a small headland—impossible except at a very low tide—passing between cliffs and some oddly shaped sea stacks, and then enter a tiny cove at the base of the next headland. Getting around this obstacle requires either a minus tide or a fair degree of athleticism. At a low point in the headland, a rope (no ladder this time, just a rope) hangs down to the beach. Hikers must *pull* themselves up this wickedly steep 100-foot incline on what amounts to a mini mountain climb. This is a challenge for all but the fittest hiker. Once on top, a path drops steeply back to the beach on the other side of the headland. Having survived all this, you now make an easy 0.3-mile beach walk north toward rushing Mosquito Creek.

The inland alternative to the beach trail, which should be the choice of all hikers except at very low tide, is longer and less dramatic but also less strenuous and safer. The forested route passes a waterless camp about 100 feet past the junction and then begins a tiring series of small ups and downs, a pattern that will continue all the way to Mosquito Creek. Views are limited in the dense forests, but your ears should get a treat from listening to the cheerful songs of winter wrens. This tiny brown bird is rarely seen but somehow belts out a song at a decibel level that is out of proportion to the bird's size. The wren sings in all seasons, even in the depths of the Northwest's dreary winters, hence this bird's name. The trail crosses several small creeks and muddy sections, the worst ones spanned by wooden boardwalks or flat-topped logs.

WARNING: These wooden surfaces provide almost no traction for boots and are especially slippery when wet.

Continuing north, the trail loses more elevation than it gains as it works along the top of the cliffs above the beach and provides occasional views to the Pacific Ocean. On a forested bench just before you descend the final 50 feet to Mosquito Creek, you will pass several good camps and an outhouse. If the camps here don't suit you, there are also good sites on the beach on either side of the creek. From here you will enjoy outstanding sunsets and views to prominent Alexander Island, a flat-topped landmark about 1.2 miles offshore.

WARNING: After heavy rains, the wade across Mosquito Creek can be treacherous. If the weather has made this stream a major challenge, then you'll be in for a rude surprise at even larger Goodman Creek (2.5 miles ahead), which may not be crossable at all in such situations.

TIP: The ford of Mosquito Creek is easier at low tide. If you're uncertain about whether to camp on the north or the south side of the stream, the decision may be dictated by when the tides are more favorable.

North of Mosquito Creek is a welcome stretch of wide, smooth, easy-walking sand. The beach slowly arcs to the northwest and is occasionally interrupted by large sea stacks that rise out of the sand. About 1.6 miles up the beach from Mosquito Creek, a particularly large sea stack sprouts a growth of evergreens on top that looks like spiked hair.

About 2.2 miles north of Mosquito Creek, you will come to a 60-foot-tall rock with a small hole in it. On the *south* side of this rock is the easily overlooked start of the inland trail leading to the ford of Goodman Creek.

GOODMAN CREEK SIDE TRIP: Before you go inland it's worth taking a side trip north along the beach another 0.3 mile to the scenic rocks and tidepools around the mouth of Goodman Creek. The creek is over 20 feet deep at its mouth and cannot be crossed, which explains why the inland detour is necessary.

From the beach, the inland trail climbs through trees over a low ridge, and then drops to the sometimes-intimidating ford of Goodman Creek. This crossing is a simple wade in midsummer, but for the rest of the year it's anywhere from calf to waist deep, so it will get your heart pounding despite the cold water.

TIP: Even though the crossing is inland, it's much easier at low tide because the water gets backed up at high tide.

Good camps can be found on either side of the creek. To relocate the trail after the ford, look for a tiny orange marker about 50 feet downstream from the crossing. You barely have time to put your boots back on before coming to the much less intimidating ford of Falls Creek, a simple jump by midsummer. About 150 feet upstream from the crossing, the creek drops over a small cliff, giving the stream its name.

From Falls Creek you gain about 200 feet to the top of a woodsy ridge before dropping down the other side.

TIP: Listen for the loud, staccato call of pileated woodpeckers in these woods.

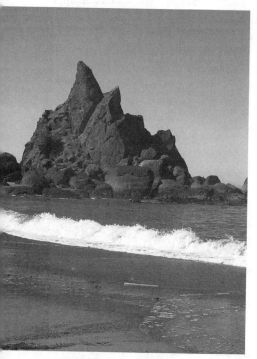

Pyramid north of Toleak Point
photographed by Douglas Lorain

As you descend you will pass some excellent overlooks of the next beach to the north. The trail down to this beach is rather steep, but it includes one sand ladder and some wooden steps to make the descent easier.

Once you reach the beach, it's an easy stroll north to Toleak Point, a low, sandy headland. Several good camps are in this vicinity, with fresh water available from Jackson Creek on the south side of the point. A toilet and an A-frame emergency shelter are also about 100 feet up a trail just on the north side of Jackson Creek.

Continuing north from Toleak Point, you follow an attractive arcing beach past a distinctive pyramid-shaped rock to Strawberry Point, where you cross a low, sandy neck of land connecting a large rock to the rest of the continent. There is a spacious camp here but no water for most of the year. At Strawberry Point you may see deer tracks in the sand or harbor seals hauled out on the nearby rocks to sun themselves.

North of Strawberry Point another lovely, arcing beach leads to a low- to medium-tide headland, followed by a short stretch of sand to the excellent camps and emergency trail shelter at Scott Creek. Cliff-edged Scotts Bluff is just north of the creek and can be rounded only at very low tide. If this isn't feasible, you must opt for the inland trail that starts near the Scott Creek shelter. The short inland path climbs fairly steeply in woods, sometimes on newly installed wooden steps, and then descends a sand ladder back to the shore at a narrow beach of sand and rocks. This beach is very scenic, with lots of sharp offshore rocks, but it's only 0.4 mile long. It ends at a rocky little cove near a prominent pinnacle with a single tree on top. There is a tiny creek here if you need water.

NOTE: If the tides block access to this cove, you can reach it by scramble ropes that lead very steeply over a small headland just south of the cove.

Now you must climb inland past Taylor Point, which cannot be rounded at any tide. The winding up-and-down trail climbs several sets of wooden stairs as it makes its way through the dense forests.

WARNING: Like other inland routes, this one has many muddy quagmires and lots of exposed roots.

You drop to a fair camp beside a tiny year-round creek, then climb to a larger camp. From here you descend several sections of steep trail and sand ladders to Third Beach. At the south end of this beach you can see a waterfall dropping down to the sand.

Walk north on this lovely beach of packed sand for 0.5 mile to a creek about 0.2 mile before the picturesque cliffs of Teahwhit Head. An excellent camp beside the creek, a little above the driftwood line, is almost always occupied. The final inland trail section climbs a series of short switchbacks from the creek through Sitka spruce forests. Once it attains the level terrain above the ocean, the graveled trail gets wider and wanders through forests of western hemlock with lots of salmonberry, elderberry, sword fern, and other understory plants. You'll reach the Third Beach Trailhead 1.4 miles from where you left the beach.

POSSIBLE ITINERARY

	CAMP	MILES	ELEVATION GAIN
Day 1	Mosquito Creek	6.1	600'
Day 2	Scott Creek	6.4	400'
	Side trip to mouth of Goodman Creek	0.6	0'
Day 3	Out	4.1	700'

BEST SHORTER ALTERNATIVES •

Without a car shuttle, outstanding one-night backpacking trips are possible to either Mosquito Creek from the south or Toleak Point from the north. For a day hike, Jefferson Cove makes an excellent goal from the south trailhead.

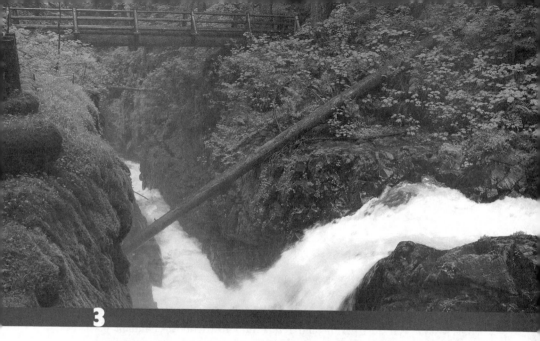

3

HIGH DIVIDE–HOH RIVER TRAVERSE

RATINGS: Scenery 10   **Solitude** 1   **Difficulty** 7

MILES: 38 (52)

ELEVATION GAIN: 5,350' (10,000')

DAYS: 4–6 (4–7)

SHUTTLE MILEAGE: 73

MAP: Custom Correct *Seven Lakes Basin–Hoh*

USUALLY OPEN: August–early October

BEST: August–early September

PERMIT: Required. As of 2019, the nonrefundable cost of a permit is $6 with an additional charge of $8 per adult in your party per night in the park. Alternatively, for $55 you can purchase an annual Olympic National Park Wilderness Pass, which covers all nightly fees for one person for the entire year. Hikers under the age of 16 are free.

Permits are limited for certain campsites on the suggested itinerary for this trip, and reservations are strongly recommended. Approximately 50% of permits for these campsites can be reserved, with the rest given out on a first-come, first-served basis.

Visit nps.gov/olym/planyourvisit/wilderness-reservations.htm for up-to-date information about quotas and reservations. Reservations are accepted in person at one of the park's wilderness information centers, online via recreation.gov, or by calling 877-444-6777. The system opens

Above: *Sol Duc Falls and a trail bridge*

photographed by Douglas Lorain

for reservations in mid-March. Changes are always likely, however, so check the park's website for the latest procedures and requirements.

RULES: Maximum group size of 12 people; groups of 7 or more must use designated group camps; no fires above 3,500 feet; camping is allowed only in designated sites in the Sol Duc/High Divide area and along the upper Hoh River Trail; bear canisters are required (free rentals available) for the High Divide area

CONTACT: Olympic National Park, 360-565-3100, nps.gov/olym

SPECIAL ATTRACTIONS

Magnificent rainforest, wildlife, wildflowers, views, glaciers

CHALLENGES

Poor weather, crowds, permit and reservation restrictions, abundant black bears, snowfields until late summer

HOW TO GET THERE

To reach the north trailhead from the west end of Lake Crescent, drive west on US 101 for 2 miles and then turn left (southwest) onto Sol Duc–Hot Springs Road, following signs to Sol Duc Valley. The good paved road passes a park entrance booth before reaching a ranger station near Sol Duc Hot Springs. The road then passes a resort and a campground before ending at a trailhead 14 miles from US 101.

The ending Hoh River Trailhead is reached by a well-marked paved road that turns left (east) off US 101 about 13 miles south of Forks. Follow Upper Hoh Road 18.5 miles to its end at the Hoh Rain Forest Visitor Center and trailhead. Overnight hikers are asked to park 0.2 mile to the west in a lot off the campground access road.

GPS TRAILHEAD COORDINATES:

Northern (Sol Duc): N47° 57.297' W123° 50.092'
Southern (Hoh River): N47° 51.618' W123° 56.068'

INTRODUCTION

Based on decades of voting with their boots, backpackers have selected this as the supreme on-trail wilderness experience in the Olympic Mountains. Every attraction that makes this range so magnificent can be seen at its best here. The hike includes the finest rainforests, best viewpoints, largest glaciers, and most colorful flower fields in the Olympics. Unfortunately, the *unwelcome* qualities of this range are also extreme on this hike. These are the most crowded backcountry trails in the Olympics. Snowfall in the high country is so heavy that many trails remain buried until late in the summer, while in the valleys, all that precipitation falls in unending volumes of rain that will test both your patience and the waterproof claims of the finest equipment. In good weather the scenery is superb, but pretty pictures don't tell the whole story.

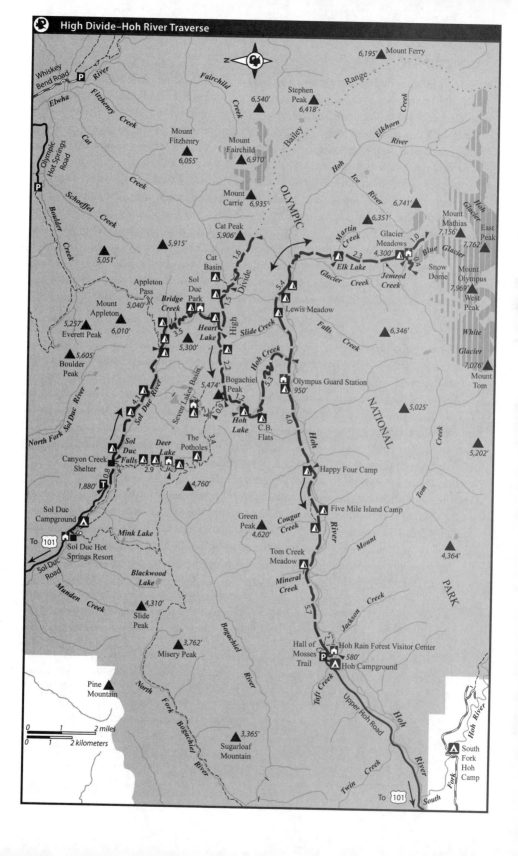

DESCRIPTION ●

The gently graded trail begins with an easy stroll through an old-growth rainforest of Douglas fir and western hemlock. At just over 0.1 mile you go straight at a junction, then at 0.8 mile reach the log Canyon Creek Shelter and a junction with the Deer Lake Trail. A short walk down the trail to the right leads to a bridge that provides an excellent view of Sol Duc Falls, an impressive, three-part, twisting cataract where the river plunges through a narrow chasm into a dark gorge.

From the junction near Sol Duc Falls, the Sol Duc River Trail bears left and continues east through luxuriant forests as it gradually climbs the valley floor. The route is rarely close to the river but crosses several small tributary creeks lined with maidenhair ferns and other water-loving plants. After passing a series of viewless, designated campsites, you keep straight at the junction with the Appleton Pass Trail at 4.9 miles and 0.3 mile later pass 7-Mile Camp. The trail passes more camps, then makes a bridged crossing of the river and begins a long, steady climb away from the stream. You cross Bridge Creek (camps) and continue climbing through attractive forests mixed with small meadows.

TIP: If you visit in mid- to late August, allow extra time to feast on juicy huckleberries.

After a spirited but short climb, you reach the excellent (but crowded) camps and seasonal ranger station at Sol Duc Park. Black bears are abundant in this area, so be sure to properly store all your food. You are likely to see bears in the meadows above the camp.

Above Sol Duc Park your trail makes an ironically bridgeless second crossing of Bridge Creek, then climbs through open parkland to tiny Heart Lake, surrounded by meadows and huckleberries. A few designated camps lie near the lake. The lakeshore and surroundings are quite popular and have been badly overused. Please respect all revegetation and closure signs to give the land a chance to recover.

Black bears are often seen on the slopes west of Heart Lake. In other parts of the country, the color phases of the American black bear range from black to light tan, but those in the Olympics are uniformly jet black. As a result, the animals are easy to spot as they lumber across the green meadows. From Heart Lake the trail ascends another 300 feet through open meadows to a ridgeline junction with the High Divide Trail.

CAT PEAK SIDE TRIP: An exceptional side trip (or day hike from a base in Sol Duc Park) leaves the main trail at this junction and turns left (east) toward the views and flowers of the Bailey Range. The path passes a spur trail to a designated (but waterless) campsite, then drops sharply down the side of a ridge to a possibly unsigned junction with a trail that descends to Cat Basin—which offers more good camps, although the area is designed for stock use and is infested with bears. Beyond this junction the up-and-down trail travels east through a saddle and along the side of a ridge. Views are usually blocked by trees, but there are enough tantalizing glimpses of Mount Olympus to keep you walking in hopes of a break in the tree cover. That break arrives not far beyond a sign saying that the trail is no longer officially maintained. The path, still good despite the lack of maintenance, breaks out into a small meadowy plateau on the side of Cat Peak, where you are treated to terrific views across the depths of the Hoh River Valley to the glacier-draped mass of Mount Olympus. Schedule extra time to enjoy this scene before returning the way you came.

Back at the junction above Heart Lake, hike west along High Divide, gaining elevation as the trail works up to this famous and spectacularly scenic ridge. From the ridgeline you can look north into a series of open meadow basins, where you will often see elk and bear—bring binoculars to get a good look. At your feet are a multitude of colorful wildflowers, including such mountain gems as avalanche lilies, bistorts, lupines, asters, and gentians, depending on the season. Most outstanding of all is the indescribable vista south to Mount Olympus, with its huge sheets of ice and radiating ridges. Between you and this peak is the deep, forested canyon of the Hoh River.

WARNING: Snow accumulates to enormous depths on the north-facing slopes of High Divide. Be prepared to crawl over snowfields well into August.

After passing a waterless camp, you reach the path's high point, literally and figuratively, just below Bogachiel Peak.

BOGACHIEL PEAK SIDE TRIP: A 0.15-mile spur trail leads to the top of this prominent knoll, where the panoramas are absolutely incredible. A fire lookout once sat atop this summit, and you have to envy the staffer who drew this assignment. Most of the Olympic Mountains, as well as a sliver of the Pacific Ocean, can be seen from here. The deep, green valleys of the Hoh, Sol Duc, and Bogachiel Rivers are separated by high snowy ridges and peaks. To the north is the huge, sloping, mostly treeless Seven Lakes Basin. Most dramatic of all, of course, is Mount Olympus, a huge mass of rock and ice to the south. Allow plenty of extra time to enjoy this vista.

TIP: Don't forget to bring a windbreaker, as the summit is often breezy.

From the Bogachiel Peak side trail, the main route goes west for 0.2 mile to a junction with the Hoh Lake Trail. To visit Seven Lakes Basin, a very worthwhile side trip, keep right at this junction and descend a ridge 0.9 mile to a junction in a saddle, where you turn right and drop into this scenic basin.

To continue your main trip from the junction below Bogachiel Peak, turn left (south) on the Hoh Lake Trail and begin the long 4,500-foot descent into the Hoh River Valley. The trail crosses attractive subalpine country with good views, as the path makes several switchbacks down to the shores of beautiful Hoh Lake, a good-size pool surrounded by heather and subalpine fir. Elk are often seen on the nearby slopes, and there are excellent designated camps for tired backpackers. The lake typically remains encased in snow and ice until midsummer.

TIP: On a clear evening, the sunset view of Mount Olympus over Hoh Lake is memorable. Take your dinner and your camera over to the lake's northeast shore to see the show.

From Hoh Lake the trail continues its long descent, much of the way through areas still recovering from a large forest fire in 1978. Dozens of switchbacks ease the grade, and a pretty waterfall at the crossing of Hoh Creek adds scenic interest. Just beyond this crossing is C. B. Flats, a grassy meadow with a group campsite and a bear wire. Alternating between forest and recovering burn areas, the path continues down through meadows and trees as it follows first the creek, then a side ridge. From the end of the ridge, the route plunges down numerous switchbacks and then rejoins the creek. The trail levels out noticeably as it reenters ancient rainforest not burned in the fire, and then leads to an intersection with the Hoh River Trail.

At this junction your choice of route will be dictated by the weather. If the rains are pouring down—something to be expected, since this is a *rainforest* after all—you should simply end the hike by turning right (west) and following the Hoh River Trail 9.7 miles to the trailhead. With good raingear and, more important, the proper frame of mind, hiking this section in the rain is both fitting and enjoyable. You won't miss any distant views—you can't see anything through the forest even on clear days—and you can appreciate the huge trees, lush mosses, and delicate undergrowth just as well in the rain as in the sun.

If the weather gods are smiling, however, you should turn left (east) at the junction and make the trip up the Hoh River Trail to the outstanding views above Glacier Meadows. The trail takes a lazy course up the valley floor, goes across a bench with views above the rushing Hoh River, and comes to Lewis Meadow, a grassy flat with good camps. The almost level trail continues through fine woods before returning to the river, which is noticeably milky-colored from glacial runoff. You pass three good camps spaced out along the river (no bear wires), then climb away from the water on short switchbacks. The trail does some ups and downs for a while, and then crosses two small creeks before dropping to a bridge over the churning Hoh River. The water races through a fern-lined slot canyon some 100 feet beneath the bridge. Downstream you can see where the relatively clear waters of the Hoh River meet the milky flow of Glacier Creek.

Now that you've left the easy valley-bottom trail behind, the path steadily climbs a slope covered with thick Douglas fir forests. Numerous fairly steep little switchbacks lead to an overhanging rock formation that gives hikers a free shower through midsummer. More climbing takes you past a hard-to-see waterfall to a crossing of Martin Creek on a footlog. A horse camp lies about 100 yards past the creek.

NOTE: This is the last place fires are permitted along the Hoh River Trail.

After a brief additional climb, you'll reach lily pad–filled Elk Lake, with an emergency trail shelter and very popular camps above its southeast shore. From Elk Lake the trail, here closed to stock, climbs fairly steeply to some nice views down to Elk Lake, north to High Divide, and west to a serrated ridge that radiates north from Mount Olympus. You hop across a small creek, then climb in forest before breaking out on a steep hillside with terrific views of the deep canyon of Glacier Creek and up to White Glacier, Snow Dome, and West Peak, the highest point on Mount Olympus (and in the entire Olympic Mountains). The trail then ducks into the woodsy canyon of small Jemrod Creek and then remains nearly level for about 0.5 mile to Glacier Meadows, which has an emergency shelter, numerous good but popular campsites, and a ranger tent a little above the camping area. The meadow itself is small but gloriously colorful, with an array of wildflowers, including glacier and avalanche lilies, lupines, bistorts, hellebores, valerian, bluebells, and many others.

SIDE TRIP TO BLUE GLACIER VIEWPOINTS: About 100 yards beyond the ranger tent, the trail splits. Both branches are well worth a visit. To the left a steep path signed UPPER BLUE GLACIER travels up a rocky gully that usually has snow for most of the summer.

WARNING: On cold mornings these steep snowfields can be icy and dangerous.

The trail becomes faint but eventually tops out on the lateral moraine above massive Blue Glacier. This overlook also provides superb vistas of Mount Olympus and Snow Dome. On clear days (definitely the exception, rather than the rule) the sight of huge fields of snow and ice is remarkable.

TIP 1: Bring binoculars to watch climbers making their way across the glacier.

TIP 2: Don't forget to bring a wide-angle lens; you'll need it.

The other trail from the fork above Glacier Meadows is the better-maintained Terminus Trail. It briefly descends to a creek, and then climbs numerous switchbacks through boulders to an excellent viewpoint. From here you can look down on the crevasses and smooth, polished rocks at the toe of Blue Glacier; up to Snow Dome, Blizzard Pass, and West Peak; and off to the north along the canyon of Glacier Creek. *Outstanding!*

To complete your hike, descend from Glacier Meadows 7.7 miles along the Hoh River Trail back to the junction with the Hoh Lake Trail, and continue straight (west). As the Hoh River Trail goes down the valley, it passes through perhaps the most magnificent temperate rainforest in North America. The dominant tree is Douglas fir, with increasing numbers of Sitka spruce, western hemlock, western red cedar, and big-leaf maple as you continue down the valley. Enormous old giants up to 300 feet tall and 11 or more feet in diameter compete for attention with young saplings; draping mosses; an understory of salmonberry, thimbleberry, and vine maple; and a ground cover of delicate ferns, mosses, oxalis, vanilla leaf, and other plants. Only in the redwood forests and sequoia groves of California will you find forests as awe-inspiring as this. In those more southerly woods, however, each tree puts on a solitary show of magnificence. Here the mass of trees and shades of green are all tangled together. You can walk for miles, and the only brown you'll see is the trail because the rest of the ground, the tree trunks, and even the rocks are all covered with a thick mat of green ferns, lichens, and mosses. In fact, the biomass (the total weight of living and dead biological material) in this forest may be the highest anywhere on the planet. In terms of animals you should keep an eye out for elk and salamanders, but birds are rather rare, with only a few species like Steller's jay, American robin, ruffed grouse, and winter wren to break the quiet of the forest. The trail is almost level, losing elevation so gradually that you're unlikely to even notice.

WARNING: On the rare hot summer day, it can be muggy and uncomfortable on this low-elevation path.

Heading west from the Hoh Lake junction, you pass some huge trees and come to the many excellent camps near Olympus Guard Station, a historical wood cabin now used as a ranger station in summer. The trail then does some ups and downs across a hillside, where young trees are growing to replace the silver snags at the lower edge of a fire scar. You soon pass a camp marked by a post showing a tent symbol and a mileage—7.8. It's easy to keep track of your mileage on this trail, as numerous camps are marked in this manner, each showing the remaining distance to the Hoh River Trailhead. Unlike the major camps shown on the map, however, these smaller camps have no bear wires.

At the 5.7-mile mark you reach Happy Four Shelter and a short side trail to some good camps near the river. As you continue down the valley from Happy Four, the forest gets even denser and grander. Shortly beyond a rare opening in the trees beside the river, the trail splits. The high water route loops to the right around Five Mile Island, while the main trail goes left and crosses a beautiful meadowy flat. River-level flats like this provide a nice contrast to the dense, conifer woods farther away from the water. Here you'll find grassy open areas and lots of deciduous trees, like big-leaf maple, alder, and cottonwood, that put on a lovely display of color in mid-October. These river flats are good places to look and listen for elk. Five Mile Island also has scenic camps with a bear wire.

With all the rain that falls here, you would expect the trail to be muddy, and it is in a few places. Overall, though, the National Park Service has done an excellent job of installing bridges, boardwalks, and raised gravel paths that keep the trail generally dry and in good shape. Below Five Mile Island you cross several creeks and pass more small camps as the trail generally remains in the forests away from the river. The last large camp with a bear wire is at Tom Creek Meadow, at the 2.9-mile mark.

Shortly beyond Tom Creek Meadow, you cross Mineral Creek below a twisting water-fall and continue down the trail past several small camps. As you approach the Hoh River Trailhead, day hikers increase in number and eventually crowd the trail almost as much as the plant life crowds the forest floor. The trail finishes by going straight at junctions with the extremely busy Spruce and Hall of Mosses Nature Trails, and then a paved section of trail takes you to the visitor center and parking lot.

POSSIBLE ITINERARY

	CAMP	MILES	ELEVATION GAIN
Day 1	Sol Duc Park	6.5	1,900'
Day 2	Hoh Lake	5.3	1,400'
	Side trip to Cat Peak	6.2	1,500'
	Side trip to Bogachiel Peak	0.3	100'
Day 3	Elk Lake	10.7	1,700'
Day 4	Olympus Guard Station	6.0	150'
	Side trip to Blue Glacier viewpoints	7.4	3,050'
Day 5	Out	9.1	200'

BEST SHORTER ALTERNATIVE

The very popular High Divide Loop from the Sol Duc Trailhead is a superb one- or two-night backpacking choice.

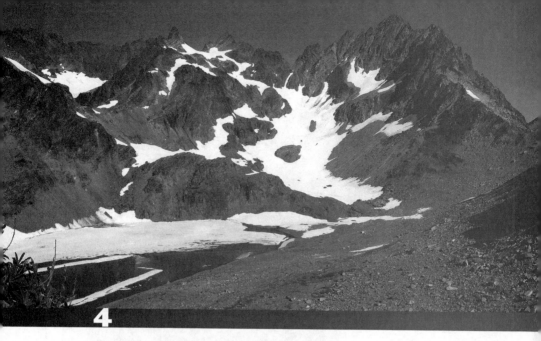

4

ENCHANTED VALLEY–
LACROSSE BASIN LOOP

RATINGS: Scenery 10   **Solitude** 4   **Difficulty** 7
MILES: 59 (66)
ELEVATION GAIN: 10,350' (12,900')
DAYS: 5–7 (5–8)
SHUTTLE MILEAGE: n/a
MAP: Custom Correct *Enchanted Valley–Skokomish*
USUALLY OPEN: Late July–October
BEST: Late July–early August/mid- to late October
PERMIT: Required. As of 2019, the nonrefundable cost of a permit is $6 with
an additional charge of $8 per adult in your party per night in the park.
Alternatively, for $55 you can purchase an annual Olympic National Park
Wilderness Pass, which covers all nightly fees for one person for the entire
year. Hikers under the age of 16 are free. Permits are unlimited, and reserva-
tions are not needed for this area.
RULES: Maximum group size of 12 people; no fires above 3,500 feet; bear
canisters are required (free rentals available) where you cannot hang food at
least 12 feet high and 10 feet out from a tree trunk
CONTACT: Olympic National Park, 360-565-3100, nps.gov/olym

continued on page 46

Above: *Mount Anderson from the Anderson Glacier viewpoint*
photographed by Douglas Lorain

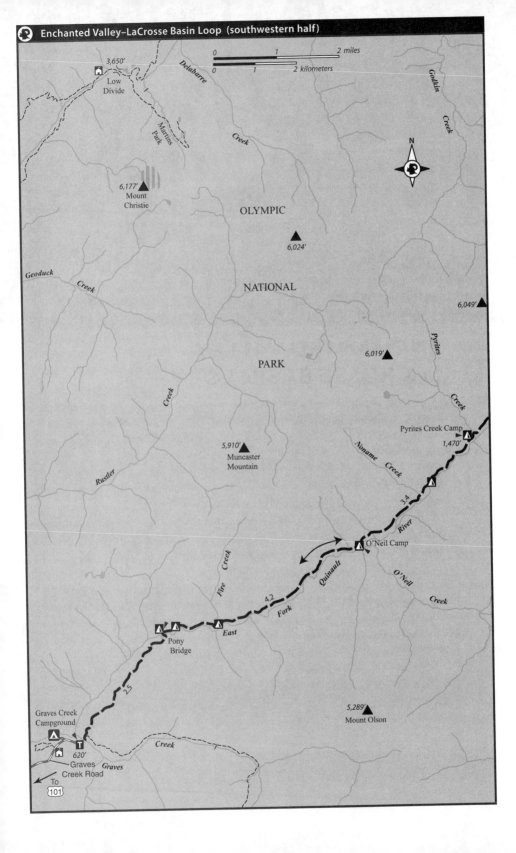

0   1   2 miles

0   1   2 kilometers

Delabarre

Goldin Creek

3,650'
Low Divide

Martins Park

Creek

6,177' ▲
Mount Christie

OLYMPIC

6,024' ▲

Geoduck Creek

NATIONAL

6,049' ▲

N

Pyrites Creek

6,019' ▲

PARK

Pyrites Creek Camp
1,470'

Creek

Noname Creek

5,910' ▲
Muncaster Mountain

3.4

Rustler

River

Quinault

O'Neil Camp

O'Neil Creek

Fire Creek

4.2

Fork

East

Pony Bridge

East

5,289' ▲
Mount Olson

2.5

Graves Creek Campground

620'
Graves Creek Road

Graves

Creek

To
101

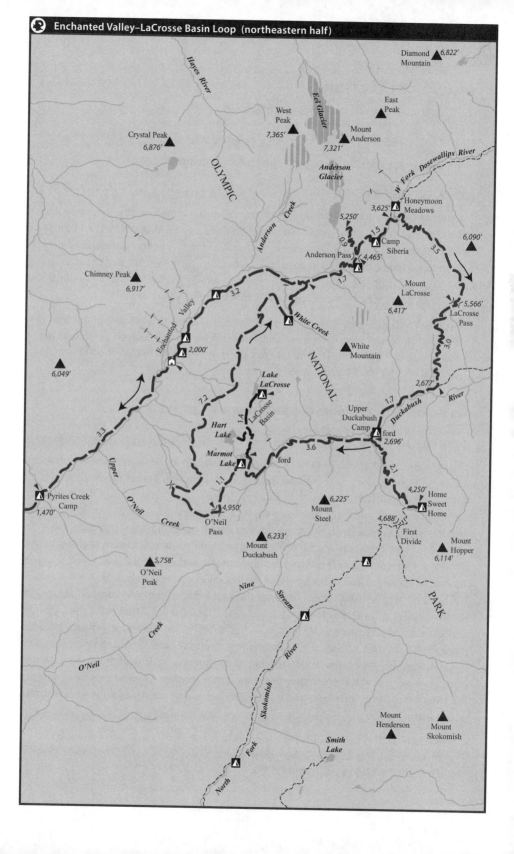

Diamond Mountain ▲6,822'

West Peak ▲ 7,365'

Eel Glacier

East Peak ▲

Mount Anderson ▲ 7,321'

Crystal Peak ▲ 6,876'

OLYMPIC

Anderson Glacier

W Fork Dosewallips River

Honeymoon Meadows

3,625'

5,250'

6,090' ▲

Anderson Creek

Chimney Peak ▲ 6,917'

1.5

Camp Siberia

Anderson Pass 4,465'

0.9

3.5

Enchanted Valley

3.2

White Creek

1.7

Mount LaCrosse ▲ 6,417'

5,566' LaCrosse Pass

2,000'

1.4

White Mountain

NATIONAL

3.0

6,049' ▲

Lake LaCrosse

7.2

Hart Lake

LaCrosse Basin

Upper Duckabush Camp

1.7

Duckabush

2,677'

River

ford 2,696'

Upper

Marmot Lake

ford

3.6

2.1

3.3

1.1

4,250' Home Sweet Home

O'Neil

Creek

4,950'

O'Neil Pass

▲6,225' Mount Steel

4,688',

Pyrites Creek Camp 1,470'

Duckabush

First Divide

Mount Hopper ▲ 6,114'

▲6,233' Mount Duckabush

5,758' ▲

O'Neil Peak

PARK

Nine

Stream

O'Neil

Creek

River

North

Fork

Skokomish

Mount Henderson ▲

Mount Skokomish ▲

Smith Lake

continued from page 43

SPECIAL ATTRACTIONS

Wildlife, diverse terrain, wildflowers, fall colors

CHALLENGES

Black bears are common—properly store all food; marginally crowded

HOW TO GET THERE

From Hoquiam, drive north on US 101 for 37 miles, almost to the southwest end of Lake Quinault. Turn right (northeast) onto South Shore Quinault Road, and after 2.2 miles pass the Quinault Wilderness Information Center, where you can obtain a permit. Continue northeast on the main road as it eventually changes from pavement to gravel and travels through lush rainforests. The narrow, winding route ends at a trailhead just past Graves Creek Campground, about 19.5 miles from US 101.

NOTE: The final few miles of this road are particularly prone to washouts, often closing the road to vehicles for months or even years. Hikers are still allowed to walk in, but you should call 360-565-3131 or visit nps.gov/olym to check the latest conditions to see just how far you'll have to walk.

GPS TRAILHEAD COORDINATES: N47° 34.365' W123° 34.209'

INTRODUCTION

If we were forced to select our favorite backpacking trip in the Olympic Mountains, this would be it. Amid glorious mountain scenery, the trip samples every major environment in the range, from lush rainforests to glaciers. There is also plenty of wildlife—including marmots, deer, elk, and black bears—to enjoy. The route runs alongside a strikingly beautiful stream and climaxes in the most sublime alpine basin in the entire range. Last, but certainly not least, it visits spectacular Enchanted Valley, where a historical chalet is well situated for viewing the surrounding meadow, peaks, and waterfalls. With good weather, this hike is about as close to backpacking perfection as you are likely to find.

The East Fork Quinault River Trail leads through a magnificent rainforest dominated by western hemlocks with a few western red cedars and Douglas firs. Beneath the thick canopy, the light-starved undergrowth of vine maple, huckleberry, bunchberry, and sword fern adds more shades of green. Roosevelt elk inhabit these forests and are often seen by quiet hikers.

Of course, this area earns its designation as a rainforest by drowning in nearly 14 feet of rain annually, so you should come prepared for the wetness. Even when it's not raining, the trees often create their own precipitation by peppering the forest floor with droplets of condensation.

WARNING: This trail includes many short ups and downs that don't show up on contour maps. The total elevation gain is actually quite substantial despite what appears on the map to be a gentle climb.

DESCRIPTION ●

The trail starts by crossing Graves Creek on a bridge and following a long-abandoned road. Just 0.1 mile from the trailhead is a junction with the Graves Creek Trail. You bear left (northeast) on the main trail and climb past massive trees, some over 250 feet tall and as much as 8 feet in diameter. The old road ends after 2 miles at a dilapidated picnic table. Beyond this point the route follows a footpath and rapidly descends to the river at Pony Bridge, which spans the stream above lovely moss- and fern-lined cliffs. On the other side of the bridge are two good campsites, the first of many pleasant riverside camps spaced out over the next several miles. The camps here do not have bear wires.

Settling into a pattern of small ups and downs, the trail climbs away from the loudly cascading stream as you travel through marvelous cathedral forests. In addition to the forests, the tour includes crossings of numerous side creeks, passes a few nice campsites, and makes frequent visits to the beautiful waters of the East Fork Quinault River. Stands of big-leaf maple, whose leaves turn a glorious mottled yellow in late October, shade much of the path. There are only limited views of the surrounding country, and the trail is often muddy, but the abundance of intimate natural scenery ensures that it's never tedious. Listen for bugling elk in the fall. At 6.7 miles you cross a usually dry creek and immediately reach the signed spur trail to O'Neil Camp.

The up-and-down pattern is a little less pronounced now as you continue up the valley through forests composed mostly of Douglas firs and western red cedars. Riverside camps are frequent, and numerous spots afford the opportunity to rest beside the river and soak in the scenery. The path crosses Noname Creek on a hiker's footlog and continues upstream to the excellent designated camps on either side of cascading Pyrites Creek, spanned by a log footbridge.

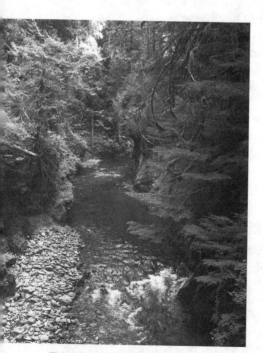

The gorge upstream from Pony Bridge
photographed by Douglas Lorain

Above Pyrites Creek the East Fork Quinault River Trail goes gradually uphill, often across river flats under a leafy canopy of alder and maple. The route crosses the river on a hikers-only suspension bridge and 0.5 mile later arrives at Enchanted Valley, where the forests abruptly open up into a mix of meadows and deciduous trees. This place has a classic mountain setting, with towering, snow-streaked cliffs rising nearly 5,000 feet to the top of Chimney Peak to the west. At the head of the valley are the dark ramparts and white glaciers of Mount Anderson, while to the east rise the forested ridges around O'Neil Pass. Countless cascading waterfalls streak down the cliffs and ridges, giving this wonderland its other common name: Valley of 10,000 Waterfalls (probably an over-statement, but not by much). Excellent designated camps are located a little beyond the Enchanted Valley chalet, a picturesque, two-story log building built in 1930. This historical structure was once used as a wilderness hotel and is now maintained by volunteers to serve as an emergency hiker's shelter and seasonal ranger station.

WARNING: Black bears are common in the Enchanted Valley, as they are in many parts of the Olympics. Hang all food and garbage on the provided bear wires or use a bear canister.

NOTE: Avalanches in 1999 toppled many trees in Enchanted Valley, opening more views but cluttering the valley floor with downed timber.

The East Fork Quinault River Trail continues up the valley past the stock camp and climbs a bit to an upper meadow where there are more good hiker camps.

TIP: These sites are just as scenic and less crowded than those near the chalet.

From here you go up and down in forests and above gravel bars near the river as you gradually gain elevation. The trail climbs fairly steeply in woods above the stream, as the canyon curves to the right (east). Openings in the forest provide nice looks at the pinnacle of West Peak, the highest point on Mount Anderson. The trail crosses frothing White Creek on a narrow, log footbridge over a small gorge with waterfalls both above and below the crossing. More climbing and several switchbacks lead you up through avalanche meadows to a jumbled rockslide. The O'Neil Pass Trail, the return route of the recommended lollipop loop, meets your route here.

Your route goes left from this junction and climbs steeply through open meadows with good views and lots of huckleberries and wildflowers. You will notice spirea, yarrow, arnica, valerian, paintbrush, pearly everlasting, bistort, columbine, hellebore, cow parsnip, and many other species. Numerous short switchbacks ease the grade of this ascent, but it's still a long haul, especially on hot summer afternoons.

Once you finally reach Anderson Pass, a mix of meadows and forest in a narrow gap with a small pond and campsite, the views are rather disappointing. To improve on this situation, drop your pack and take the very rewarding 0.9-mile one-way side trip up the Anderson Moraine Trail.

ANDERSON GLACIER VIEWPOINT SIDE TRIP: The path goes to the left (north) from Anderson Pass and switchbacks steeply up open slopes, which are carpeted with huckleberries that provide a treat for the taste buds in August and early September and a treat for the eyes in mid- to late October when the leaves turn bright red. You pass a small pond, then make a final steep scramble over rocks and heather to the top of a large moraine overlooking Anderson Glacier, formerly a large ice sheet but one that has obviously receded considerably in recent decades. At the foot of the diminished glacier is a large meltwater lake, usually covered with ice and snow for most of the summer. The dramatic scenery here includes marvelous vistas southwest to Enchanted Valley and across the East Fork Quinault River Canyon to Mount LaCrosse.

After returning to Anderson Pass, you hike northeast past a small tarn and descend the West Fork Dosewallips River Trail. The trail drops to Anderson Pass Camp, locally called Camp Siberia due to the cold winds that commonly blow through here, and then continues its forested descent to Honeymoon Meadows. There are good camps and a usually empty ranger cabin here. At the west end of this flat meadow is a junction with the LaCrosse Pass Trail.

WARNING: Honeymoon Meadows is still another favored spot for the ubiquitous black bears of the Olympics. Store your food properly at night and anytime you're away from camp.

From the junction in Honeymoon Meadows, turn right (southeast) on the LaCrosse Pass Trail, which immediately crosses West Fork Dosewallips River and then a second stream coming down from LaCrosse Pass. The trail makes a long, moderately steep, switchbacking climb through forests with only occasional brief glimpses of the surrounding terrain. After about 2 miles you break out of the forest into a huge sloping meadow with terrific views and a liberal display of colorful wildflowers. Craggy Mount LaCrosse rises to the southwest, and towering Mount Anderson dominates the skyline to the northwest. At your feet are acres of false hellebore, valerian, buttercups, avalanche lilies, and a host of other blossoms. These are some of the finest mountain meadows you will find anywhere. The joyous path makes a long sidehill ascent all the way to a ridge just above LaCrosse Pass. In addition to the now-familiar northerly vistas, LaCrosse Pass has equally striking views south and west to Mounts Hopper, Steel, and Duckabush.

The deep valley immediately below you is the canyon of the Duckabush River. With a goal of reaching this stream, the trail makes an interminably long descent into this canyon. Short switchbacks, numbering in the hundreds, ease the grade but not the monotony. The viewless route has no water and can be a long, hot, dry climb when coming up from the Duckabush side (which is why it is recommended that you begin from the Dosewallips side, as described here). The 3,000-foot descent finally ends at a junction with the Duckabush River Trail, where you turn right (west).

This river trail travels through some impressive old-growth forests of Douglas fir, western hemlock, and grand fir, generally staying well away from the water. After 1.7 miles the trail crosses the river. There is usually a logjam here, but if not, you'll have to make a knee-deep ford. Immediately after the crossing you come to Upper Duckabush Camp and a junction. A bear wire here serves as a reminder of the presence of bruins in these mountains.

HOME SWEET HOME SIDE TRIP: A worthwhile side trip leaves the Duckabush River Trail here and climbs fairly steeply south for 2.1 miles to a lovely meadow with the charming name of Home Sweet Home. A short side trail leads to several small but excellent campsites. Flowers choke the meadow and there are superb views, especially looking west to Mount Steel. From Home Sweet Home adventurous hikers can continue climbing another 550 feet to First Divide and follow scramble trails to Mount Hopper and beyond.

Back at Upper Duckabush Camp, the Duckabush River Trail goes west (upstream) across slopes with a mix of forests and brushy areas as the river, now just a good-size creek, gradually curves to the south. The trail climbs away from the stream and then loses a little elevation to a ford of the creek.

WARNING: In early summer this crossing can be wet and rather treacherous.

The route then rapidly gains elevation on its way to a junction beside tiny Marmot Lake, which features good camps, a picturesque island, and a lovely meadow setting.

LAKE LACROSSE SIDE TRIP: From the junction on the southeast shore of Marmot Lake, a not-to-be-missed side trail climbs a series of short, steep switchbacks north into the open terrain of outstandingly beautiful LaCrosse Basin. This path passes a fine viewpoint of the long, deep canyon of the Duckabush River and soon reaches a junction. To the left (west) a trail goes 0.2 mile to Hart Lake, in a steep, rocky basin. To reach an even more scenic destination, however, keep right (north) at the junction, and follow this trail over small rocky knolls, past patches of twisted mountain hemlock, over a lovely little creek, and through absolutely gorgeous meadows to Lake LaCrosse. This slender lake has a spectacular setting surrounded by meadow slopes and alpine peaks, with wildflowers and heather adding color to the scene. To the south rises distinctive Mount Duckabush, which perfectly catches the evening light for photographs. The lake often remains frozen well into July, but once ice-free it can hold its own with any lake in Washington for beauty. A good camp lies in a patch of trees above the northeast shore of the lake.

TIP: Look for wildlife in this area. One morning, just before dawn, I sat in my tent and watched 51 elk walk quietly past—an unforgettable experience.

To exit LaCrosse Basin, return to Marmot Lake, then turn west and make a long, fairly gentle climb to 4,950-foot O'Neil Pass. The way is mostly through open meadows, so the hiking is very scenic. Views from the pass are pleasant, but not as good as they will be in the miles to come. From O'Neil Pass the trail gradually loses elevation as it crosses a rocky hillside above the headwaters of Upper O'Neil Creek, then curves away from this stream and contours across an open slope to a ridgeline saddle with terrific views across the East Fork Quinault River Valley. From this saddle the trail rounds a small, steep-walled basin.

WARNING: Snow lingers in this high basin until late summer. Be prepared to traverse snowfields.

As the trail continues its long descent along the side of this ridge, you travel through forests of hemlock and Douglas fir and cross numerous avalanche chutes, some still filled with snow even in late summer. The most memorable feature of this trail, however, is the *view!* The vistas across Enchanted Valley to Chimney Peak are incredible. In addition, Mount Anderson and West Peak are often visible to the northeast, and on very clear days you'll even be able to look down the long valley of the East Fork Quinault River and spy the distant waters of the Pacific Ocean.

As the trail loses elevation, the vistas gradually become less grand and the tree cover gets thicker. The hiking is nonetheless pleasant as the trail switchbacks down a ridge and goes into a lovely little basin where you cross White Creek (good camps). Now the trail makes a forested descent for 0.7 mile to a reunion with the East Fork Quinault River

Trail below Anderson Pass. To return to your car, simply turn left (west) and descend this beautiful trail for 16.6 miles back through Enchanted Valley and along the lovely East Fork Quinault River. This is rather a long trail to redo, but it's so pretty that you won't have any complaints about hiking it again.

POSSIBLE ITINERARY

	CAMP	MILES	ELEVATION GAIN
Day 1	Pyrites Creek	10.1	1,700'
Day 2	Honeymoon Meadows	9.7	3,300'
	Side trip to Anderson Glacier	1.8	800'
Day 3	Upper Duckabush Camp	8.2	2,100'
Day 4	Lake LaCrosse	5.0	2,050'
	Side trip to Home Sweet Home	4.2	1,600'
	Side trip to Hart Lake	0.4	150'
Day 5	Enchanted Valley	12.9	700'
Day 6	Out	13.4	500'

A bear in a huckleberry patch above Anderson Pass
photographed by Douglas Lorain

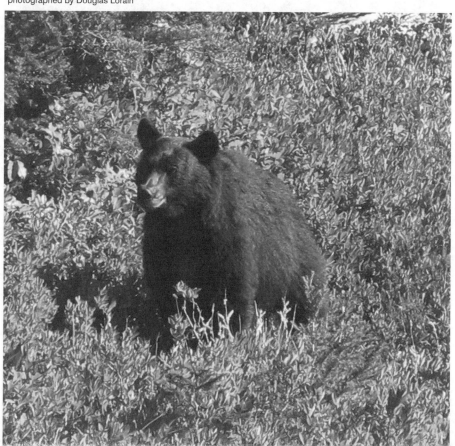

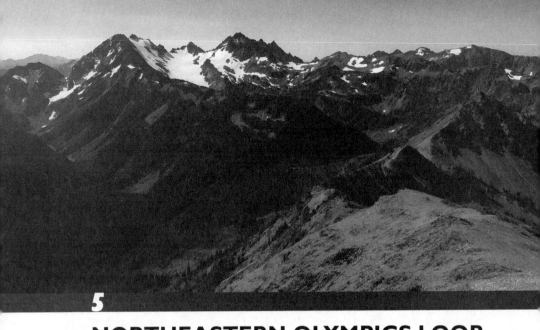

5

NORTHEASTERN OLYMPICS LOOP

RATINGS: Scenery 9 **Solitude** 5 **Difficulty** 7

MILES: 46 (55)

ELEVATION GAIN: 12,400' (14,300')

DAYS: 4–5 (4–7)

SHUTTLE MILEAGE: n/a

MAP: Custom Correct *Gray Wolf–Dosewallips*

USUALLY OPEN: Mid-July–October

BEST: Late July–mid-August

PERMIT: Required. As of 2019, the nonrefundable cost of a permit is $6 with an additional charge of $8 per adult in your party per night in the park. Alternatively, for $55 you can purchase an annual Olympic National Park Wilderness Pass, which covers all nightly fees for one person for the entire year. Hikers under the age of 16 are free.

Permits are limited for certain campsites on the suggested itinerary for this trip, and reservations are strongly recommended. Approximately 50% of permits for these campsites can be reserved, with the rest given out on a first-come, first-served basis.

Visit nps.gov/olym/planyourvisit/wilderness-reservations.htm for up-to-date information about quotas and reservations. Reservations are accepted in person at one of the park's wilderness information centers, online via recreation.gov, or by calling 877-444-6777. The system opens

Above: *View northwest from Sentinel Peak*
photographed by Mark Wetherington

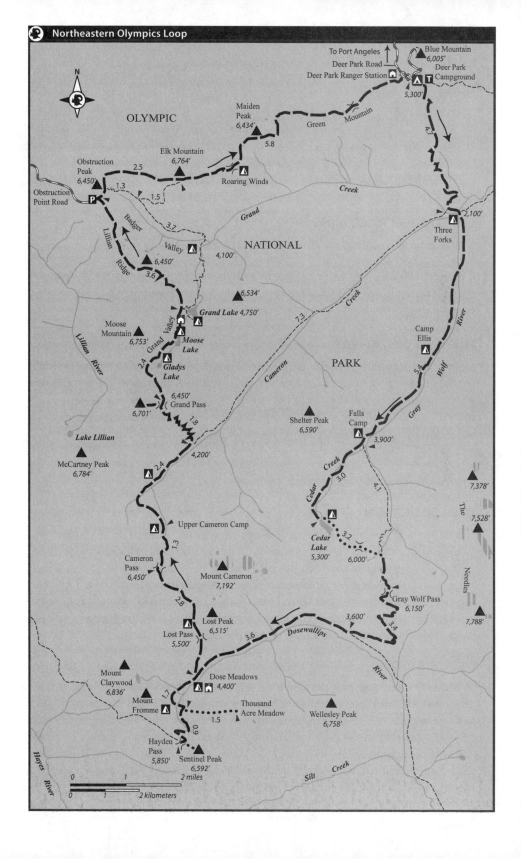

N

OLYMPIC

NATIONAL

PARK

To Port Angeles
Deer Park Road
Deer Park Ranger Station

Blue Mountain
6,005'
Deer Park
Campground
5,300'

4.1

Maiden
Peak
6,434'

Green Mountain

5.8

Elk Mountain
6,764'

Roaring Winds

Obstruction
Peak
6,450'

2.5

1.3

1.5

Obstruction
Point Road

Grand   Creek

Three
Forks
2,100'

Badger

3.7

Valley
4,100'

Lillian

6,450'

3.6

6,534'

Grand Lake 4,750'

7.3

Cameron   Creek

Camp
Ellis

Moose
Mountain
6,753'

Grand Valley

Moose
Lake

5.4

Gray   Wolf   River

2.4

Gladys
Lake

Lillian River

6,450'
Grand Pass

6,701'

1.8

Shelter Peak
6,590'

Falls
Camp
3,900'

Lake Lillian

4,200'

2.4

McCartney Peak
6,784'

Cedar   Creek

3.0

4.1

7,378'

7,528'

Upper Cameron Camp

1.3

Cedar
Lake
5,300'

3.2

6,000'

The

Needles

Cameron
Pass
6,450'

2.8

Mount Cameron
7,192'

Gray Wolf Pass
6,150'

7,788'

Lost Peak
6,515'

3,600'

3.4

Lost Pass
5,500'

3.6

Dosewallips

Mount
Claywood
6,836'

Dose Meadows
4,400'

River

Mount
Fromme

1.7

Thousand
Acre Meadow

1.5

Wellesley Peak
6,758'

60

Hayes   River

Hayden
Pass
5,850'

Sentinel Peak
6,592'

0   1   2 miles

0   1   2 kilometers

Silt   Creek

for reservations in mid-March. Changes are always likely, however, so check the park's website for the latest procedures and requirements.

RULES: Maximum group size of 12 people; no fires above 3,500 feet; bear canisters are required (free rentals available) where you cannot hang food at least 12 feet high and 10 feet out from a tree trunk

CONTACT: Olympic National Park, 360-565-3100, nps.gov/olym

SPECIAL ATTRACTIONS

Fine mountain scenery, old-growth forests, expansive views

CHALLENGES

Some very steep trails; ice and snow around Cameron Pass; black bears, especially at Dose Meadows

HOW TO GET THERE

From downtown Port Angeles, head east on US 101, and go about 4.5 miles. Turn right (south) on Deer Park Road. The road is initially paved, then changes to gravel and makes a long, twisting climb all the way to the Deer Park Campground and trailhead, 16 miles from US 101. Late fall–late spring, the road is closed at the park boundary.

NOTE: Trailers are not recommended on Deer Park Road.

GPS TRAILHEAD COORDINATES: N47° 56.941' W123° 15.497'

INTRODUCTION

This excellent loop trip explores the less-well-known northeastern Olympic Mountains. While far from arid, this part of the range is drier than the peaks to the west, so there are no glaciers or grand rainforests on this trip. You *will* enjoy, however, many miles of high ridges with fine views, lovely streams, lots of wildflowers, plenty of wildlife, and a greater degree of solitude. The hike has several steep sections and one high, snowy pass, but the excellent scenery is ample compensation. The loop is equally scenic in either direction but is described clockwise to avoid a long, tough uphill at the end of the trip.

DESCRIPTION

Begin by hiking east past Deer Park Campground through an attractive mix of wild-flower meadows and open subalpine-fir forests, where you'll be treated to wonderful views of the distant peaks. After just 0.2 mile turn right (south) at a junction and begin a long 3,300-foot descent that will test even the strongest knees. The route plunges down a forested ridge at a consistent, moderately steep grade. Views are limited, but the forest is attractive, and regular switchbacks help to break up the monotony. Eventually your knees and jammed toes get a break as the trail bottoms out at a junction with the Cameron Creek Trail.

Your route turns left (east) and immediately comes to the old trail shelter and possible campsite at Three Forks. This shelter sits in a tiny meadow and is a pleasant spot to eat lunch and tend to any foot problems from the long descent. Continuing downstream, you cross the Gray Wolf River on a log and soon reach a junction with the Gray Wolf River Trail. Wolves (gray or otherwise) no longer inhabit the Olympic Mountains, but their former presence is honored in the name of this strikingly beautiful stream.

You turn right (south) at this junction and hike upstream. For the most part, this is an enjoyable walk through forests of cedar, hemlock, and fir. Views are infrequent and feature only forested hillsides across the canyon, but the lovely river is often visible and always a joy. The route includes a few small ups and downs but generally makes a gradual climb of the valley. After 1 mile you cross the river and continue upstream past Camp Ellis and a series of avalanche openings. About 5.4 miles from the junction near Three Forks is a small opening that provides a good place to camp. On the less positive side, the campsite contains the remains of Falls Shelter, which burned down as a result of arson in 2006.

From the Falls campsite you have a choice of trails. The shorter and easier option is to continue straight up the Gray Wolf River Trail as it climbs into increasingly open forests and meadows, crossing the stream several times on its way to Gray Wolf Pass.

Persons experienced in cross-country travel might consider a more challenging and arguably more scenic option to Gray Wolf Pass that follows the irregularly maintained Cedar Lake Way Trail. The poorly marked route begins in the meadow just beyond Falls campsite and makes a spirited climb up the valley of Cedar Creek. The trail is rough in spots, but you should be able to follow it fairly easily through the trees. Once the route emerges from the forest and enters an area of wet shrubs and meadows, it becomes less distinct, but experienced hikers should have no problem. Views of the surrounding peaks are very pleasant, and wildflowers crowd the meadows and stream banks. Near the head of the valley, the stream curves southeast and the trail goes through a small area of open woods before emerging at Cedar Lake. At 21 acres, this is one of the largest subalpine lakes in the Olympic Mountains, filling a large basin surrounded by 7,000-foot peaks. The best camps are near the outlet.

The return to the Gray Wolf River Trail from Cedar Lake requires cross-country hiking. Follow the northeast shore of Cedar Lake to the lake's southeast end, and then begin to climb increasingly open, multilevel meadow slopes.

TIP: Be sure to look back to Cedar Lake from time to time for ever-improving views of the lake and surrounding basin.

Your goal is the low point in the ridge to the southeast. Once you reach this pass, scramble downhill and to the right (southeast) through forests, meadows, and boulders to two small ponds. From here, contour cross-country southeast another 0.5 mile, and you should reach the Gray Wolf River Trail in a little meadow basin near the head of the stream.

By whatever route you choose, the final mile to Gray Wolf Pass follows the Gray Wolf River Trail as it climbs steadily up rocky slopes (and probably a few snowfields) to the 6,150-foot pass. From this grandstand there are fine views of the Gray Wolf Valley, numerous peaks, and the deep Dosewallips River Valley to the south. Yes, you're going *all the way down there.*

Now brace your knees for a long 2,550-foot switchbacking drop to the Dosewallips River. Along the way the scenery changes from meadows, to high-elevation forest, to lower-elevation old-growth trees. Views and water are both limited until you reach the junction at the bottom. Turn right on the Dosewallips Trail and begin to travel up this very enjoyable path on open, meadowy slopes that provide excellent vistas of the surrounding cliffs and mountains.

The path enters large Dose Meadows 3.6 miles from the Gray Wolf River Trail junction. The meadows showcase wildflowers, good camps, a ranger tent that is intermittently staffed in the summer, and a junction with the Lost Pass Trail. Perhaps the most outstanding feature of Dose Meadows is its view of the distinctive pinnacle called Mount Fromme to the west-southwest.

WARNING: Black bears favor this meadow, so properly store all food, and camp away from game trails.

SIDE TRIP TO HAYDEN PASS: After you've made camp, there is an excellent side trip you can make from Dose Meadows. You begin by climbing the path going south and west toward Hayden Pass. Travel around the head of a basin, then cross the Dosewallips River (only a creek by this point, but still enough to get your feet wet), and continue climbing to a series of lovely meadow benches with more good camps. From here experienced hikers might consider taking an unmarked side route that goes east over a ridge and drops to the huge sloping expanse of Thousand Acre Meadow. The name overstates things a little, but the meadow is large by anyone's standards. Wildflower lovers can stay happy for hours.

The main destination of your side trip is Hayden Pass. To reach it, continue climbing south on the main trail, make a simple rock-hop across the creek, and climb steadily on switchbacks.

WARNING: The north- and east-facing slopes here are often covered with dangerous snowfields until late summer.

The path tops out at Hayden Pass, on the side of prominent Sentinel Peak, and provides fine views west to the canyons of the Hayes and Elwha Rivers.

TIP: While not a casual stroll, if you felt comfortable taking the Cedar Lake Way Trail, you might want to attempt summiting Sentinel Peak southeast of Hayden Pass. A steep route exists up the relatively stable talus, and there is minimal exposure. The terrific view is well worth the effort.

Back at Dose Meadows, fill up on water and turn north on the trail to Lost Pass. This path was clearly built by someone of the-shortest-distance-between-two-points mentality who felt switchbacks were for sissies. Fortunately, although it is dry, the climb is relatively short and mostly in the shade. Once on top, there is much to enjoy. Pink heather and a colorful array of other flowers liven up the foreground, and views extend from nearby Lost Peak to more distant Mount Claywood, Wellesley Peak, and Sentinel Peak.

From Lost Pass the route makes a scenic traverse around the west side of Lost Peak before entering a beautiful alpine basin. Wildflowers brighten the sloping meadow between Lost Peak and Mount Cameron, and sights include not only these nearby summits but also

Mount Claywood and the Lost River Valley. A small but attractive campsite lies in a clump of subalpine firs near the crossing of a small creek.

Your tour now makes a long sidehill climb of an open slope to Cameron Pass. Views improve as you climb, eventually extending west all the way to the snowy summit of Mount Olympus and south to Mount Anderson with its glacier-filled north bowl. At 6,450 feet, Cameron is one of the highest trail passes in the Olympic Mountains. Evidence to support this statement is immediately apparent because, on the east side of the pass, hikers must negotiate large snowfields. By late summer the snow melts and reveals ice that may be even more difficult to cross.

TIP: Because the descent can be rather treacherous, those not comfortable with snow and ice travel should ask a ranger about conditions before starting their trip.

After descending about 800 feet of snow, you should be able to relocate the trail at the base of a scree slope and make an easier transit of the more level parts of Cameron Basin. This is one of the most spectacular subalpine basins in the range (which is really saying something), and it contains a wealth of wildflowers, including glacier lilies, pasqueflowers, bistorts, and lupines. Distant vistas are superb, but the most photogenic landscapes are back up to the nearby cliffs of Mount Cameron.

The trail descends through the multiple levels of Cameron Basin, passing the excellent campsites at Upper Cameron Camp before reentering forest. Your route then drops steadily into Cameron Creek Valley, crossing several headwater creeklets amid lush vegetation along the way. The trail turns northeast and follows the north bank of the creek through forests and brushy areas of alder, willow, and salmonberry, with increasingly restricted views and a few mediocre campsites.

Now the trail contours briefly away from the creek, gains a bit of elevation, and reaches a junction with the Grand Pass Trail. Turn left (northwest) and prepare for a rigorous and mostly shadeless climb, as you gain almost 2,250 feet in 1.8 miles. Any way you do that math, it comes out awfully steep! Countless small switchbacks were put in to give the impression that the trail engineers weren't totally sadistic (personally, I'm not buying it). The advantage, of course, of steep trails is that you get to the high-elevation views and scenery more quickly. Just below the top at Grand Pass, the trail enters an attractive region of partial forest, rocks, and steep heather fields. Good views extend back toward McCartney Peak and the area around Cameron Pass.

SIDE TRIP TO PEAK 6,701: For even broader views, from Grand Pass take the unofficial but perfectly good trail that goes west and in 0.3 mile climbs steeply to the top of a 6,701-foot knoll. From here you can see most of the Olympic Mountains, including Mount Olympus, Mount Anderson, and the remote Lillian River Valley.

From Grand Pass the trail drops past an icy pond, then through a barren region of snowfields and rocks in the upper reaches of Grand Valley. Tiny alpine wildflowers brighten the small meadows, while marmots whistle their high-pitched alarms from practically every rock. There are also nice looks at the peaks that tightly enclose this narrow valley.

NOTE: You are now entering the Grand Valley quota area, so your permit must allow you to camp here if that is your plan. Reservations are strongly advised.

The trail makes an irregular descent down the valley, often in rocky areas, past tiny and meadow-rimmed Gladys Lake (camps), and then down to much larger Moose Lake. This long, deep lake was not named for the animal, which has never inhabited the Olympics, but for a man whose last name was Moose. Side trails lead to lovely designated campsites near this very scenic lake. Just below the lake is a seasonal ranger tent.

A little farther down the valley are a junction and a choice of trails. Your decision will probably be dictated primarily by the weather. To the right (east), a trail drops to shimmering and green-tinged Grand Lake (fine camps) and continues steeply down the forested canyon of Grand Creek, twice crossing its flow. The trail passes an attractive 40-foot waterfall along the way to a nice sheltered camp near the crossing of Badger Creek. From the stream crossing, the path ascends sloping Badger Valley through a string of scenic meadows to the head of the valley. Like Moose Lake, Badger Valley's name seems more than a little peculiar, as badgers don't live in these mountains. Supposedly, it was named after a horse whose owner called the animal Badger. In upper Badger Valley you keep right (east) at a junction and steeply climb a rocky hillside for 1.5 miles to a junction with the Obstruction Point–Deer Park Trail near the summit of Elk Mountain. In bad weather this lower-elevation alternative is the superior choice.

If the weather is favorable—don't count on it—a more spectacular option from Grand Valley is to turn left (north) at the junction above Grand Lake and climb increasingly open slopes in a series of 25 switchbacks. The route hits a ridgeline, then turns west and continues its tiring 1,600-foot ascent to just below the top of a 6,450-foot high point with 360-degree views. To the east is the deep, forested canyon of Grand Creek. To the west is the Lillian River Valley and distant Mount Olympus. To the north is Hurricane Ridge, and at your feet are tiny wildflowers amid the rocks. It's a real top-of-the-world kind of place. The popular trail continues north along Lillian Ridge, much of the way above timberline, as it crosses talus slopes and large areas of tundralike vegetation. Views are continuously marvelous. The trail ends at the road-end trailhead below Obstruction Peak.

Obstruction Peak from the Grand Ridge Trail on Elk Mountain
photographed by Douglas Lorain

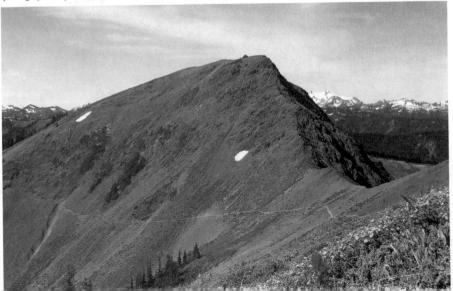

WARNING: Lillian Ridge is quite exposed, making it windy and downright uncomfortable, or even dangerous, in bad weather.

To complete your tour, turn northeast from Obstruction Peak, following the trail back to Deer Park. Originally, park promoters planned to construct a road along this high route connecting Hurricane Ridge with Deer Park. Fortunately, these plans never came to fruition, so hikers can now enjoy these wonderful views at a more respectful pace. The shadeless route is above timberline for most of the way, and the excellent views are too numerous to list.

WARNING: This trail has very little water. Carry at least 2 quarts.

Start by looping to the north, going straight at a junction at 0.2 mile with a side trail that drops toward Badger Valley, and traversing steep slopes to the high view-packed ridgeline of Elk Mountain. At the east end of this ridge are some steep slopes covered with shale and a junction with the trail coming up from Badger Valley, the alternate route from Grand Valley.

Continuing east, the trail makes an undulating descent to a saddle holding usually dry but wildly scenic Roaring Winds Camp. You turn north and quickly regain about 600 feet of the recently lost elevation. The trail goes up to Maiden Peak, loops around the east end of this high point, and drops again, first steeply and then less dramatically, to the long up-and-down ridge called Green Mountain. Views are more limited on this lower ridgeline, but they are still terrific. Especially noteworthy are the views north to Port Angeles, the Strait of Juan de Fuca, and Canada's Vancouver Island. The route makes another uneven descent through forest and old fire scars to a saddle west of Deer Park. The last mile follows an old road uphill to the Deer Park Ranger Station. From here you simply hike east on the road a final 0.2 mile to your car.

POSSIBLE ITINERARY

	CAMP	MILES	ELEVATION GAIN
Day 1	Falls Shelter	10.1	1,800'
Day 2	Dose Meadows (via Cedar Lake)	13.2	3,800'
Day 3	Dose Meadows		
	Day hike to Hayden Pass and Thousand Acre Meadow	8.2	1,600'
Day 4	Grand Valley	10.7	4,300'
	Side trip to Peak 6,701	0.6	300'
Day 5	Out (via Obstruction Peak)	11.9	2,500'

BEST SHORTER ALTERNATIVES

From the trailhead at Obstruction Point, you can make a reasonable day hike along the first part of Grand Ridge to view-packed Elk Mountain. A point-to-point trip along Grand Ridge from Obstruction Point to Deer Park makes an excellent one-night backpacking trip that samples this area's high ridges. For another short but popular overnight option, visit and explore Grand Valley from the Obstruction Point trailhead (reservations are highly recommended).

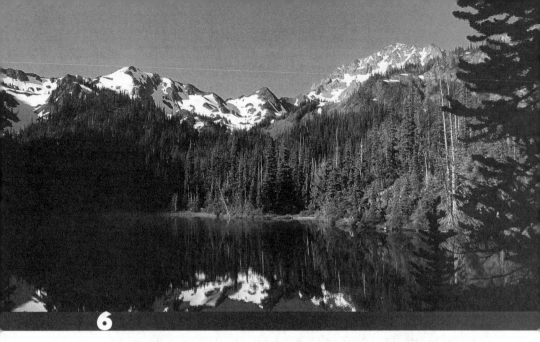

6

DUNGENESS–MARMOT PASS LOOP

RATINGS: Scenery 8   **Solitude** 6   **Difficulty** 6

MILES: 30 (44)

ELEVATION GAIN: 6,600' (10,500')

DAYS: 3–6 (3–6)

SHUTTLE MILEAGE: 4

MAP: Custom Correct *Buckhorn Wilderness*

USUALLY OPEN: Mid-July–mid-October

BEST: Mid-July–early August

PERMIT: No, for most of the trip, simply sign in at the trailhead. If you camp in Royal Basin or at Home Lake in Olympic National Park, you must purchase an overnight permit. As of 2019, the nonrefundable cost of a permit is $6 with an additional charge of $8 per adult in your party per night in the park. Alternatively, for $55 you can purchase an annual Olympic National Park Wilderness Pass, which covers all nightly fees for one person for the entire year. Hikers under the age of 16 are free.

Permits are limited for certain campsites on the suggested itinerary for this trip, and reservations are strongly recommended.

Visit nps.gov/olym/planyourvisit/wilderness-reservations.htm for up-to-date information about quotas and reservations. Reservations are accepted in person at one of the park's wilderness information centers, online via recreation.gov, or by calling 877-444-6777. The system opens

Above: *Royal Lake*

photographed by Douglas Lorain

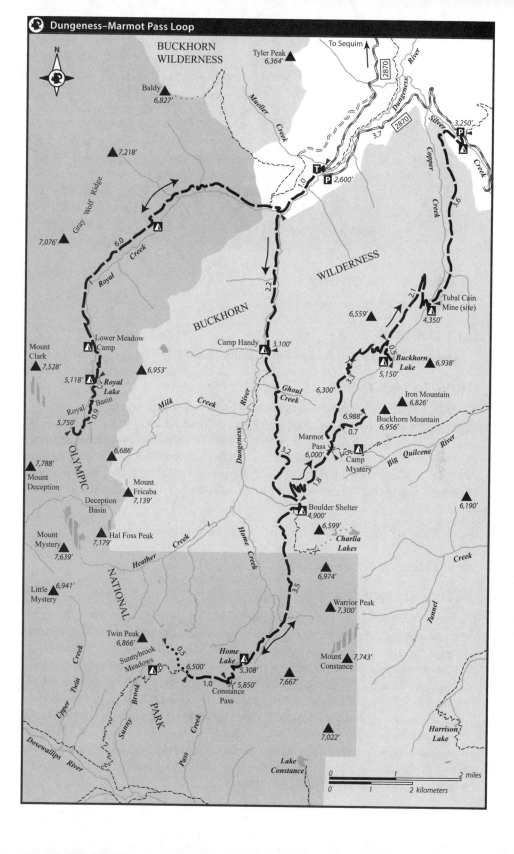

Dungeness–Marmot Pass Loop

BUCKHORN
WILDERNESS

To Sequim

Tyler Peak
6,364'

Baldy
6,827'

7,218'

7,076'

Gray Wolf Ridge

6.0

Royal Creek

Lower Meadow
Camp

Mount
Clark
7,528'

5,118'

*Royal
Lake
Basin*

5,750'

0.9

Royal

6,686'

OLYMPIC

7,788'
Mount
Deception

Mount
Fricaba
7,139'

Deception
Basin

Mount
Mystery
7,639'

Hal Foss Peak
7,179'

Heather

Little
Mystery
6,941'

NATIONAL

Twin Peak
6,866'

Sunnybrook
Meadows

0.5

6,500'

1.0

Upper Twin Creek

Dosewallips River

Sunny

PARK

Brook

Pass

Creek

Home Creek

Milk Creek

Dungeness River

Ghoul Creek

Camp Handy
3,100'

2.2

3.3

6,300'

6,988'

Marmot
Pass
6,000'

3.2

1.8

0.7

Camp
Mystery

Boulder Shelter
4,900'

6,599'

*Charlia
Lakes*

6,974'

3.5

Warrior Peak
7,300'

*Home
Lake*
5,308'

7,667'

Mount
Constance
7,743'

5,850'
Constance
Pass

7,022'

*Lake
Constance*

WILDERNESS

6,559'

2.1

Tubal Cain
Mine (site)
4,350'

Copper Creek

Silver Creek

3,250'

P

3.7

3.6

2870

Dungeness River

2870

2,600'

T
P

1.0

0.5

*Buckhorn
Lake*
5,150'

6,938'

Iron Mountain
6,826'

Buckhorn Mountain
6,956'

Big Quilcene River

6,190'

Tunnel Creek

Harrison
Lake

BUCKHORN

N

| 0 | | 1 | | 2 miles |
| 0 | 1 | | 2 kilometers | |

for reservations in mid-March. Changes are always likely, however, so check the park's website for the latest procedures and requirements.

Permits are unlimited for Home Lake, but for Royal Basin you *must* have a reserved permit. No first-come, first-served permits are given out for this limited-use area.

RULES: No dogs allowed in the national park; camping allowed only at designated sites in the Royal Creek drainage

CONTACTS: Olympic National Forest, Hood Canal Ranger District, 360-765-2200, fs.usda.gov/main/olympic; Olympic National Park, 360-565-3100, nps.gov/olym

SPECIAL ATTRACTIONS

Great mountain views, wildflowers

CHALLENGES

Permit limits and restrictions for Royal Basin side trip

HOW TO GET THERE

From Sequim, take US 101 east about 2.7 miles to a junction near milepost 267.2. Turn right (south) onto paved Palo Alto Road, proceed 8.3 miles to a prominent fork, and then veer right (southwest) onto gravel Forest Service Road 2880, following signs to Dungeness Forks Campground. After 1.7 miles, bear left (south) at a junction onto FS 2870, and then drive 8 miles to the Dungeness Trailhead parking lot just after a bridge. If you have a second car, leave it 3.7 miles farther along FS 2870 at the Tubal Cain Trailhead.

NOTE: You'll need a Northwest Forest Pass to park at this trailhead.

GPS TRAILHEAD COORDINATES: N47° 52.651' W123° 08.221'

INTRODUCTION

When Olympic National Park was established in 1938, its boundaries were rather arbitrary, usually following neither recognizable natural features nor any other discernible pattern. As a result, some of the region's most spectacular wildlands, which should logically have been included in the park, were left out of the protected zone. One such area is now preserved in the Buckhorn Wilderness, which abuts the northeast boundary of the national park. Here, travelers will discover spectacular alpine ridges, rugged peaks, clear streams, acres of wildflowers, and superb views that are nearly the equal of anything in the park itself. Unlike in the park, however, here hikers will encounter fewer restrictions on travel, can obtain a permit for free, and generally see fewer people. This loop explores the best of this wilderness and includes two long but terrific side trips to even more wonders just over the border in Olympic National Park.

DESCRIPTION ••

Although the Dungeness Trail parking lot is on the east side of the Dungeness River, the trail actually begins on the west side of the road bridge. So cross the bridge, sign in at the register, and then climb two short switchbacks before heading south along the river trail. The travel here is both easy and enjoyable, with little elevation gain and plenty of shade under the canopy of a relatively open forest of Douglas fir and western hemlock with a few Pacific yews growing beneath the larger evergreens. Unlike the much wetter rainforests of the western Olympic Mountains, the ground cover here is fairly sparse, with just a scattering of vanilla leaf, bunchberry, Pacific rhododendron, Oregon grape, and a few ferns amid a patchwork of moss and downed logs. The dominant sounds come from the nearby Dungeness River, with its soothing river music. At the 1-mile point is a junction with the Royal Basin Trail.

ROYAL BASIN SIDE TRIP: Royal Basin's multileveled alpine bowl features some of the finest scenery in Olympic National Park, and for those who can snag a coveted overnight permit (reservations required) it really should not be missed. Really strong hikers can visit it as a long day hike without the need for a permit, but the place deserves more time than that to be fully appreciated.

To reach this paradise, turn right (northwest) at the junction just before the log bridge over Royal Creek, climb two quick switchbacks, and then go straight (west) at a junction with the Lower Maynard Burn Trail. From here the trail sets off on a long uphill. Along the way you pass a campsite and several avalanche chutes that offer enticing glimpses of the high peaks all around. At 5.3 miles things briefly level out at a lovely wildflower-covered meadow, where the signed Lower Meadow Camp is located. Just beyond this landmark you cross a log over Royal Creek and climb five more switchbacks to Royal Lake. Surrounded by 7,000-foot peaks and encircled by a scenic path, this mountain gem makes a great lunch stop or (with a reserved permit) you can spend the night at the designated campsites above the west shore.

For the side trip's ultimate highlight, however, keep hiking from the designated camping area to a lush, flat upper meadow. From there a steep path ascends past a waterfall and up an often-snowy gully to rolling Upper Royal Basin. This wildflower-filled paradise offers small ponds for exploring and incredibly photogenic views of jagged Mounts Clark and Deception. It was a long hike to reach this goal, but you'll be glad you made the effort.

For the main loop, you bear slightly left (south) at the Royal Basin turnoff onto the less heavily traveled Dungeness Trail, immediately cross a log bridge over large Royal Creek, then resume your joyful riverside ramble. The route is entirely in forest and has no views, but it's very pleasant, and you always have the river for company. There are countless spots along the way where you can visit the clear water, either for some fishing or to take a quick dip in one of the cold pools. After 1.7 miles you cross the river on a log bridge, then go up the east bank another 0.5 mile to a trail fork. The trail to the right (downhill) goes 125 yards to Camp Handy, a comfortable spot on the river with a wooden shelter and space for several tents.

Camp Handy marks the end of the easy river walk and the start of your climb to the high country. The well-graded trail goes up the forested hillside east of the river, rapidly leaving the sounds of cascading water. After 0.5 mile is a fork. The old Heather Creek Trail goes right (downhill), but you angle left (southeast), following a sign to Marmot Pass, and resume climbing. Rhododendrons up to 10 feet tall line the trail here, so expect abundant pink blossoms in early summer. You hop over tiny Ghoul Creek at 4.1 miles (despite the name, there is nothing scary about the crossing), then steadily climb to the loop's first nice viewpoint (excluding the Royal Basin side trip) at around 5 miles. From here you can look down into the heavily forested canyon of the Dungeness River, see across to Mount Fricaba, and look southwest to Little Mystery and several unnamed peaks west of Constance Pass.

As you continue to gain elevation, the views become more frequent and include the rugged crags of 7,639-foot Mount Mystery and the snow-streaked spires of even taller Mount Constance to the south. Closer at hand you may also notice the forest now includes such higher-elevation species as western white pine and Pacific silver fir. Flowers such as yarrow, twinflower, beardtongue, lupine, and pipsissewa have also become common. At 6.4 miles is a junction with the Marmot Pass Trail, which goes sharply left and is the return route of this hike. For now, go straight (southeast) and in just 50 yards come to an avalanche-swept basin with a small creek, nice camps, and a sturdy wooden structure called Boulder Shelter.

CONSTANCE PASS SIDE TRIP: Before completing the loop, you won't want to miss the long side trip to Constance Pass, either as a day hike from a base camp at Boulder Shelter or as an overnight at Home Lake. To reach it, go left at the junction with the short dead-end side path to Boulder Shelter, following a small sign saying HOME LAKE.

The Constance Pass Trail climbs away from Boulder Shelter for 0.1 mile, and then comes to a fork. The route to the left (south) is the unmaintained Charlia Lakes Way Trail, a steep but easy-to-follow path that leads to a grand ridgetop viewpoint and then a very steep scramble down to the austere Charlia Lakes (another excellent day hike goal). The main trail goes right (southeast) at the Charlia Lakes junction and for the next 2 miles makes a very scenic up-and-down traverse. Views along the way are nearly continuous and always superb, especially to the west of an alpine ridge that includes Mount Fricaba towering over the green chasm of Heather Creek. Partway along this section, you pass a sign marking your entry into Olympic National Park. Dogs are not allowed beyond this point. Flowers are abundant along this trail in July and early August. Depending on the local microhabitat, you should look for fireweed, yarrow, pearly everlasting, tiger lily, tall larkspur, Jacobs ladder, snowberry, beardtongue, lupine, valerian, paintbrush, thistle, columbine, stonecrop, and other blossoms too numerous to list. As for wildlife, you stand a good chance of spotting marmots, deer, and maybe even a black bear.

The traverse ends with a mostly downhill crossing of a large talus slope at the base of the towering, dark mass of Mount Constance. From here you climb in stunted forest, meadows, and rocky areas, gaining some 650 feet to tiny Home Lake, where there are campsites (an Olympic National Park permit is required) and a nice view up to the bare slopes of an unnamed peak to the west. Unfortunately, underground seepage causes the water level of Home Lake to drop considerably by late summer, giving it that bathtub-ring appearance.

The trail just touches Home Lake before resuming its uphill assault on Constance Pass, another 500 feet higher. The trail is steep, but the rewards are considerable, with great views of Mount Constance as you climb. The only trees at these high elevations are a few scattered subalpine firs, which leaves plenty of room for open meadows that are ideal habitats for a kaleidoscope of colorful wildflowers. Look for partridge foot, phlox, bistort, pink heather, and, in wetter areas, elephant head and grass-of-Parnassus.

Once at Constance Pass the views to the south over the Dosewallips River to distant Mount Anderson are breathtaking. Believe it or not, however, even better and loftier viewpoints are yet to come because, instead of descending from Constance Pass, the trail turns right (west) and climbs even higher along an alpine ridge. The often-steep path soon takes you past the last of the wind-whipped trees and into a land of rocks and meadows, from which you can see west to Mount Olympus with its large, sparkling glaciers and east across the hazy lowlands of Puget Sound to Mount Rainier. Hundreds of summits in the Olympic Mountains come into view, and those familiar with the range can spend hours identifying them all.

From the high point of this ridge, the trail drops to the flowery wonderland of Sunnybrook Meadows. If you prefer to stay in the highlands, leave the trail on the ridgetop and wander cross-country along a wide alpine ridge to the northwest, passing several more outstanding viewpoints. Especially noteworthy are the views of Mount Mystery and Mount Deception to the northwest. Unfortunately, the hiking gets rocky and difficult after about 0.5 mile, so unless you have climbing gear and experience, it's time to turn around.

WARNING: The high country above Constance Pass is very exposed. Avoid this area during bad weather—it is potentially dangerous, and you won't see anything anyway.

Once you've had your fill of the scenery around Constance Pass, return the way you came to Boulder Shelter.

To complete the loop back from Boulder Shelter, turn northeast and head up the trail to Marmot Pass. The climb begins in open forests of subalpine firs and whitebark pines, then leaves the trees and crosses huge open slopes with lots of wildflowers. Cinquefoil, yarrow, owl's clover, buckwheat, onion, white heather, larkspur, harebell, paintbrush, and lupine are especially abundant. Also common here are mats of ground-hugging juniper. The views are breathtaking, especially south to Mount Constance and west to both Mount Deception and an aptly named group of peaks called The Needles. After climbing for 1.8 very scenic miles, you reach a junction at Marmot Pass, where you turn left (northwest) and ascend even higher on the view-packed slopes of Buckhorn Mountain.

SIDE TRIP TO BUCKHORN PEAK: A relatively easy and very worthwhile scramble trail leaves the main route just 120 yards from Marmot Pass and goes 0.7 mile to the top of a butte just west of Buckhorn Mountain, where the views seem to go on forever.

Even without that side trip, however, the main trail is a superbly scenic high route, which ranks as one of the best in the state. After completing its circuit of the west side of

Buckhorn Mountain, the trail tops out on an above-timberline ridgetop, from which you can see east into the valley of Copper Creek and across to lofty Iron Mountain.

For the next 0.6 mile the trail descends along a wonderfully scenic ridgetop using 18 short switchbacks to reach a saddle. You then drop off the east side of the ridgeline, traveling through a mix of lovely meadows and open forest. Occasional switchbacks keep the grade from becoming too steep. At every break in the trees, you enjoy excellent views to the south of the peaks at the head of Copper Creek.

After 10 downhill switchbacks, an unsigned but obvious trail goes sharply right (southeast). This 0.5-mile path leads to tiny and woodsy Buckhorn Lake, which has a rocky and sloping shoreline. If you are looking to camp, the best site is where the trail crosses a small creek about 0.2 mile before you reach the lake. The return route goes straight (northeast) at the Buckhorn Lake junction and traverses very gradually downhill across an open, grassy slope with wide views and abundant wildflowers. After one long and then two short switchbacks, you come to a good camp at the crossing of Copper Creek. The rusted equipment near this camp is all that remains of the long-abandoned Tubal Cain Mine.

After crossing the creek, the trail descends briefly beside the stream and then begins a long but very gentle downhill traverse of the west side of a ridge. The entire way is in forest, with increasing numbers of showy rhododendrons as you go north. Several tiny creeks along the way provide water. The only significant point of interest comes about 0.5 mile below the Copper Creek crossing, where a 50-foot side trail forks to the right (uphill) to an old mine tunnel. This tunnel is worth a quick look, but it's too dangerous to explore. Once the trail finally rounds the end of the ridge, it drops to a log bridge over Silver Creek, where there is a shelter and possible campsite, and almost immediately thereafter comes to the Tubal Cain Trailhead. With two cars, your hike is over; otherwise, it's a pleasant 3.7-mile, mostly downhill road walk back to the Dungeness Trailhead.

POSSIBLE ITINERARY

	CAMP	MILES	ELEVATION GAIN
Day 1	Royal Lake	7.0	2,400'
	Side trip to Upper Royal Basin	1.8	700'
Day 2	Boulder Shelter	11.4	2,500'
Day 3	Boulder Shelter		
	Day hike to ridge above Constance Pass	10.0	2,300'
Day 4	Buckhorn Lake	5.7	1,600'
	Side trip to Buckhorn Peak	1.4	900'
Day 5	Out (excluding road walk)	6.2	100'

BEST SHORTER ALTERNATIVE •

Doing either a really long day hike or (better) a one-night backpacking trip into Royal Basin is highly rewarding.

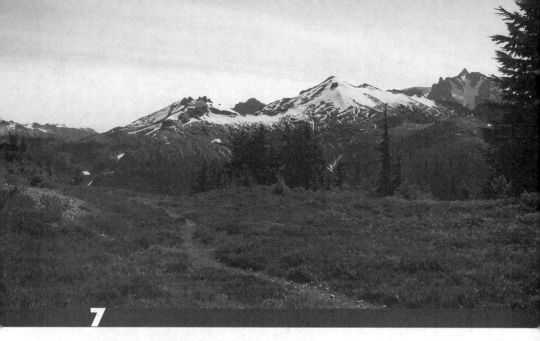

NORTHERN NORTH CASCADES LOOP

RATINGS: Scenery 9   **Solitude** 4   **Difficulty** 8

MILES: 48 (56)

ELEVATION GAIN: 10,550' (13,500')

DAYS: 3–5 (4–6)

SHUTTLE MILEAGE: n/a

MAPS: Green Trails *Mt. Shuksan (#14)* and *Mt. Challenger (#15)*

USUALLY OPEN: Late July–September

BEST: August

PERMIT: Required. As of 2019 they are free but limited. About 60% of the available campsites can be reserved in advance—highly recommended—with the rest given out on a first-come, first-served basis. Reservation requests should be submitted between March 15 and April 15 for the summer season. Reservation requests can only be made online; a $20 nonrefundable fee applies to reserved permits. Walk-up permits can be obtained on the first day of the trip or up to one day before. See nps.gov/noca/planyourvisit/backcountry-reservations.htm for full details. Pick up permits (whether reserved in advance or a walk-up permit) from the wilderness information center in Marblemount, or, more conveniently for this trip, at the Glacier Public Service Center.

Above: *Looking southeast from Copper Ridge*

photographed by Mark Wetherington

RULES: Camping allowed only at a restricted number of designated sites; no fires at higher-elevation camps; maximum group size of 12
CONTACT: North Cascades National Park, 360-854-7200 ext. 515; in summer, contact the park's wilderness information center, 360-854-7245, nps.gov/noca

SPECIAL ATTRACTIONS

Great mountain views, old-growth forests

CHALLENGES

Camping restrictions; rugged trail; black bears are common in this area—hang or store all food properly

HOW TO GET THERE

From Bellingham, drive east on WA 542 for 22.9 miles to Kendall. Turn right (east) to continue on WA 542, and go another 10.8 miles to the small community of Glacier, where you can pick up a backcountry permit at the Glacier Public Service Center. From there continue east on WA 542 for another 13 miles to a bridge over the North Fork Nooksack River. Just before crossing the river, turn left onto Forest Service Road 32. Keep left at a fork in the road after 1.5 miles and continue on FS 32 to the road-end trailhead, about 5.4 miles from the state highway.

NOTE: You'll need a Northwest Forest Pass to park at this trailhead.

GPS TRAILHEAD COORDINATES: N48° 54.606' W121° 35.562'

INTRODUCTION

Nowhere is the rugged beauty of the North Cascades on better display than it is here. Everything seems to be on a larger-than-life scale. There are big trees, huge glaciers, incredibly deep canyons, impossibly steep ridges, and vast views. For variety, the trip visits a fire lookout and uses a unique hand-powered cable car to make a stream crossing.

You must begin by obtaining the required backcountry permit. This is somewhat more complicated than that simple statement would imply. To protect the land, the National Park Service severely restricts the number of available campsites (see "Permit" on the previous page). If you successfully make a reservation—no small accomplishment given the booming popularity of this area—you must still visit a ranger station in person to convert your reservation to an active permit.

TIP: If unsuccessful with an advanced reservation, you might still be able to secure a walk-up permit. To improve your chances of obtaining a permit, start on a weekday and be as flexible as possible about your schedule.

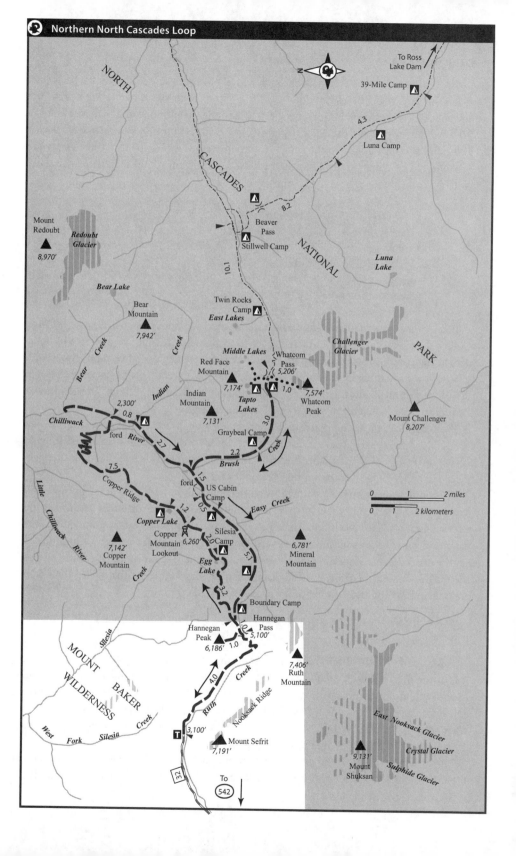

NORTH

CASCADES

NATIONAL

PARK

MOUNT

BAKER

WILDERNESS

To Ross
Lake Dam

39-Mile Camp

4.3

Luna Camp

8.2

Beaver
Pass

Stillwell Camp

10.1

Luna
Lake

Mount
Redoubt
8,970'

Redoubt
Glacier

Bear Lake

Bear
Mountain
7,942'

Twin Rocks
Camp

East Lakes

Challenger
Glacier

Bear Creek

Indian Creek

Middle Lakes

Red Face
Mountain
7,174'

Whatcom
Pass
5,206'

Indian
Mountain
7,131'

Tapto
Lakes

1.0

7,574'
Whatcom
Peak

Mount Challenger
8,207'

Chilliwack

2,300'
0.8

ford   River

2.7

Graybeal Camp

3.0

Brush   Creek

2.2

Little Chilliwack River

7.5

Copper Ridge

1.5

ford

US Cabin
Camp

1.2   0.5

Easy   Creek

7,142'
Copper
Mountain

Copper Lake

Copper
Mountain
Lookout
6,260'

Silesia
Camp

2.0

5.1

6,781'
Mineral
Mountain

Egg
Lake

3.2

Creek

Boundary Camp

Hannegan
Pass
5,100'

Hannegan
Peak
6,186'

1.0
1.0

7,406'
Ruth
Mountain

Silesia   Creek

4.0

Ruth   Creek

Nooksack Ridge

3,100'

West   Fork   Silesia   Creek

T

542

To
542

Mount Sefrit
7,191'

East   Nooksack Glacier

Crystal Glacier

9,131'
Mount
Shuksan

Sulphide Glacier

0   1   2 miles
0   1   2 kilometers

DESCRIPTION •

The trail begins as a gentle path through a lovely forest beside Ruth Creek. Occasional avalanche-caused openings provide tantalizing glimpses of the surrounding peaks. The first mile's easy warm-up hiking gives way to a moderate climb as the path works away from the valley floor, and the scenery improves with views of the icy summits of Nooksack Ridge and Ruth Mountain to the south. Your climb eases where the trail travels near the edge of a lovely heather and wildflower meadow. From the meadow the trail makes a short switchbacking ascent to forested Hannegan Pass.

> **HANNEGAN PEAK SIDE TRIP:** Don't miss the superb side trip from this pass to Hannegan Peak. The moderately graded trail goes north for 1 mile through forest and then meadows and heather, gaining 1,100 feet to the summit. Tremendous views are your reward for this exertion, as you can look to horizons filled with the glacier-clad summits of Mount Baker, Mount Shuksan, and dozens of less well-known but no less impressive summits.

Back at the pass, you continue east and descend in moderate switchbacks into the Chilliwack River Valley. The route emerges from the trees to enter a large area of boulders at the head of this basin, where several sloping avalanche chutes support a wealth of wildflowers, especially tall, pink fireweed. The trail enters North Cascades National Park about 1 mile below the pass near a junction beside Boundary Camp. The Chilliwack River Trail, the return leg of your loop, drops to the right.

From the Boundary Camp junction you bear left (northeast) and begin a long, uneven climb. Numerous switchbacks ascend through forest, with frequent breaks that provide ever-improving views. Eventually the trail attains the glorious ridgetop meadows and gardens of Copper Ridge—ample compensation for all that sweat.

The ridge itself is inviting enough, with delicate wildflowers, meadowy bumps, and scattered trees, but you probably won't notice any of these subtle features because of the overwhelming views. No human-made skyline can compare with this grandeur, as icy crags and snowy ridges fill the sky in every direction. The distinctive high summit to the southwest is Mount Shuksan, while Bear Mountain and distant Mount Redoubt rise to the northeast, and the rugged Picket Range can be seen to the southwest. To the north are a seemingly infinite number of icy peaks in Canada.

WARNING: Despite all the visible snow and ice, there is surprisingly little water available along the ridge. Carry at least 2 quarts.

After about 1 mile of up-and-down wandering, you'll reach a junction with the side trail dropping to tiny Egg Lake, about 200 feet below in a grassy meadow. This pond is pleasant, although not really all that impressive by North Cascades standards. Three approved campsites are situated beside Egg Lake, so if this is where your permit allows you to camp, you will need to drop down to the lake for the night. Somewhat better views are found at tiny Silesia Camp on the ridge above.

The wonderful and easy ridgetop walk continues for another mile before you tackle the 1,000-foot climb to Copper Mountain Lookout, usually staffed by a friendly ranger. The ranger's friendliness is no doubt enhanced by the view from the front porch. To call the scene *spectacular* just doesn't do it justice. The vistas range from the deep, forest-covered canyons of the Chilliwack River and Silesia Creek to towering Mount Baker above the southwest horizon, its volcanic majesty draped in glacial white. Countless impossibly rugged peaks and spires are visible in two countries and, best of all, not a single road despoils the view.

TIP: With a compass and a good contour map, you can spend hours identifying distant landmarks.

From the lookout, the trail loses some elevation, contours a bit through more meadows, and then drops in a series of switchbacks to the shores of Copper Lake. This deep pool is set in a tightly enclosed glacial cirque and has the last permitted campsites along the ridge.

TIP: Views from Copper Lake are limited. If this is your destination for the night, spend any spare hours at the lookout before coming down to make camp.

To continue the tour, hike north on the ridge trail along an up-and-down course. Views along this section are less frequent and typically feature the cliffs of the ridge itself rather than distant vistas, but they are still excellent. Eventually the trail leaves the ridge and makes a long, often steep switchbacking descent through forests and rocky areas to a crossing of the Chilliwack River.

WARNING: There is no bridge here, and the river does an admirable job of fulfilling the chilly part of its name, but the ford is not especially dangerous.

You may have to search a bit to relocate the trail on the opposite bank.

Shortly beyond the ford is a junction with the Chilliwack River Trail, where you turn right (southwest) and gradually climb the forested valley. The trail passes inviting Indian Creek

Campsite at Indian Creek
photographed by Mark Wetherington

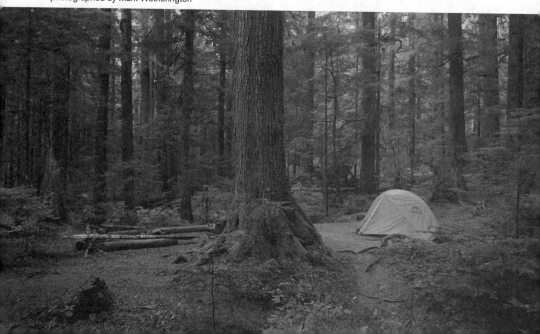

Camp, then continues south through an old-growth forest with lots of interesting understory plants and mushrooms. The stream itself is only occasionally visible through the trees.

About 2.7 miles from Indian Creek Camp, you'll reach a junction with the Brush Creek Trail. The route back to Hannegan Pass goes straight, but for now you turn left (southeast) and steadily climb this large side valley, often through brushy areas.

WARNING: So much dew collects on the overhanging vegetation here that just walking through on a sunny morning can soak you as thoroughly as one of the North Cascades' frequent rainstorms. Bring gaiters and good rain pants.

Views are limited along this forested route, but the hiking is pleasant. After 2.2 miles you arrive at Graybeal Camp, a good potential choice for a base camp location.

TIP: The bouldery banks of Brush Creek near the camp provide some exceptionally photogenic views of Whatcom Peak to the east.

WARNING: The trees and snags around Graybeal Camp are disturbingly unstable. Set up your tent away from snags.

Plan to spend at least one day exploring spectacular Whatcom Pass, one of the scenic climaxes of North Cascades National Park. From Graybeal Camp the trail climbs steadily out of the lower valley, working up the north side of the headwall basin of Brush Creek. Views up to distinctive Whatcom Peak are especially noteworthy as you climb out of deep forest, through sloping meadows, and into an area of stunted Alaska yellow cedars and subalpine firs. If the weather is favorable, small but very scenic Whatcom Camp, a little below the west side of Whatcom Pass, is a terrific place to spend a night enjoying the majesty of this spectacular location. Fires are prohibited.

SIDE TRIP TOWARD WHATCOM PEAK: Once you reach the pass, the joys have only just begun because explorations from here are relatively easy and highly rewarding. To the south a sometimes-rugged climber's route works up a ridge toward the awesome cliffs and crags of Whatcom Peak. Panoramas of the surrounding peaks and the massive, U-shaped valley of Little Beaver Creek to the east defy description—even photographs fail to do them justice. Eventually the scramble route is best left to mountaineers, but from the high vantage point at the end of hiker access, you are treated to an up close look at massive Challenger Glacier.

SIDE TRIP TO TAPTO AND MIDDLE LAKES: North of the pass are even more rewarding rambles. Bring a good contour map and make your way northwest on boot-beaten routes around stunted trees and through meadows for about 1 mile to a rocky area holding the scenic Tapto Lakes (possible camps, with an off-trail camping permit). Another good destination is quiet Middle Lakes, reachable by a sidehill scramble over talus slopes east of Tapto Lakes. The view near Middle Lakes across Little Beaver Valley to the enormous white expanse of Challenger Glacier is superb. The lake itself sits in a meadowy cirque on the side of aptly named Red Face Mountain (the red is from exposed volcanic rocks). Scramblers can climb higher on the side of Red Face Mountain for even better views.

After returning down Brush Creek to the junction with the Chilliwack River Trail, turn left (upstream and southwest) and wander up and down through the dense forest. After 0.8 mile the trail splits, giving you a choice of methods to cross the Chilliwack River. The branch to the right leads to a ford, but a more interesting option goes to the left and uses a cable car. It's a fairly easy hand-over-hand system to pull yourself across in a metal car.

Continuing up the west bank, the trail stays mostly in the trees, with only occasional meadows providing glimpses of the stream and surrounding ridges. At the first of these meadow openings is US Cabin Camp, a pleasant campsite just 0.5 mile upstream from the cable car.

Above this camp the shady valley-bottom route is relatively gentle, although it is rarely level. As the path curves gradually west, the slope of the climb becomes more noticeable and then picks up significantly as the trail aims to regain the high country around Hannegan Pass. You pass Copper Creek Camp, then continue the steady ascent through deep forests. Eventually you return to Boundary Camp and the avalanche meadows in the headwall basin of the Chilliwack River. Here you meet the Copper Mountain Trail. Go left (southwest) and return to your car the way you came—over Hannegan Pass and then down Ruth Creek to the trailhead.

VARIATION

An epic traverse of the North Cascades can be made by starting at the Hannegan trailhead and ending at Ross Lake Dam. Take the hike as described as far as Whatcom Camp and Tapto Lakes. From there descend east from Whatcom Pass along Little Beaver Trail to Big Beaver Trail. Turn south, cross over Beaver Pass, and continue through beautiful old-growth cedar forest to 39 Mile Camp and Ross Lake Dam. While this trip leaves nothing to be desired in the scenery department, logistically it is a bit inconvenient, as it requires a car shuttle of 127 miles each way.

POSSIBLE ITINERARY

	CAMP	MILES	ELEVATION GAIN
Day 1	Silesia Camp	8.2	3,200'
	Side trip up Hannegan Peak	2.0	1,100'
Day 2	Indian Creek Camp	11.5	1,700'
Day 3	Whatcom Camp	7.9	2,900'
	Side trip toward Whatcom Peak	2.0	1,000'
Day 4	US Cabin Camp	10.6	150'
	Side trip to Tapto and Middle Lakes	3.4	850'
Day 5	Out	10.1	2,600'

BEST SHORTER ALTERNATIVE

A day hike up to Hannegan Peak is fun, scenic, and worthwhile. We must warn you, however, that the views from the top will leave you feeling unfulfilled, and you'll soon be planning to take the longer backpacking trip.

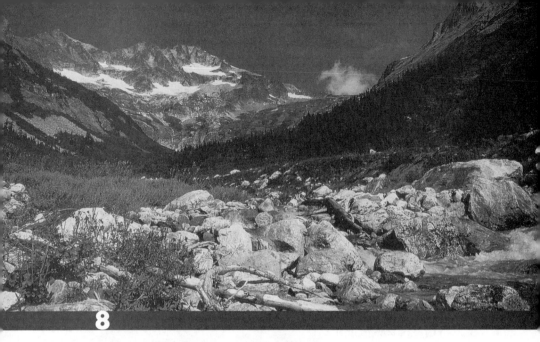

SOUTHERN NORTH CASCADES LOOP

RATINGS: Scenery 9   **Solitude** 5   **Difficulty** 6

MILES: 66 (81)

ELEVATION GAIN: 14,200' (15,800')

DAYS: 5–10 (7–10)

SHUTTLE MILEAGE: 8

MAPS: Trails Illustrated *North Cascades National Park (#223)*; Green Trails *Diablo Dam (#48), Mt. Logan (#49), McGregor Mtn. (#81),* and *Stehekin (#82)*

USUALLY OPEN: Mid-July–early October

BEST: August

PERMIT: Required. As of 2019 they are free but limited. About 60% of the available campsites can be reserved in advance, with the rest given out on a first-come, first-served basis. Reservation requests should be submitted between March 15 and April 15 for the summer season. Reservation requests can only be made online; a $20 nonrefundable fee applies to reserved permits. Walk-up permits can be obtained on the first day of the trip or up to one day before. See nps.gov/noca/planyourvisit/backcountry-reservations.htm for full details. Pick up permits (whether reserved in advance or a walk-up permit) from the wilderness information center in Marblemount (if you are coming from the west) or the Methow Valley Visitor Center in Winthrop (from the east).

Above: *Mount Logan from North Fork Bridge Creek*
photographed by Douglas Lorain

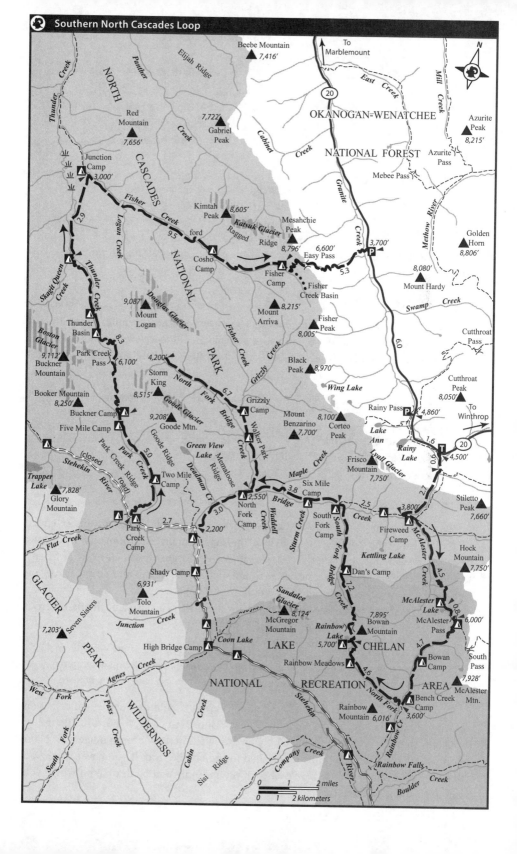

To
Marblemount

OKANOGAN-WENATCHEE

NATIONAL FOREST

N

Beebe Mountain
▲ 7,416'

East Creek

Mill Creek

20

Azurite
Peak
▲ 8,215'

Elijah Ridge

Panther Creek

Thunder Creek

NORTH

Red
Mountain
▲ 7,656'

7,722'
▲ Gabriel
Peak

Cabinet Creek

Creek

Azurite
Pass

Mebee Pass

CASCADES

Junction
Camp
▲ 3,000'

29

Fisher Creek

Logan Creek

9.5

Kimtah
Peak ▲

8,605'
Katsuk Glacier
Ragged Ridge

ford

Mesahchie
Peak

8,796'

6,600'
Easy Pass

3,700'
P

5.3

Granite Creek

Methow River

Golden
Horn
▲ 8,806'

8,080'
▲ Mount Hardy

Skagit Queen Creek

Thunder Creek

NATIONAL

Cosho
Camp

Fisher
Camp

Fisher
Creek Basin

Swamp Creek

Cutthroat
Pass

9,087'
▲ Mount
Logan

Douglas Glacier

Mount
Arriva

▲ 8,215'

Fisher
Peak
▲ 8,005'

6.0

Boston
Glacier

Thunder
Basin

PARK

Fisher Creek

Grizzly Creek

Cutthroat
Peak
▲ 8,050'

To
Winthrop

9,112'
Buckner
Mountain

Park Creek
Pass

8.3

6,100'

4,200'

Storm
King

North Fork

Black
Peak ▲ 8,970'

Wing Lake

Rainy Pass
P

4,860'

Booker Mountain
▲ 8,250'

Buckner Camp

8,515'
Goode Glacier

9,208'
Goode Mtn.

Goode Ridge

Bridge Creek

Grizzly
Camp

Mount
Benzarino
▲ 7,700'

8,100'
Corteo
Peak

Lake
Ann

Rainy
Lake

20

4,500'

Five Mile Camp

Green View
Lake

Walker Park

Memaloose
Ridge

Maple Creek

Frisco
Mountain
7,750'

Lyall Glacier

1.6

T

2.7

Stiletto
Peak ▲ 7,660'

Trapper
Lake
▲ 7,828'
Glory
Mountain

Park Creek Ridge

(closed

Stehekin River

road)

Two Mile
Camp

Deadman Cr.

5.0

3.0

2,550'
North
Fork
Camp

Waddell Creek

Bridge

Sturm Creek

3.8

Six Mile
Camp

2.5

South
Fork
Camp

3,800'

Fireweed
Camp

McAlester Creek

Hock
Mountain
▲ 7,750'

2.7

2,200'

Park
Creek
Camp

Flat Creek

Shady Camp

6,931'
Tolo
Mountain

Junction Creek

Sandalee
Glacier

8,124'
McGregor
Mountain

South Fork Bridge Creek

Dan's Camp

Kettling Lake

1.2

7,895'
Bowan
Mountain

4.5

McAlester
Lake

0.8

McAlester
Pass

6,000'

GLACIER

7,203'
▲ Seven Sisters

High Bridge Camp

Coon Lake

LAKE

Rainbow
Lake
5,700'

Rainbow Meadows

CHELAN

4.7

Bowan
Camp

South
Pass

▲ 7,928'
McAlester
Mtn.

PEAK

Agnes Creek

West Fork

Pass Creek

WILDERNESS

NATIONAL

RECREATION

North Fork

Rainbow
Mountain 6,016'

Stehekin River

4.6

AREA

Bench Creek
Camp
3,600'

South Fork

Sisi Ridge

Cabin Creek

Company Creek

Rainbow
Mountain

Rainbow Cr.

River

Rainbow Falls

Boulder Creek

0   1   2 miles

0   1   2 kilometers

RULES: Camping allowed only at a restricted number of designated sites; no fires at higher-elevation camps; maximum group size of 12
CONTACT: North Cascades National Park, 360-854-7200 ext. 515; in summer, contact the park's wilderness information center, 360-854-7245, nps.gov/noca

SPECIAL ATTRACTIONS

Ruggedly beautiful mountain scenery, easy road access

CHALLENGES

Black bears are common—store all food properly; camp-raiding chipmunks; a few rattlesnakes in lower elevation areas

HOW TO GET THERE

Take WA 20 to Rainy Pass, then continue southeast another 1.6 miles to the heavily used Bridge Creek Trailhead. Hikers with two cars should leave the second one at the well-marked Easy Pass Trailhead off WA 20, about 6 miles north of Rainy Pass on the west side of the road.

NOTE: You'll need a Northwest Forest Pass to park at these trailheads.

GPS TRAILHEAD COORDINATES:
Southern (Bridge Creek): N48° 30.300' W120° 43.146'
Northern (Easy Pass): N48° 35.274' W120° 48.174'

INTRODUCTION

The rugged beauty of the North Cascades is on spectacular display in this extended loop hike. The route samples nearly all of the range's many environments, from low-elevation eastside forests of ponderosa pine to low-elevation westside forests of fir and hemlock. In between, towering peaks surround high snowy passes and deep basins. You can also expect to see big trees and tiny wildflowers, lumbering black bears and scurrying chipmunks, rushing streams and quiet mountain lakes. There just isn't much missing from this wonderful hike.

WARNING: Good raingear, including gaiters and waterproof boots, are essential in the North Cascades, even if it doesn't rain. Dew often covers the thick brush and grasses that crowd many trails. Just hiking through on a sunny morning can get you soaked.

Start by picking up the required backcountry permit from the wilderness information center in Marblemount or the Methow Valley Visitor Center in Winthrop. The use of available campsites is strictly regulated. Rangers do their best to accommodate your plans but must work around the limits established to protect the land. If you haven't reserved your sites in advance, plan to arrive early in the morning and be flexible on where you want to go and are willing to camp.

DESCRIPTION ••

The hike starts with a short drop from the trailhead to a meeting with the Pacific Crest Trail (PCT). Go straight (southeast), following the PCT as it makes a pleasantly gradual descent through forests and leaves the highway sounds behind. About 0.6 mile from the trailhead, you come to a junction where you go straight on the PCT, cross Bridge Creek, and soon enter North Cascades National Park.

As you continue down the trail, you make a forested, uneven, and rather uneventful descent to a prominent junction at 3.3 miles.

TIP: Hikers with limited time can go straight (west) here, following the PCT along Bridge Creek. This shortcut misses some wonderful scenery but takes one to two days and considerable climbing off your trip.

Opting for the longer, more scenic option, you turn left (east), cross Bridge Creek, and walk through popular Fireweed Camp.

TIP: Hikers who are setting a more leisurely pace should camp here the first night.

A little beyond this camp you bear right (southeast) at the junction with the Twisp Pass Trail and begin a sustained climb above splashing McAlester Creek. A meadow opening about 1.8 miles from Fireweed Camp provides views of the surrounding ridges, only a small taste of what is to come.

Now you enter the Lake Chelan National Recreation Area and begin climbing away from the creek. The last mile of the climb follows a series of switchbacks before the trail levels off just before McAlester Lake. While not as dramatic as some other lakes in the

Buckner Mountain from Thunder Basin
photographed by Douglas Lorain

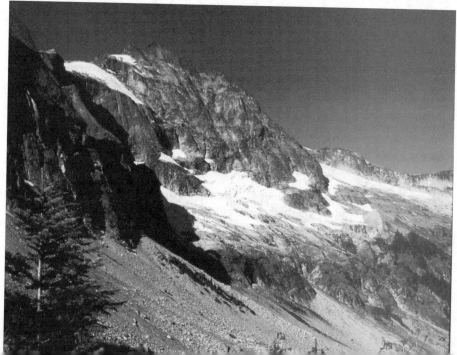

North Cascades, this scenic pool sits beside a lovely meadow and offers good fishing. The horse and hiker camping areas are reached by a short side trail on the north side of the lake.

From McAlester Lake the trail makes a short climb to the meadows, larches, and flowers around McAlester Pass, where you'll find a small approved camp.

TIP 1: Look for black bears on the nearby slopes, especially during the berry season in August.

TIP 2: A worthwhile side trip for energetic hikers goes southeast from McAlester Pass to the fine views from South Pass.

Brace your knees for a sustained downhill, as the trail makes a fairly steep descent from McAlester Pass into the canyon of Rainbow Creek. Switchbacks ease the initial miles, and numerous views of the surrounding peaks provide impressive diversions. Near the bottom of the first major descent, the path levels off beside Rainbow Creek and travels below a bouldery area before crossing the stream. You pass Bowan Camp shortly after the creek crossing and continue losing elevation into a drier eastside forest that includes a few ponderosa pines.

Upon reaching Bench Creek Camp, whose tent sites are dug out of the side of a hill, you turn right (east) at a junction and make a quick descent to a crossing of Rainbow Creek. The trail now makes a determined effort to regain all of that lost elevation. After numerous forested switchbacks, the trail rounds the canyon mouth and levels off somewhat near the creek. As you approach the head of the canyon, you'll reach large and very attractive Rainbow Meadows, which is an inviting lunch or overnight stop with large wooden picnic tables made from logs. Beyond the meadows the trail once again climbs, this time in a series of switchbacks over an open talus slope. Like most such areas in the Pacific Northwest, these rocks are home to a healthy population of pikas. These cute little guinea pig–like creatures spend their brief summers gathering food for the coming winter and squeaking at passing hikers. Given their small size and shy nature, they are more often heard than seen.

At the top of the rocky slope, the trail enters a lovely little vale and soon reaches Rainbow Lake, with a designated camping area on the south shore.

WARNING: The deep waters of this beautiful mountain lake remain very cold all summer long. Swimming is invigorating, to say the least.

Granite peaks and ridges rise on three sides of the lake, making this a choice camp spot.

TIP: For a truly outstanding outlook of Rainbow Creek Canyon, continue about 100 yards on the trail that goes past the campground's outhouse to a low ridge. This overlook makes a wonderful spot to cook dinner and watch the sunset.

Reluctantly leaving this mountain jewel behind, you climb a series of steep switchbacks to a large sloping meadow. The trail traverses a hillside along this meadow and tops out at a high pass overlooking the immense canyon of South Fork Bridge Creek. To the north you'll be able to see hundreds of distant peaks crowding the skyline.

From the pass you drop in a series of fairly steep switchbacks, then cross a large rocky area as you descend to the marshy headwall basin of the canyon. The meadow here contains a bonanza of water-loving wildflowers and affords neck-craning views of Bowan

Mountain and other surrounding peaks. Below this meadow the trail reenters forest, passes small Dan's Camp, and continues to lose elevation. Occasional breaks in the trees provide wonderful vistas of McGregor Mountain to the west. Eventually the trail bottoms out and crosses good-size Bridge Creek on a log bridge to pleasant South Fork Camp. The trail then climbs 100 feet up the opposite bank to where you rejoin the PCT.

NOTE: Hikers who skipped the side loop to McAlester and Rainbow Lakes will reach this point after an easy 2.5-mile hike down the PCT from Fireweed Camp.

Your route turns left (west) on the PCT and crosses a series of mostly open, south-facing slopes above Bridge Creek.

WARNING: The trail here can be uncomfortably warm on sunny days.

In the canyon below, Bridge Creek cascades along amid cottonwoods, firs, and pines. You pass a side trail dropping to Six Mile Camp and continue to the narrow side canyon of Maple Creek, spanned by a short swinging bridge. Beyond Maple Creek the path travels through an attractive area of rocky slopes, ponderosa pines, and canyon views. It then passes a junction with the Walker Park Trail and switchbacks down 0.3 mile to North Fork Camp. This choice spot sits on a bench just above the confluence of Bridge Creek and North Fork Bridge Creek, both beautiful clear streams.

WARNING: A larcenous population of chipmunks has learned how to raid food here by climbing down thick bear ropes to backpackers' food bags. If you didn't bring a bear-resistant canister, use a more distant tree limb or a narrower cord that the little thieves can't climb down.

NORTH FORK BRIDGE CREEK SIDE TRIP: Unless you are really strapped for time or the rains have set in, plan to spend a day at North Fork Camp and make the outstanding side trip up North Fork Bridge Creek, one of this trip's scenic highlights. Begin by returning to the Walker Park Trail junction and turning north. The well-graded but often overgrown and rough path gradually wanders up the mostly wooded slopes on the east side of the stream. Frequent openings in the tree cover provide tantalizing views of Memaloose Ridge to the west. You pass Walker Park Camp, and then continue another mile to the crossing of Grizzly Creek at Grizzly Camp.

TIP: To keep your feet dry, look for a log crossing of this stream about 100 yards downstream from the horse ford.

As you continue upstream, the gently graded path begins to climb intermittently, and views to the west of towering Goode Mountain and Storm King improve. A small meadow about 1 mile past Grizzly Creek has gorgeous views of these two peaks and marks the start of the truly outstanding scenery. Just past this meadow, the trail climbs past a hard-to-see waterfall and then continues through a series of increasingly dramatic meadows. Tall, glacier-clad peaks tower above you as the trail alternates between short climbs and meadow rambles. The tread gradually becomes more overgrown with brush and grasses and eventually disappears entirely amid the flowers.

TIP: Near where the trail peters out, photographers should make a side trip to the creek for nice shots over the stream to Mount Logan and other peaks at the head of the basin.

Be sure to pull yourself away from this paradise while you still have enough time to return to camp.

Back on the PCT at North Fork Camp, you cross Bridge Creek on a substantial bridge, then climb along the south bank.

WARNING: Rattlesnakes are occasionally seen at these lower eastside elevations. Watch your step.

Even though the trail parallels Bridge Creek and goes downstream, it gains a frustrating amount of elevation to a point high above the stream before finally leveling off and dropping to a trailhead on an old gravel road. Before the road was washed out in floods in 2003, National Park Service shuttle buses made regularly scheduled trips along this road. The road is now closed to all traffic, serving instead as a wide trail. Fortunately, the road walk is pleasant and relatively short.

To continue your trip, turn right (west) on the road, now rapidly being reclaimed by shrubbery, and immediately walk over the bridge spanning Bridge Creek.

TIP: About 100 feet downstream from the bridge, a scenic waterfall located among sculpted rocks is well worth a look.

Above Bridge Creek the narrow gravel road passes a side trail to Goode Ridge after 100 yards (a rugged but beautiful possible side trip), then leads upstream through forests and lush riparian shrubbery beside the lovely Stehekin River.

Shortly after crossing Park Creek, about 2.7 miles from Bridge Creek, look for Park Creek Camp and the signed Park Creek Trailhead on the right (north). You leave the road here and follow this path as it initially goes gently up a wooded slope but soon begins climbing in earnest. Switchbacks ease the grade, and a rocky promontory about 1.3 miles from the start provides a good rest stop with excellent views. A little beyond this overlook the trail rounds a ridge, where you are treated to nice views of the slotlike gorge of Park Creek, then continues to a crossing of Park Creek at tiny Two Mile Camp. The climb now eases somewhat, as the trail alternates between forests and open areas above the east bank of Park Creek. You pass through a series of wet meadows choked with willows before reaching first Five Mile Horse Camp, then Five Mile Hiker Camp, and finally the restored Buckner Camp.

NOTE: This is the last legal camp on the south side of Park Creek Pass, a goal that is still over 2,000 feet above.

Beyond Buckner Camp the trail soon leaves Park Creek and begins to switchback up the east side of the canyon. The sometimes-steep route requires frequent rest stops, and the ever-improving views provide an excellent excuse. A little over 1 mile from Buckner Camp, the trail tops a low rise and enters the beautiful, sloping meadows below Park Creek Pass. For the next mile the route makes a joyful climb through these lovely alpine gardens before crossing a trickling creek in a meadow basin.

TIP 1: Look for black bears here, especially during berry season in August.

TIP 2: The rolling meadowy ridges west of the trail make for an easy and rewarding cross-country ramble. The payoff for this side trip is a dramatic view of nearby Buckner and Booker Mountains.

After a final push you'll reach Park Creek Pass, a rocky divide that remains snow-filled for much of the summer. The vistas north from this pass into Thunder Creek Canyon and west to the huge glaciers and cliffs of Buckner Mountain are overwhelming.

Now the trail crosses a bouldery hillside above the low point in the pass, and then makes a long descent into Thunder Basin, passing countless fine viewpoints along the way. About 2.8 miles from the pass is Thunder Basin Camp. The hiker's camping area here has been periodically closed in recent years due to bear activity.

The gently graded trail passes the Thunder Basin horse camp and closely follows the lovely clear headwaters of Thunder Creek. Shortly after the horse camp, you cross the stream on a log.

WARNING: This crossing can be confusing because a false trail continues straight, without crossing the log. If you find yourself on a track that rather suddenly peters out, backtrack about 50 feet to the log, then cross the creek to the correct path on the other side.

Climb briefly away from the creek before beginning a long switchbacking descent through forests of ever-larger trees to the lower valley of Thunder Creek. Just before you cross a bridge over cascading Thunder Creek, you reach inviting Skagit Queen Camp. The tour now makes several ups and downs but generally descends through impressive old-growth forests. Not long after crossing a small creek, the trail begins a sometimes steep and tiring 900-foot climb along a ridge to the east. Views are limited until you reach a rocky promontory near the top of the climb. After topping the ridge, the path continues a short distance to a junction with the Fisher Creek Trail. To reach Junction Camp, keep straight for about 100 yards to where a marked side trail leads to the camping area.

TIP: For an excellent evening view, continue a little beyond the most northerly of the designated campsites here to a rocky overlook.

The quickest and easiest exit from Junction Camp is to continue north down the Thunder Creek Trail. This route passes through lovely old-growth forests and eventually reaches Colonial Creek Campground on Diablo Lake. The *recommended* route is more strenuous than the Thunder Creek Trail, but it's also more scenic and usually less crowded. To take this route, hike east on the rougher Fisher Creek Trail as it follows an up-and-down course along the south bank of its namesake stream. The route is mostly in viewless forest, but the hiking is still enjoyable amid lush vegetation. You cross Logan Creek, milky with glacial silt, and then continue along Fisher Creek, now crystal clear and strikingly beautiful. Eventually the trail crosses the stream (no bridge), makes a short detour downstream, and then continues upstream. You pass Cosho Camp and shortly thereafter begin a forested climb, generally staying well above Fisher Creek. Rather abruptly, the path breaks out of the trees into a large brushy meadow with good views. Particularly noteworthy is the view to the west back down the canyon to square-topped Mount Logan and large Douglas Glacier. About 0.5 mile from the start of these meadows is a strip of trees holding Fisher Camp.

> **FISHER CREEK BASIN SIDE TRIP:** A worthwhile side trip from Fisher Camp follows the main trail upstream for 0.2 mile to where it turns left (north) and begins climbing. You leave the main trail here and turn right (southeast) onto an unmarked but easy-to-follow use path that continues up the canyon. After about 0.6 mile of mostly level hiking, the path rounds a bend and enters scenic Fisher Creek Basin, where the meandering creek is surrounded by meadows, flowers, and towering peaks. The prominent pointed summit at the head of this basin is Fisher Peak.

To complete your trip from Fisher Camp, you climb a mostly open slope in a seemingly endless series of fairly steep switchbacks. Views down Fisher Creek Canyon grow more dramatic as you climb. Eventually the switchbacks end as the trail contours the final 0.4 mile to Easy Pass, where camping is strictly prohibited to protect the area's fragile alpine gardens.

The trail now steeply descends the rocky gorge of tiny Easy Pass Creek. This descent starts by crossing talus slopes and then continues into brushy meadows and finally forest. The steep trail is hard on the knees, but after a week in the North Cascades, you'll be accustomed to the ups and downs of these mountains. At the bottom, the trail crosses Granite Creek, which is usually spanned by a narrow log. If not, the hiker must make a chilly ford or search for a log crossing downstream. After the crossing, the trail climbs a short distance to the Easy Pass Trailhead on WA 20. If you have only one car, the trip must end with a hitchhike or a 7.6-mile walk up the busy highway over Rainy Pass and down to the Bridge Creek Trailhead.

VARIATIONS

As mentioned in the text, you can shorten the trip by either skipping the horseshoe loop down to McAlester and Rainbow Lakes, or by going straight down Thunder Creek and skipping the Fisher Creek and Easy Pass section of the hike.

POSSIBLE ITINERARY

	CAMP	MILES	ELEVATION GAIN
Day 1	McAlester Lake	7.8	2,000'
Day 2	Rainbow Lake	10.1	2,700'
Day 3	North Fork Camp	11.2	800'
Day 4	North Fork Camp		
	Day hike up North Fork Bridge Creek	13.8	1,400'
Day 5	Buckner Camp	10.5	2,100'
Day 6	Junction Camp	11.2	3,100'
Day 7	Fisher Camp	9.5	2,100'
	Side trip to Fisher Creek Basin	1.2	200'
Day 8	Out (excluding the road walk)	5.3	1,400'

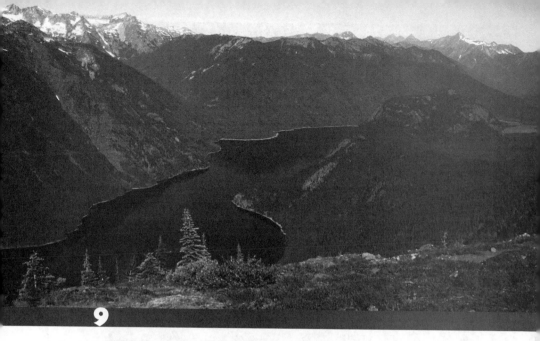

9

WESTERN PASAYTEN–ROSS LAKE LOOP

RATINGS: Scenery 8   Solitude 5   Difficulty 8

MILES: 80 (107)

ELEVATION GAIN: 17,600' (25,200')

DAYS: 7–11 (9–14)

SHUTTLE MILEAGE: n/a

MAPS: Green Trails *Ross Lake (#16), Jack Mountain (#17), Pasayten Peak (#18),* and *Mt. Logan (#49)*

USUALLY OPEN: Mid-July–October

BEST: Early to mid-August

PERMIT: Required. For the Pasayten Wilderness section they are free, unlimited, and available at the trailhead. Permits are limited only for the section in the Ross Lake National Recreation Area. During the summer camping season (May 15–September 30), you can reserve sites at the designated camps along the East Bank Trail bordering Ross Lake. About 60% of the available campsites can be reserved in advance, with the rest given out on a first-come, first-served basis. Reservation requests should be submitted between March 15 and April 15 for the summer season. Reservation requests can only be made online; a $20 nonrefundable fee applies to reserved permits. Walk-up permits can be obtained on the first day of the trip or up to 1 day

Above: *Ross Lake and views west from Desolation Peak*
photographed by Douglas Lorain

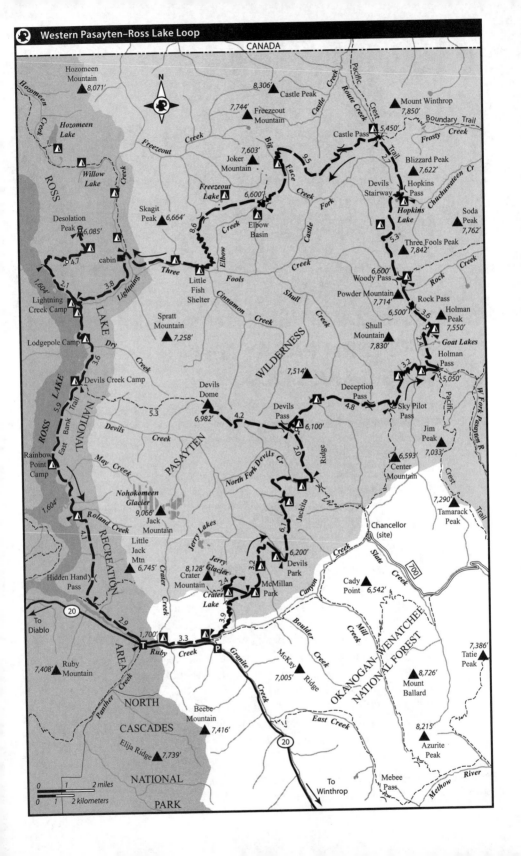

before. See nps.gov/noca/planyourvisit/backcountry-reservations.htm for full details. Pick up permits (whether reserved in advance or a walk-up permit) from the wilderness information center in Marblemount (if you are coming from the west) or the Methow Valley Visitor Center in Winthrop (from the east).

RULES: Maximum group size of 12 people and 18 stock in Pasayten Wilderness; camp only at designated sites and maximum group size of 12 people in Ross Lake National Recreation Area

CONTACTS: Ross Lake National Recreation Area: North Cascades National Park, 360-854-7200 ext. 515; in summer, contact the park's wilderness information center, 360-854-7245, nps.gov/noca. Pasayten Wilderness: Okanogan-Wenatchee National Forest, Methow Valley Ranger District, 509-996-4000, fs.usda.gov/main/okawen.

SPECIAL ATTRACTIONS

Wildflowers, good views, solitude

CHALLENGES

Some rough and sketchy trails; a (very) few grizzly bears; long, difficult trip with no opportunity to resupply

HOW TO GET THERE

Take WA 20 to the well-marked East Bank Trailhead, just west of the Panther Creek bridge. The trailhead is about 19.5 miles west of Rainy Pass and 12.4 miles east of the Diablo turnoff. Parking is on the north side of the road.

GPS TRAILHEAD COORDINATES: N48° 42.474' W120° 58.626'

INTRODUCTION

The vastness of the Pasayten Wilderness is enough to make lovers of true wilderness jump for joy. Stretching more than 50 miles east to west, and a full 20 miles north to south, this sanctuary is one of the largest designated wilderness areas in the United States. Many long trails, most only lightly used, explore this backcountry, and although the scenery is generally more subdued than that of the rugged peaks to the west, the solitude and flowers are ample reward for the long miles. The trails connect to form huge loop trips, all major backpacking adventures. The western Pasayten loop is arguably the best in the entire wilderness and provides a glorious sampling of what this area has to offer.

DESCRIPTION

From the popular East Bank Trailhead the path drops 0.2 mile in switchbacks to a cable suspension bridge over the swift, clear waters of Ruby Creek. Several signs here discuss the colorful gold-mining history of this area. Immediately on the other side of the bridge is a trail junction. The East Bank Trail, the return leg of your loop, goes left (northwest), but your present route turns right (east) on the less heavily used Ruby Creek Trail. As you travel upstream the path goes up and down through a dense forest of Douglas fir, western hemlock, and western red cedar. On several occasions the trail provides easy access to the creek, although the stream is closed to anglers. About 0.9 mile from the Ruby Creek bridge, you make a bridged crossing of Crater Creek and leave the Ross Lake National Recreation Area. A good campsite sits less than 100 feet beyond this small creek.

TIP: This camp does not require a National Park Service permit and is a good choice for hikers who got a late start.

Above the camp the woodsy trail continues upstream. Although the path is quite close to the busy highway across the creek, most of the traffic noise is drowned out by the pleasant sound of rushing water. You'll pass a couple more decent camps before arriving at a dilapidated wooden cabin and good camps across from the Canyon Creek Trailhead parking area on the other side of Ruby Creek.

Just 150 yards beyond the wooden cabin is a junction with the Canyon Creek Trail.

NOTE: The log bridge that this trail once used to cross the creek has been washed out. Unless it has been replaced, hikers are forced to make a cold and potentially difficult ford to reach the nearby Canyon Creek Trailhead.

Your route goes straight (northeast) and immediately begins a long 3,300-foot climb on the Devils Park Trail. This can be a tough uphill with heavy packs, but trees provide plenty of shade, and water is available from two trickling creeks near the beginning. The consistent uphill grade is kept reasonably moderate by 60 mostly short switchbacks. At the seventh switchback you enter the Pasayten Wilderness and soon leave the last of the car sounds behind. After 45 more switchbacks you cross a very welcome creek below a cascading waterfall. The switchbacks finally end, but the uphill continues as you cross a forested hillside to a small creek and a junction. The main loop trail goes straight (northeast).

CRATER LAKE SIDE TRIP: Before continuing with the loop, first you'll want to allow time for a fine side trip that turns to the left (west) and climbs moderately steeply to Crater Lake. This very shallow, fishless pool is rimmed by cliffs, wildflower meadows, and larches; it's well worth a visit.

TIP: If you want to camp here, you'll find that those sites near the lake are too fragile and exposed to be recommended. Instead set up your tent at a scenic spot on the outlet creek about 0.1 mile below Crater Lake.

Ambitious hikers can go beyond the lake on one of two steep and unmaintained boot paths leading to glorious high viewpoints (both former lookout sites) on the ridges both west and east of the lake.

Back on the main trail, you pass a good camp just 100 feet beyond the Crater Lake junction and then enter the mostly flat expanse of McMillan Park. This lovely area is typical of the Pasayten high country and is a good example of what makes hiking here such a joy. The park is a gorgeous mix of shallow ponds, scattered subalpine firs, and open meadows with a wealth of wildflowers. There are yarrow, pussytoes, tiger lilies, Sitka valerian, arnica, lupine, aster, pasqueflowers, paintbrush, cinquefoils, heather, pearly everlasting, and countless others. The mountains here may be less craggy and spectacular than those in North Cascades National Park to the west, but the hiking here is generally easier and a lot more colorful.

After gradually losing elevation to reach a superior campsite at the north end of McMillan Park, the trail turns east and climbs fairly steeply along a wide, mostly open ridge. The ridge offers excellent views from here, especially to Crater and Jack Mountains to the west and Ragged Ridge in the distance to the south. Near the top of the ridge you curve south and gradually make your way to Devils Park, another large, sloping wildflower garden. Shortly after you enter the park, you'll pass some good camps beside a wooden trail shelter. Several more good camps appear farther along the trail, although water there dwindles to a tiny trickle by late summer. To exit Devils Park, follow the trail as it loops to the north and gradually ascends an open hillside. The wildly scenic trail now spends a lot of time climbing the side of Jackita Ridge, but the views, flowers, and huckleberries are so abundant that you probably won't even notice the sweat. After topping out on a spur ridge, the path steeply switchbacks down a large scree slope.

WARNING: Steep snowfields linger here into midsummer, and once they melt, the loose rocks make walking treacherous. Take it slowly.

The path now contours through open forests and then tops another spur ridge and descends into a meadowy creek basin with reliable water and a good campsite. From this basin you ascend a huckleberry-covered hillside to the top of a third and final spur of Jackita Ridge. There are excellent views here of the rounded summits to the north and the rugged cliffs and glaciers of Jack Mountain to the west.

The trail now drops very steeply, losing 1,000 feet in woods and flowery meadows to a rock-hop crossing of North Fork Devils Creek. From here you turn upstream and regain all of the elevation you just lost. The first part of the climb occurs in rocky avalanche meadows with stunted trees and limited shade. The second half of the climb is often extremely steep and rugged (it's rough going), but it passes a good campsite, and there is shade while you hike. The route tops out in a meadow high on the western slopes of Jackita Ridge at a poorly marked junction where you bear left (north).

After two full days of difficult up-and-down hiking, you deserve a break, and the trail finally gives it to you. The next 2 miles are an easy, mostly level traverse along the side and top of Jackita Ridge. The panoramas to the west of Jack Mountain, Mount Terror, the Picket Range, and distant Mount Baker are expansive and enchanting. Not so enchanting is the abundance of flies, but that's all part of hiking in this part of Washington.

The joyous hike continues north to a junction at Devils Pass. There is a camp here with water from a spring about 0.2 mile to the east. Better camps are found near a broken-down trail shelter in a meadowy basin southeast of the pass. You can reach this basin by going east on the trail toward Sky Pilot Pass for 0.1 mile to an obvious but unsigned fork. Veer right and drop down to the meadow with its shelter and nearby spring.

WARNING: Horse parties often camp here, so it may be a bit aromatic.

DEVILS DOME SIDE TRIP OR EAST BANK EXIT: From Devils Pass you have a choice. If you want a shorter loop hike, turn west on the popular trail to Devils Dome and Dry Creek Pass. This path follows a long scenic ridge, and then loses a knee-challenging 5,300 feet to a junction with the East Bank Trail above Ross Lake. From there you turn south and return to your car via the East Bank Trail for a total loop distance of about 43 miles.

TIP: Even if you don't take this shorter loop, it's well worth a side trip at least as far as Devils Dome to enjoy the dream-lovely ridgetop gardens and the great views.

For a full experience of the vast Pasayten Wilderness, turn east at Devils Pass, and veer left (northeast) at the fork leading down to the meadow camp mentioned previously. The trail contours gently across open slopes for 1.3 miles to a good camp in a wide, sloping basin. By late summer of dry years, there may be no water here, but usually you can count on a couple of trickling creeks in the rocky ravines a few hundred yards ahead. From the camp the trail continues to contour gently or gradually lose elevation through forests and small meadows, then makes a few short switchbacks and descends more noticeably to heavily forested Deception Pass. The easy hiking is now over as you steadily climb some 900 feet to rather disappointing Sky Pilot Pass. At the junction here, the trail to Chancellor, an old mining settlement, turns sharply right (south) and goes uphill, while your trail curves only slightly to the right and goes downhill.

WARNING: Don't be misled by the obvious path going uphill to the left. It simply dead-ends after passing a dry campsite.

Your route makes one quick switchback, then gradually descends or remains level on a traverse of a partly forested hillside. A little over 1 mile from Sky Pilot Pass, you hop across a pretty little creek and come to a fine camp on the creek's north bank. From here it's all downhill as you drop in five unevenly spaced switchbacks through forest to a simple log crossing of Canyon Creek. A mediocre camp lies beside this stream. From Canyon Creek you make a short, gradual ascent through forest to Holman Pass, a low woodsy saddle where you meet the Pacific Crest Trail (PCT).

At Holman Pass you turn left (north) on the PCT and begin a long, very gradual sidehill ascent. The route is in the trees at first but then leads through meadows with good views of Shull Mountain to the west. The PCT is almost always gently graded, and this stretch is no exception as you make four lazy switchbacks up to a large meadow with great views and acres of wildflowers. A tiny spring provides water for a nice, scenic campsite here.

TIP: From here you can make an easy and enjoyable cross-country side trip of about 0.5 mile to the tiny Goat Lakes, in a small, meadowy cirque to the south.

The PCT continues north, making a gradual uphill traverse on the west side of a ridge to Rock Pass. The views here are breathtaking, especially north to Powder Mountain and Three Fools Peak, and down the curving valley of Rock Creek. A former section of the PCT goes straight from the pass, but the official trail goes right (southeast) and descends three long switchbacks across steep meadows and scree. The trail then contours across open slopes and begins to climb in short switchbacks. The larch-studded meadows here are alive with alpine wildflowers, including both pink and white heather, phlox, partridge foot, and the tiny blue flowers of Cusick's speedwell. At one of the switchbacks you reunite with the former section of the PCT, and a little later you come to the poorly marked junction with a trail going east down Rock Creek. Stick with the main trail and climb more short switchbacks to the rocky defile of Woody Pass. There is an adequate camp just before the trail reaches Woody Pass, but you'd have to melt snow for water.

Your tour now returns to the west side of the divide and makes an easy contour that provides fine views. To the northwest are Joker and Freezeout Mountains and Castle Peak, while to the west are the icy crags of North Cascades National Park, and in the southwest Jack Mountain reappears. The PCT rounds a spur ridge, then gently climbs above a meadowy basin, into which you could descend to water and camps.

The trail now climbs to a high point on the ridge with more superb views, including large parts of E. C. Manning Provincial Park in Canada. From here you descend a narrow ridge at a place called Devils Stairway and switchback down a rocky slope. Below you are the clear waters of circular Hopkins Lake. Near the bottom of the switchbacks, an obvious spur trail leads to this scenic lake, which has a very good camp above its northern shore and lots of hungry trout.

Hopkins Lake is home to a population of very tame mule deer. You will see them in your camp in the evening and probably hear them stomping around for most of the night. The deer have learned to listen for backpackers getting up at night to relieve themselves; then they come rushing to the spot to enjoy the newly formed "salt lick." Hopkins Lake is also the traditional last campsite for PCT thru-hikers. In mid- to late September there are often several camped here, and it's fun to listen to them reminisce about their long journey.

The main PCT continues a short distance beyond the Hopkins Lake spur trail to Hopkins Pass. A faint and abandoned trail goes to the right here, but your route stays straight (north). The next 2.7 miles go by very quickly as you gradually lose elevation to Castle Pass.

TIP: Stock up on water at any of the small creeks along the way to Castle Pass. You will need lots of it in the many dry miles to come.

There are two junctions at Castle Pass. The first is with the Boundary Trail, which goes uphill to the right (east) on its way to the Pasayten River. You turn left (west) and 0.1 mile later reach the second junction in a tiny meadow. A camp with water lies a few hundred yards north on the PCT. From Castle Pass the PCT continues straight on its way to Canada, but your route turns left (southwest) at a small cairn in the middle of the meadow, about 75 feet past where the sign points to Ross Lake.

You're now on a little-used path officially called the Castle Pass Trail but more often referred to as the Three Fools Trail. Hikers may naturally be curious about the origin of a name like that. As the story goes, three young prospectors had traveled a considerable distance up the canyon of a creek now named in their honor before they discovered that the "hot tip" they had been given was nothing more than a ruse to lure them away from a more productive claim on Ruby Creek.

The remote and rugged trail includes many seemingly unnecessary ups and downs, but the scenery is excellent, and there's a good chance that you'll have the route all to yourself. The path (often incorrectly shown on maps) starts with a fairly steep uphill to a high meadow; then it briefly crosses a burn area. Watch for lots of birds here, including several kinds of woodpeckers, pine siskins, and various warblers. You now drop steeply a few hundred feet to a saddle in the ridge, enjoying fine views of pointed Castle Peak as you hike.

For the next few miles the trail makes several steep little ups and downs with only occasional gentler stretches. Most of the way is in meadows or burned areas where wildflowers and views are abundant as you travel along the top of a wonderful ridge separating Castle Creek to the north from the Three Fools Creek drainage to the south.

WARNING: The route is very exposed and almost always windy. In good weather it's glorious, but in rain or snow it may be dangerous and probably shouldn't even be attempted until the weather improves.

Eventually the ridge turns north, where you'll get terrific views of Freezeout and Joker Mountains and the large basin of Big Face Creek. The trail makes a very scenic sidehill traverse, then descends 27 badly overgrown switchbacks into this basin to a rock-hop crossing of Big Face Creek.

WARNING: The path here receives only irregular maintenance and is often overgrown, so it may be difficult to follow.

Big Face Creek is your first reliable water since before Castle Pass, a distance of about 7 miles. If you want to camp here, a fair campsite lies about 0.1 mile before you reach the creek. The trail now goes up and down through forests and meadows well above the creek as it slowly curves into the next canyon. Once you enter this canyon, you must tackle a dry, unrelentingly steep, 1,700-foot climb. Most of the way is in a brushy meadow completely exposed to the sun, so your pace will likely slow to a crawl. Also keep in mind that black bears and even a few grizzlies live in this area, and frequent large piles of bear scat serve as proof of a healthy bruin population. It's very hard to see ahead of you in the thick brush, so you may feel more comfortable making noise as you hike and carrying bear spray.

Gradually the terrain becomes more alpine, with much less brush, more wildflowers, and better views. Keep left (west) at a switchback, where a climber's trail heads to Joker Mountain. A final series of easier, meadowy switchbacks takes you to a high pass with good views to the west of Mount Baker and the countless glacier-clad peaks of the North Cascades.

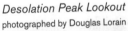

Desolation Peak Lookout
photographed by Douglas Lorain

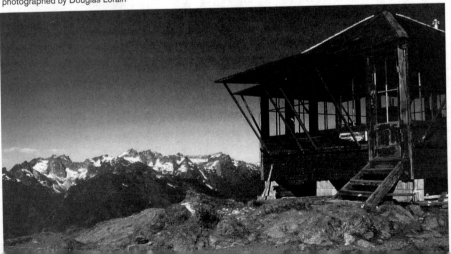

TIP: For the nearest water and scenic camps, leave the trail at the pass and drop about 500 feet to the water and spacious rolling meadows of Elbow Basin to the west. These scenic camps are worth the extra effort because the trail stays high and dry for the next 6 miles.

From the pass above Elbow Basin, the trail goes first northwest and then west along an open ridge covered with immense grassy meadows and wildflowers. The route is extremely scenic, with outstanding panoramas. In places the path may be lost amid the greenery, but if you look for small cairns and generally stay on the south side of the crest, you should be fine. At a low point in the divide you'll be able to look down on Freezeout Lake, which can be reached by a steep scramble route and has some decent camps. Shortly beyond the Freezeout Lake overlook, you descend a rocky section to another long saddle.

Now the *downhill* begins. It's well over 3,000 feet down to Three Fools Creek, and it will probably seem like more. Climbing this section is exhausting, which is one reason I recommend a counterclockwise loop. It all starts deceptively gently amid huckleberries and open forests, then the pace picks up and the switchbacks begin. There are about 50 of them, and they are all short and rather steep. Fortunately the trail is easy to follow, although you must push through some brushy areas. As you descend, the forest cover changes rapidly from high-elevation subalpine fir and mountain hemlock to predominately Douglas fir, joined by western red cedar and western hemlock at the canyon bottom.

You finish the downhill and turn downstream while you are still a few hundred feet above cascading Three Fools Creek in a deep cleft below you. About 0.8 mile later you make two more switchbacks and come to the creek above a nice camp at small Little Fish Shelter. This is your first on-trail water since Big Face Creek.

Now the route follows the clear stream as you go up and down and fight through thickets of vine maple, thimbleberry, and alder that are rarely cleared by trail crews. Before long you come to a confusing spot where it looks like the trail might cross the creek, but a quick look at the map shows that it doesn't. Instead you stay on the maddeningly overgrown north bank of the stream, pass a nice creekside camp, and then climb steeply away from the water. From here you traverse a wooded hillside with many small ups and downs and enter the Ross Lake National Recreation Area at a sign pointing the other way and identifying the Pasayten Wilderness. The trail then descends through a tunnel of hemlocks and cedars to a junction with the much-better-maintained Lightning Creek Trail.

You turn left (west), cross Lightning Creek on a log bridge, and immediately come to a well-built log cabin. The trail climbs again in dense forests, gaining about 500 feet before leveling off with only minor ups and downs. The route traverses a hillside, mostly in forest but sometimes through open, rocky areas of shale, where you'll have pleasant views of the heavily forested slopes across the canyon. At one of these openings, you get your first good look west to Ross Lake. From here the route goes rather steeply down an open hillside sprinkled with Douglas firs and ponderosa pines; the hillside offers frequent views of fjordlike Ross Lake and its surrounding peaks. Just before the lake is a junction with the East Bank Trail.

To reach Lightning Creek Camp veer left (downhill and south), make one more switchback, and, about 100 yards before reaching the suspension bridge over Lightning Creek, turn back to the right (west). This path leads to the popular camp with its picnic tables, fire pits, and sturdy metal bear boxes to keep critters out of your food. The camp is well located but not really all that pleasant because it has lots of mosquitoes throughout the hiking season, noisy powerboats are present on the reservoir, and the camp is often inhabited by even noisier boat-in campers. Another problem is that the designated tent pads are filled with loose sand, which tends to get into everything and gives little for tent stakes to hold onto. A freestanding tent is preferable. The camp is a good spot, however, for watching and listening to loons on the lake and screech owls hooting at night.

DESOLATION PEAK SIDE TRIP: If the weather is good, plan on spending a day at Lightning Creek to make the long but very rewarding day hike up Desolation Peak. To reach it, hike north on the scenic trail along Ross Lake for 2.1 miles to a junction with a boater's shortcut trail. Turn right (east) and climb a myriad of short, moderately steep switchbacks up the western slopes of Desolation Peak. Numerous excellent views of the lake and craggy peaks to the west provide good excuses for needed rest stops. Once you reach the generally open north-south crest of the mountain, you turn left (north) at the spur heading to Desolation Camp and climb another mile to the summit. From both the upper parts of the trail and the staffed lookout building on top, you'll enjoy absolutely smashing views! There is always, of course, the large, blue swath of Ross Lake some 4,500 feet below you, but also to the south is Jack Mountain with large Nohokomeen Glacier on its north flank, and Snowfield Peak with the even larger Neve Glacier covering most of its north side. To the southwest are Mount Prophet, the Picket Range, and small parts of Mount Shuksan and Mount Baker. As you look west, notice the Little Beaver Valley, the Mox Peaks, and Mount Spickard. To the north are the sheer spires of Hozomeen Mountain and an infinity of peaks in Canada. Finally, to the east and southeast stretches the enormous Pasayten Wilderness, in which you can pick out many familiar landmarks and much of the route you traveled earlier in this hike. The lookout here is famous in literary circles as the one-time summer abode of Jack Kerouac, who wrote memorably about the view he enjoyed from the summit.

NOTE: Black bears are common on Desolation Peak. If you want to spend the night at tiny and waterless Desolation Camp, the National Park Service requires that you use a bear canister because the trees are too short to properly hang your food.

Once you've had your fill of the scenery from Desolation Peak, which on clear days could take several hours, return to Lightning Creek Camp.

To complete your trip, hike south on the East Bank Trail and cross the impressive arcing bridge over the Lightning Creek backwater of Ross Lake. On the south side of the bridge are more lakeshore campsites. The East Bank Trail goes through attractive mixed woods of maple, alder, cedar, and Douglas fir for most of the rest of your hike, usually well away from the lake. The hiking is generally uneventful but pleasant as you rarely gain or lose much elevation, and the miles go by rapidly. You pass a spur trail to Lodgepole Camp, and then climb into the woods and cross Dry Creek on a flat-topped log before coming to the next landmark at a four-way trail junction. To the right (west) a short path leads down to Devils Camp, while to the left (east) is the trail going up to Devils Dome. This junction is the end of the shorter loop option mentioned earlier in the text. Your route goes straight (south), loses a bit of elevation, and makes a bridged crossing of the quiet, cliff-walled grotto where the waters of Devils Creek meet the reservoir.

The next couple of miles are the most dramatic along the entire East Bank Trail, as the path has been carved and blasted out of the steep hillsides and sheer cliffs just a few feet above the lake's deep waters. The views across the lake are wonderful.

TIP: Hike this section early in the morning when the lighting is better for views and photos across the water. Avoid the afternoon, as these exposed slopes can get extremely hot.

The path eventually works away from the shore and passes the spur trail to Rainbow Point Camp. Most of the remaining route stays in forest, as the trail gradually climbs inland away from the lake. You will often travel through open, parklike forests with moss carpeting the ground and an abundance of vine maple. These conditions create lovely dappled sunshine and lots of good fall colors in October. A log footbridge takes you over May Creek, whose slightly silty water is the result of runoff from Nohokomeen Glacier. On the south bank of the creek is an equestrian camp. Just 1.3 miles later is boisterous Roland Creek with its pleasant camps for hikers in the trees near the clear stream. The uphill is more noticeable now as you gain about 800 feet over the next 3 miles. Gradually the trail levels off in dense western-hemlock forests, goes through indistinct Hidden Hand Pass, and descends to a four-way junction, where you will once again hear the sounds of traffic on WA 20. To the right (west) is a spur trail to Ross Lake. The Little Jack Mountain Trail goes sharply to the left (east). Your tour veers slightly left (southeast) and follows a wide and gently graded old roadbed for 2.7 miles back to the bridge over Ruby Creek. To return to your car, simply cross the bridge and climb 0.2 mile to the trailhead.

VARIATION

As mentioned in the text, a satisfying shorter version of this trip is the 43-mile loop via Devils Dome.

POSSIBLE ITINERARY

	CAMP	MILES	ELEVATION GAIN
Day 1	McMillan Park junction	7.2	3,900'
Day 2	Devils Park	3.2	1,300'
	Side trip to Crater Lake and viewpoint (morning)	4.8	1,800'
Day 3	Devils Pass	8.1	2,700'
Day 4	Devils Pass		
	Day hike to Devils Dome	8.4	1,300'
Day 5	Spring camp near Goat Lakes	10.4	2,200'
Day 6	Castle Pass	11.6	2,000'
Day 7	Elbow Basin	10.0	2,800'
Day 8	Lightning Creek Camp	12.9	1,200'
Day 9	Lightning Creek Camp		
	Day hike to Desolation Peak	13.6	4,500'
Day 10	Roland Creek	9.5	600'
Day 11	Out	7.0	900'

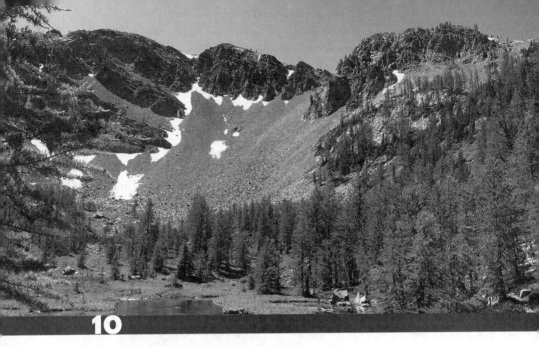

10

BUCKSKIN RIDGE–
PTARMIGAN PEAK LOOP

RATINGS: Scenery 8   **Solitude** 9   **Difficulty** 10

MILES: 52

ELEVATION GAIN: 13,300'

DAYS: 4–6

SHUTTLE MILEAGE: n/a

MAPS: Green Trails *Pasayten Peak (#18)* and *Washington Pass (#50)*. It is strongly advised that you also either print from the internet or obtain a copy of the 1:24,000 USGS maps for the off-trail section, specifically *Tatoosh Buttes* and *Mount Lago*. Unfortunately, the trail locations on all of these maps (Green Trails and USGS), especially along Buckskin Ridge, are frequently wrong, and often by a lot.

USUALLY OPEN: July–October

BEST: Mid- to late July/late September–early October

PERMIT: None required

RULES: Maximum group size of 12 people and 18 stock

CONTACT: Okanogan-Wenatchee National Forest, Methow Valley Ranger District, 509-996-4000, fs.usda.gov/main/okawen

Above: *A shallow pond south of Buckskin Lake*
photographed by Douglas Lorain

SPECIAL ATTRACTIONS •••••••••••••••••••••••••••••••••••••••

Outstanding mountain scenery, amazing views, lots of solitude

CHALLENGES •••

Many miles of rough and sketchy trails; a long section of off-trail travel with one short but extremely steep and difficult section that is only for experienced cross-country hikers

HOW TO GET THERE ••••••••••••••••••••••••••••••••••••••

From Winthrop, head 13.5 miles northwest on WA 20 to the well-signed turnoff for Mazama. Turn right (east) onto Lost River Road and proceed 0.4 mile to a four-way junction, where you turn left (northwest) and drive 6.6 miles to the end of the pavement. Now on Forest Service Road 5400, drive 2.4 miles on good gravel, and then turn right (north), following signs to Harts Pass. This road is sometimes quite narrow (be very wary of oncoming traffic), badly washboarded, and rough at times, so take it slow. After 9.8 miles you reach a junction just before Harts Pass. Keep right, then turn right again just 0.1 mile later, now on FS 600. Drive 1.6 miles to the Slate Pass trailhead at the second road switchback. Parking is limited.

NOTE: You'll need a Northwest Forest Pass to park at this trailhead.

GPS TRAILHEAD COORDINATES: N48° 43.938' W120° 40.092'

INTRODUCTION ••

This wonderful loop usually provides days of complete solitude despite an abundance of outstanding scenery. The reasons for the lack of crowds are some rugged and often sketchy trails and a long off-trail section between Tatoosh Buttes and Butte Pass. Most of the cross-country travel is straightforward and relatively easy walking over alpine tundra and rocks, but some steep talus slopes and one short section of extremely steep travel with loose rocks ensure that this trip is strictly for experienced hikers looking for a challenge and to really get away from it all. The rewards are many, but the difficult travel ensures that you'll earn those rewards.

NOTE: Most of this trip is either cross-country or on remote trails that are infrequently maintained, steep, brushy, and/or quite rocky. As a result, it's almost never possible to hike at a fast pace. Plan on shorter than normal daily mileages.

DESCRIPTION ••

Amid glorious alpine scenery with vistas, scattered subalpine fir trees, and open wildflower-covered slopes, the trail climbs briefly to reach Slate Pass, where you enter the Pasayten Wilderness. From here you can soak in the enormity of this vast preserve and spy Slate Peak Lookout less than a mile to the northwest. The trail then descends three switchbacks to a beautiful larch-studded basin. At the lower end of this basin, near 0.7 mile, is a junction and the start of the loop.

continued on page 98

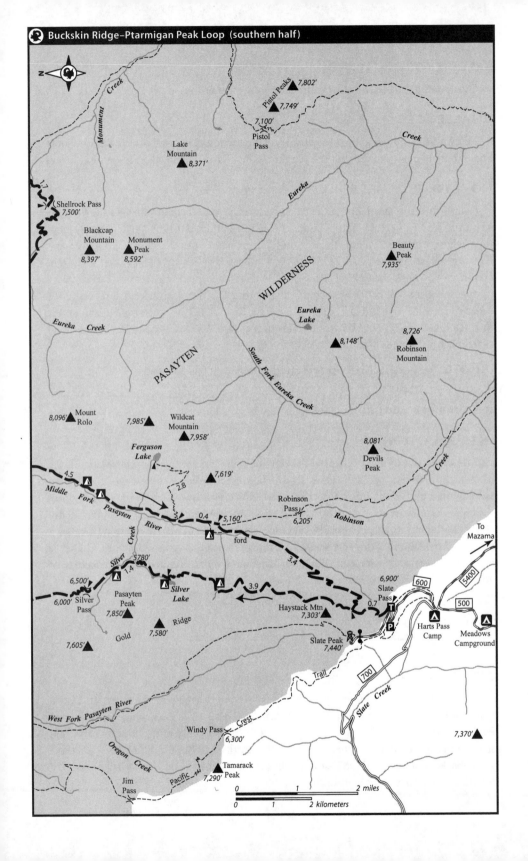

N

Monument Creek

Pistol Peaks ▲ 7,802'
▲ 7,749'
7,100' ✕
Pistol
Pass

Lake
Mountain
▲ 8,371'

Creek

17

Shellrock Pass
7,500'

Eureka

Blackcap
Mountain   Monument
▲   ▲ Peak
8,397'   8,592'

WILDERNESS

Beauty
▲ Peak
7,935'

Eureka Creek

*Eureka
Lake*

PASAYTEN

8,726'
▲
Robinson
Mountain

South Fork Eureka Creek

▲ 8,148'

8,096' ▲ Mount
Rolo

7,985' ▲   Wildcat
Mountain
▲ 7,958'

8,081'
▲
Devils
Peak

*Ferguson
Lake*

▲ 7,619'

Creek

4.5   🏕   🏕

Middle   Fork   Pasayten   River

2.8

0.4 ▶ 5,160'

Robinson
Pass
6,205'

Robinson

To
Mazama

🏕
ford

3.4

Silver   5780'
1.4

6,500'
▲

Pasayten
Peak
6,000' Silver
Pass   7,850' ▲

*Silver
Lake*   🏕

🏕   3.9

6,900'
Slate
Pass

600

5400

0.7
T
P

500

🏕
Harts Pass
Camp

🏕
Meadows
Campground

7,605' ▲

7,580'

Gold   Ridge

Haystack Mtn
7,303'

Slate Peak
7,440'

West Fork Pasayten River

700

Slate Creek

7,370' ▲

Windy Pass
6,300'

Crest

Oregon   Creek

Jim
Pass

Pacific

▲ Tamarack
Peak
7,290'

0   1   2 miles
0   1   2 kilometers

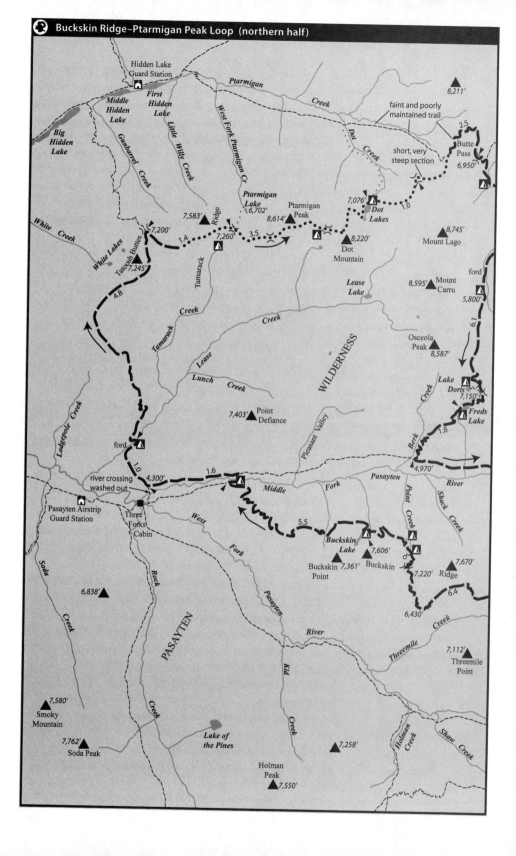

continued from page 95

Middle Fork Trail goes right (downhill and east), and the recommended loop returns that way. For now, you bear left (north) on Buckskin Ridge Trail. This route goes along with many minor ups and downs as it explores the lovely high meadows and partly forested slopes of Gold Ridge. The hiking is a joy, with plenty of wildflowers and pleasant scenery. Just after you hop over a splashing little creek at 3.5 miles, you pass a nice one-tent campsite on your right (east). This is a very scenic and enticing option, especially for those who got a late start. Another 1.1 miles, including a fairly steep little uphill and a switchbacking downhill, take you to the unsigned but obvious junction with the spur trail going left (west) to Silver Lake. Don't miss this 100-yard one-way side trail because this shallow lake is backed by ruggedly scenic peaks and has fine campsites.

The Buckskin Ridge Trail goes right (north) at the Silver Lake turnoff and switchbacks downhill for 0.6 mile beside the outlet creek of Silver Lake to a hop-over crossing of the multibranched stream. You then climb through forest to a mediocre campsite on the left (west) just before the crossing of small Silver Creek. A steady uphill in forest and through charming glades then leads to Silver Pass. Good views extend northwest from here to a variety of scenic ridges and valleys.

You now face a steep downhill, which is accomplished in more than a dozen rocky switchbacks. After bottoming out, you make an up-and-down traverse in forest and view-packed little meadows for 0.8 mile, then tackle a brutally steep 950-foot climb mostly in a strip meadow fully exposed to the afternoon sun. Following that challenge, the narrow tread traverses to the north-northwest with countless steep little ups and downs.

WARNING: Green Trails and USGS maps are inaccurate and significantly understate both the distance and the elevation gain between Silver Pass and Buckskin Lake.

After a more extended, but blessedly gradual, downhill on a high open slope, you round a side ridge, then switchback steeply down into a rocky basin with an abundance of alpine larches and no water. Atop the next little side ridge, the trail turns east and back uphill, employing numerous well-graded switchbacks to ascend a partly forested slope. Looking west-southwest you'll enjoy fine views of towering Jack Mountain in the distance. You finally top Buckskin Ridge at 7,220 feet. Rather frustratingly, you top out well above two lower passes on either side, which seem like they would have made better places for the trail to cross the ridge. Putting aside this oddity, from this high viewpoint you will enjoy expansive vistas to the east of pyramid-shaped Osceola Peak.

Your next goal is a deep basin on the east side of the ridge. After first descending to the lower pass to the north, the trail drops rather steeply in 14 switchbacks to the basin floor. Here you'll discover spring water, a couple of shallow ponds, and excellent views back up to the peaks rimming the basin. The second (lower) pond offers a nice and very scenic campsite above its east side near the outlet.

You make a short climb away from the second pond, and then rapidly lose 200 feet before leveling out not far from a small and easily overlooked lake on your right with a possible campsite. The trail then goes up and down to the north for about 0.6 mile, rounding a sharp ridge along the way to reach long and skinny Buckskin Lake (12.4 miles). Camping at one of the excellent sites near the outlet allows you to fully appreciate the fine scenery of this lake, highlighted by the impressive cliffs of an unnamed butte to the south.

Resuming its northward course, the trail crosses the outlet creek to Buckskin Lake, then turns right (downhill and east) and gradually descends two switchbacks. You then continue descending as you cross an open slope with inspiring views up and down the forested valley of Middle Fork Pasayten River.

The trail contours around a rocky slope to cross a tiny but usually reliable creek, then climbs away from this creek, first in two quick switchbacks, followed by a gradual uphill traverse. Soon you're once again contouring across view-packed open slopes, happily striding along on an easy trail with your head on a swivel, enjoying all the fine scenery. After about 0.4 mile of this fun, the trail reenters forest and begins a long, uneventful, and generally viewless descent. Although the contour maps indicate several distinct switchbacks, on the ground it's much less obvious, as the trail snakes around in 20 or so rounded turns and meanders. At the bottom, you intersect a well-used horse trail paralleling the Middle Fork Pasayten River, 5.5 miles from Buckskin Lake.

Going straight (north) here would take you to a lower crossing of the Middle Fork that is still shown on most maps. A 2016 landslide, however, took out this bridge and left behind a potentially difficult ford. For a better alternative, turn sharply right (south) and gently descend for a little less than 0.2 mile to a nice campsite just before a crossing of the river. In late 2018 a volunteer trail crew installed a new bridge here, allowing for an easy and dry crossing. About 150 yards up the east bank is a junction.

The Robinson Creek Trail goes right (south), but you should turn sharply left (north), following a small sign saying TO TATOOSH BUTTES. This very gentle route begins along the edge of an old burn area (expect blowdown), but soon enters unburned forest and meanders northward for 1.3 miles to a junction. The lower river crossing, where the old bridge was obliterated by the 2016 landslide, sits to the left, but you turn right (northeast) on Tatoosh Buttes Trail. This path gently climbs through forest for 0.7 mile, then enters an old burn filled with brush, snags, and usually plenty of blowdown. After 0.2 mile of this unpleasant and shadeless task, you reach the high bank above clear Lease Creek. The trail then turns upstream for 0.1 mile to a bridgeless crossing. Lots of downed logs across the flow offer options for a dry crossing, or you can make a simple ford. A poor, shadeless, one-tent campsite appears on the left immediately after you cross the creek.

NOTE: Lease Creek is your last reliable water source for several tough uphill miles, so be sure to stock up here.

The often-faint trail cuts left immediately after crossing Lease Creek, then switchbacks and sets off on a long uphill with no shade (due to the burned trees) or water. Try to make this climb in the cool of the morning. A total of 17 switchbacks of varying length and increasing steepness take you all the way up to the open ridgetops and meadows of the Tatoosh Buttes—a worthy reward for your efforts. Views from here seem endless over a vast territory of roadless and scenic terrain. The vista to the south of the Lease Lake cirque and the snow-streaked crags of Mounts Carru and Lago looks especially dramatic. You'll happily amble along, gradually gaining elevation through this wonderland to a point about 4.8 miles from Lease Creek, where you reach a ridgetop high on the slopes of Tatoosh Buttes. To the south rises the nearby rugged pyramid of Ptarmigan Peak, and to its right the towering crag of Osceola Peak in the distance. Here begins the long off-trail portion of this trip.

WARNING: If the weather is threatening, do not attempt this off-trail section, which is largely above timberline and very exposed.

Things start off very easy as you turn right (south) and pick up an easy-to-follow use trail that crosses open terrain dotted with trees and offering stunning views. The trail disappears after 0.4 mile, but things remain easy as you cross tundra slopes on the side of Tamarack Ridge to a broad saddle about 1.4 miles from the official trail. From here it is simple to drop into the lovely basin to the west, which usually has water and is a very scenic place to camp.

At the saddle you are right beneath a very rugged side summit of Ptarmigan Peak and are standing smack in the middle of some of Washington's best scenery, with countless rugged peaks, ridges, and canyons visible in all directions. A potential side trip from here steeply drops 500 feet down the east side of the ridge to small Ptarmigan Lake. Unfortunately, much of the area surrounding this lake was burned in a huge 2017 fire, reducing the lake's scenic appeal.

Back at the saddle, your off-trail adventure now calls for you to climb a fairly gentle slope of rock and tundra to a low point in an orange-tinged ridge that extends northwest from Ptarmigan Peak. Once at this high saddle, you turn left (southeast) and carefully climb a narrow ridgeline, gaining nearly 500 feet before you leave this ridge and head south.

WARNING: Goat paths that cross the slope before you have climbed the recommended 500 feet may look inviting, but they are often dangerously steep and difficult to safely negotiate. It is much better to stick with the ridgeline climb and not turn south until you are crossing very high on the rock-and-tundra western slopes of Ptarmigan Peak.

TIP: If you are so inclined, from this high route it's a straightforward, nontechnical, and highly rewarding scramble to reach the top of Ptarmigan Peak. Needless to say, the views are amazing!

Once on the ridgeline south of Ptarmigan Peak, you descend easy slopes to the saddle between Ptarmigan Peak and Dot Mountain. Here you'll find a shallow snowmelt pond. Camping here would be extremely scenic, but also completely exposed to the wind and weather. For a better camping option, climb the gentle ridge toward Dot Mountain, gaining about 150 feet, to a relatively flat area on the east side of the peak. Peak baggers can easily summit Dot Mountain from here. In the basin southeast of the peak are the two sparkling Dot Lakes. Descending to those lakes is quite steep, but it's perfectly reasonable for experienced hikers as you dig your heels into loose scree and carefully navigate talus slopes into the larch-filled basin. In general, the easiest course is to go east from the high flat area on Dot Mountain along a descending ridge for about 0.2 mile, then drop to the lakes where the way down becomes a little less steep.

The Dot Lakes are stunning! They are backed by snow-streaked cliffs and peaks and offer superb potential campsites, especially near the east end of the lower lake. In very late September and early October, the thousands of alpine larch trees that fill this basin ensure that the Dot Lakes can rival anywhere in Washington for fall colors. Luckily this beauty spot escaped (just barely) the ravages of the huge 2017 fires that touched Ptarmigan Lake and scorched some 100,000 acres of land to the east.

All by themselves the Dot Lakes make this trip worthwhile. But you can't stay here forever (darn those pesky limits on vacation days), so pack up your gear and consider your next options. The safest course is to go east, slowly picking your way steeply down through the burn zone over rocks and lots of annoying downed logs along Dot Creek to the bottom of the canyon. Here you must look very carefully to pick up the indistinct and almost never maintained Ptarmigan Creek Trail. You then turn right (south) and make the long climb through miles of burned deadfall to Butte Pass. This route is slow, tedious, and not much fun (OK, it really isn't *any* fun), but it's doable for any patient and experienced hiker.

For very confident, athletic, and experienced off-trail enthusiasts (and I *really* mean it—only if you qualify on all those counts should you consider this), there is a second alternative. Contour to the south from lower Dot Lake, staying near the edge of or slightly in the burn area and crossing moderately steep but manageable slopes. After 1 mile you come to a minor low point in a narrow ridge that extends northeast from Mount Lago.

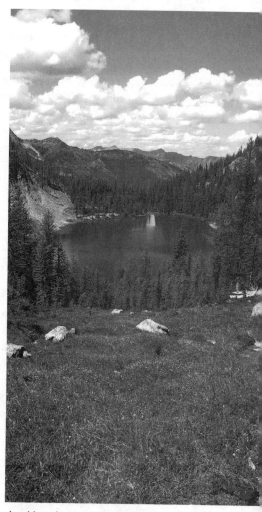

Now comes the short but very tricky part that is the crux of the entire off-trail section of this loop. *Very* carefully descend a super steep gully with loose rocks and burned snags almost directly on the north side of the ridge saddle. Use whatever handholds you can find and expect to shimmy along on your backside from time to time.

WARNING: Be extremely careful of dislodging rocks onto members of your party farther down the slope.

After about 0.15 mile the slope moderates a bit (whew!), allowing you to work your way across steep but more manageable boulder fields all the way to a relatively flat area near the head of Ptarmigan Creek. You contour around the west and south sides of this flat area, alternating between boulder hopping and forested or brushy areas. As you approach the southeast side of the flat area, look carefully for the faint Ptarmigan Creek Trail, where you reunite with the easier route from Dot Lakes mentioned previously. This path is a feast of blowdown and doesn't appear to have been maintained in recent memory, but it still makes your travel marginally easier. The path goes in and out of burn areas as it makes a switchbacking ascent to a high ridgetop, then follows the ridge to the west

Looking down on Freds Lake
photographed by Douglas Lorain

for about 0.3 mile to unsigned Butte Pass. Great views from here extend north to Ptarmigan Peak and west to Mount Lago.

Still playing hide-and-seek with burn areas, the trail steeply descends the south side of Butte Pass in a series of short switchbacks. After 0.3 mile, near the unsigned junction with the Monument Creek Trail, the tread disappears in a burn area. If you simply contour to the right for about 200 yards, however, you'll find the trail again as it heads west.

The little-used path soon leaves the burn zone for good and ascends to an extremely scenic little rocky tarn at the headwaters of Monument Creek. Mount Lago and an unnamed sharp summit to the west provide a stunning setting for this pond. It is possible to camp here, but there isn't much in the way of flat ground.

Next up is the climb to Shellrock Pass. The indistinct path—look for occasional small cairns—climbs steeply through an alpine-larch forest before leaving the trees and making a pair of switchbacks up a talus slope. The scenery and views of spiky orange-tinged peaks and nearby cliffs are amazing.

WARNING: The final stretch to the pass cuts across a steep talus slope that is difficult for stock and often has a steep snowfield across the trail well into July.

After admiring the views from Shellrock Pass, which could take a while, you begin a long series of downhill switchbacks and traverses leading to a large flat basin at the head of Eureka Creek. Once arriving there, the obscure tread crosses the creek and then continues downstream another 0.8 mile to a second crossing. Neither of these crossings have a bridge, but they are both simple fords. About 0.3 mile after the second crossing, you pass a nicely sheltered campsite in deep forest by a little tributary creek.

Soon after this campsite, the trail starts climbing again, passing through a series of openings that offer good views of Mount Rolo to the west-southwest and the long, trailless valley of Eureka Creek to the south. The trail is frequently narrow, steep, and brushy, but at least it's easy to follow as it leads you up to a rolling area with lots of heather and alpine larches. After an additional switchbacking climb, you come to an unsigned but obvious junction. The 0.25-mile one-way trail to the right (north) leads to deep and attractive Lake Doris (possible camps).

Your route goes left (west) at the junction and a little over 0.1 mile later takes you to the top of an unnamed pass. To the west you can see Pasayten Peak, Buckskin Ridge, and much of the country you walked through earlier in the trip. To the east are the rugged peaks flanking Shellrock Pass. To the north-northeast is the very tall pyramid of Osceola Peak. And nearby to the south is massive Mount Rolo.

It's all downhill from here, as 25 mostly short and rocky switchbacks lead you to oval-shaped Freds Lake. This deep, blue-green gem has fine scenery and superb campsites at its west end. If you camp here, you'll have time to appreciate this lake's good fishing and its above-average swimming options, at least in late July and August once the water warms up.

Continuing the downhill beyond Freds Lake initially involves two switchbacks, and then an extended descending traverse, followed by a series of 36 more switchbacks. At the bottom of this forested descent is a junction. You turn left (south) and stride along on this gentle, forested, mostly viewless trail, which is well maintained and gets considerable use by equestrians. For the first time on this loop, the miles go by quickly, and before you know it, you've passed good campsites after 3.2 and 3.3 miles respectively and gone 4.5 miles (with a cumulative elevation gain of only about 200 feet) to the unsigned but obvious junction with the Ferguson Lake Trail.

TIP: This is a fairly strenuous but rewarding side trip to a scenic lake if you have an extra day.

Go straight (south) and, a bit over 0.3 mile later, keep left (south) where a well-used trail goes right (west) down to a horse camp next to a sloping meadow. Not quite 0.1 mile later is another fork. The Robinson Creek Trail goes left (southeast), but you bear right (downhill and southwest), following signs to Slate Peak. This path descends a bit, then heads upstream through a meadow filled with July wildflowers to a simple, ankle-deep ford of what's left of Middle Fork Pasayten River.

Now begins an extended but always well-graded climb. As you gain altitude the forest thins out, and you encounter increasing numbers of open areas with plenty of wildflowers and ever-improving views. After hiking 2.4 miles from the Robinson Creek Trail, you make the first of what will be seven switchbacks of varying length. These take you back up into the beautiful subalpine meadows on Gold Ridge, where you return to the junction with the Buckskin Ridge Trail. Turn left (south) and retrace your steps 0.7 mile back to the trailhead.

VARIATION

If you prefer to avoid this trip's long cross-country section, you can make a different on-trail loop instead. After completing the route along Buckskin Ridge and reaching the West Fork Pasayten River, hike west on the Rock Creek Trail, climbing to the divide where you meet the Pacific Crest Trail. From there you hike south along this scenic route back to the road below Slate Peak, less than a mile from the Slate Pass trailhead.

POSSIBLE ITINERARY

	CAMP	MILES	ELEVATION GAIN
Day 1	Buckskin Lake	12.4	3,750'
Day 2	Lease Creek	8.1	350'
Day 3	Dot Lakes	9.7	4,150'
Day 4	Freds Lake	11.3	3,100'
Day 5	Out	10.8	1,950'

BEST SHORTER ALTERNATIVE

A one-night trip along Buckskin Ridge to Silver Lake or Buckskin Lake gives you a taste of the area, if not the full meal.

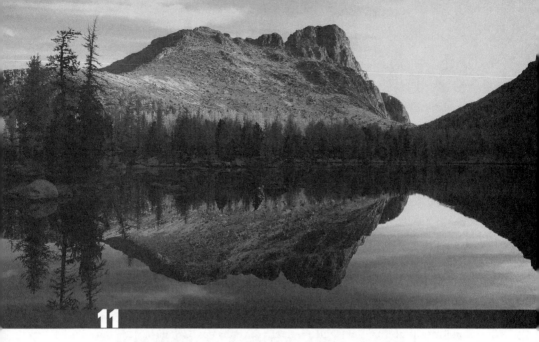

11

EASTERN PASAYTEN LOOP

RATINGS: Scenery 8   **Solitude** 8   **Difficulty** 7
MILES: 54 (60)
ELEVATION GAIN: 9,100' (11,250')
DAYS: 6–7 (6–7)
SHUTTLE MILEAGE: n/a
MAPS: Green Trails *Coleman Peak (#20)* and *Horseshoe Basin (#21)*
USUALLY OPEN: Late June–mid-October
BEST: Mid-July/late September–early October
PERMIT: None required
RULES: Maximum group size of 12 people and 18 stock
CONTACTS: Okanogan-Wenatchee National Forest: Methow Valley Ranger
    District, 509-996-4000; Tonasket Ranger District, 509-486-2186; fs.usda
    .gov/main/okawen

SPECIAL ATTRACTIONS ●●●●●●●●●●●●●●●●●●●●●●●●●●●●●●●●●●●●

Solitude, alpine wildflowers, excellent fall colors

CHALLENGES ●●

Cattle, long stretches without water, potentially difficult stream crossing, large burn
areas with little shade and blackened snags

Above: *Cathedral Peak over Upper Cathedral Lake*
photographed by Mark Wetherington

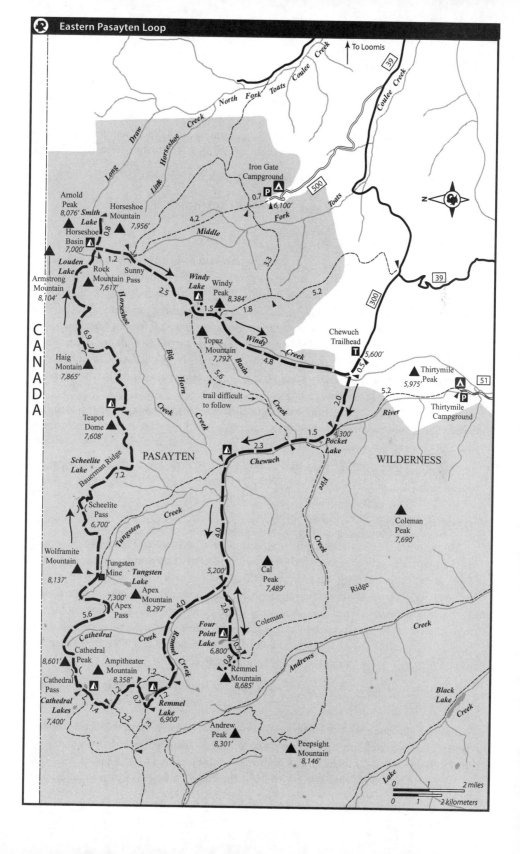

HOW TO GET THERE ••

From Loomis, drive north on Loomis-Oroville Road 2 miles. Turn left (northwest) onto Toats Coulee Road. In 4.5 miles, turn right (north), and go 1.1 miles. Veer right (northwest), and go 4.5 miles. Turn right (north), and continue for 6.5 miles. The road curves south and turns into Forest Service Road 39. Continue on this road 3.6 miles to the junction with FS 300. Drive straight approximately 3 miles up FS 300 to the Chewuch Trailhead.

NOTE: You'll need a Northwest Forest Pass to park at this trailhead.

GPS TRAILHEAD COORDINATES: N48° 52.320' W120° 00.228'

INTRODUCTION ••

Arctic tundra isn't an ecosystem normally associated with the Lower 48 states. The Pasayten Wilderness, however, hides large expanses of this unusual terrain, and you don't have to go all the way to Alaska to see it. In mid-July these rolling meadowlands support such a wealth of tiny flowers that botanists and photographers can stay happy here for weeks. In addition to tundra, this magnificent loop visits pleasant forests, fine viewpoints, and spectacular cirque lakes nestled beneath rugged granite peaks. Although a few places along the way will probably have some people, nowhere is it crowded, and for much of the way you'll probably enjoy perfect solitude. This is especially true in the fall, when not only the people are gone but so are the bugs.

If flowers don't excite you, one of the most memorable times to take this trip is the last week of September or the first week of October. The meadows then are golden brown and the beautiful Lyall "alpine" larches have turned a brilliant yellow.

WARNING: Be prepared for cold nights and the possibility of snow when hiking this late in the season.

DESCRIPTION ••

The Windy Creek Trail leaves the trailhead in a burned area and reaches a reasonably distinct junction with the Cathedral Driveway Trail after just 0.5 mile. Continue straight (northwest) onto the Cathedral Driveway Trail and cross a small bridge over modest Windy Creek. Your route continues through burned forest, which allows for decent views of the Pasayten country but does little for shielding you from the sun. After another 0.5 mile, the route begins to descend to the Chewuch River. The descent is fairly steep at times, but overall it isn't too malicious as far as wilderness trails go. Your downward trajectory terminates at a junction with the Chewuch River Trail at 2.5 miles.

WARNING: Forest fires in recent years have left large sections of blackened snags in this area and for many miles to come. Bring a hat because shade is at a premium.

From the junction your route turns right (upstream and north) on the Chewuch River Trail. Follow this trail through more burned forest past marshy Pocket Lake, a faint junction with the Fire Creek Trail, and an indistinguishable junction for the Basin Creek Trail. Many of the secondary and tertiary trails in the Pasayten have yet to fully rehab after devastating wildfires, and conditions vary from mildly frustrating to impassable and insanity-inducing. Meanwhile, the well-maintained Chewuch River Trail gently climbs along its namesake stream, and views of the river and the slopes of the mountains above provide some visual reprieve from the monotony of the burned forest. At 6.3 miles, you arrive at a trail junction near a spacious campsite at the confluence of Horseshoe Creek and the Chewuch River.

In late summer, crossing Horseshoe Creek should merely involve some strategic rock-hopping and likely won't require you to take your boots off. Above this crossing, head west, as the trail continues to parallel the river through forest in varying stages of recovery from past burns, and its gradient increases slightly. After almost 4 miles, you will reach the signed junction with the trail to Four Point Lake, where you turn left (west) to make this outstanding side trip. This trail, which receives much less maintenance than the mainline Chewuch River Trail, meanders briefly through the forest before crossing the thin channel of the Chewuch River. It then climbs steeply and enters unburned forest as it nears Four Point Lake. Take a right (north) on the obvious spur trail reached after approximately 2.5 miles of hiking to cover the final few hundred feet to Four Point Lake, one of the most scenic lakes in the Pasayten Wilderness. There are good camps among the larches and firs around this lake, as well as outstanding views of the surrounding peaks, composed mostly of beautiful white granite. Trout cruise the waters of this lake, making it a worthwhile destination for anglers as well as sightseers.

REMMEL MOUNTAIN SIDE TRIP: After setting up camp, retrace your steps some 250 feet to the main trail, then follow that path southwest for 0.7 mile to a small basin at the top of a series of switchbacks. From here leave the trail and follow the north side of the small creek as you make your way along an obvious route to the top of Remmel Mountain. Although you might encounter faded bits of trail here and there that offer some reprieve from the cross-country experience, for all intents and purposes you will be on your own for the walk-up ascent of this impressive mountain. The views from the top, which still has some debris associated with the former lookout tower once perched atop its summit, are simply unbelievable—not a road in sight!

A quick descent on the trail from Four Point Lake returns you to the Chewuch River Trail, where you turn left (northwest) and continue gaining elevation. This route is sometimes rocky, and views are once again mostly of burned forest, but it avoids steep climbs, so the walking is easy. Remmel Creek generally remains out of sight in a shallow canyon to the left. After you cross Cathedral Creek, the trail begins to climb more steadily, as the path gets narrower and more rugged, and views become more frequent as the forest thins. Remmel Creek cascades along in a narrow defile below the trail.

As the path levels out at the top of the climb, it passes a junction, crosses two small creeks, and then enters the meadow flat holding lovely Remmel Lake. Although not as dramatically scenic as Four Point Lake or Upper Cathedral Lake (yet to come), this lovely mountain pool has the advantage of being surrounded by flowery meadows and scattered trees.

WARNING: Camps here are often trampled and smelly from bovines and equines.

The trail passes along the south shore of Remmel Lake and continues to a junction. You turn right (northeast) here and follow a glorious route that begins in meadow and partial forest, then climbs to a series of huge open tundra meadows. You turn left (northwest) at an indistinct junction and continue crossing these large, gently sloping meadows.

TIP: During the July blooming period, be sure to schedule extra time to enjoy the acres of tiny blossoms that cover these fields.

At an intersection with the Boundary Trail, turn right (northeast) and continue this wonderfully scenic meadow ramble. Eventually the trail crosses through a wide saddle and begins to work around the western cliffs of Amphitheater Mountain. A little-used footpath drops to Lower Cathedral Lake, but you stick with the main trail, which contours to the shores of spectacular Upper Cathedral Lake. A forest fire in 2016 burned nearby, but it fortunately spared the high country around the lake. The towering granite cliffs of Amphitheater Mountain and prominent Cathedral Peak provide a dramatic backdrop for this lake. Larches add splashes of gold in the fall, making for lasting memories and beautiful photographs. Numerous camps give backpackers a chance to stay and bask in this scenery.

WARNING: For the next 20 miles the Boundary Trail stays fairly high, providing lots of views but very limited water, especially in the fall. Camps with water are rare, so fill every water bottle you have at Upper Cathedral Lake and refill them at every opportunity.

The Boundary Trail climbs a short distance east from Upper Cathedral Lake up open slopes to Cathedral Pass, the low point between Amphitheater Mountain and Cathedral Peak. The path then loses elevation as it rounds the headwater basin of Cathedral Creek. The views from the east side of this high basin back to the pointed spire of Cathedral Peak are especially noteworthy. Now you make a scenic traverse along the west side of a ridge before climbing to Apex Pass.

TIP: This is your last good view of Cathedral Peak, so take a minute to snap a few photos before continuing east.

From Apex Pass you make a long, gradual descent as the trail crosses the headwaters of Tungsten Creek, where there are good views of Apex Mountain to the south. Views,

Tungsten Mine buildings
photographed by Mark Wetherington

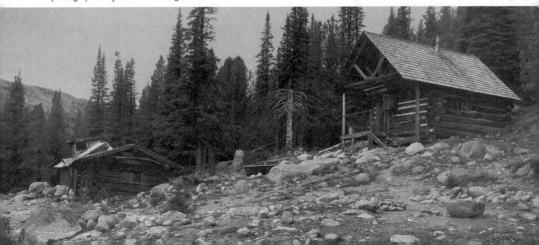

larches, meadows, and generally beautiful scenery are continuous companions here, as they will be for miles to come. Keep straight (east) at a junction near some old equipment associated with the Tungsten Mine (an old bunkhouse and another building associated with the mine are located just uphill if you have the interest and time to explore them). Then make a long, mostly level traverse of the steep hillside below Wolframite Mountain.

Your route alternates between rocky slopes and brushy areas of willows and forests as it works down to heavily forested Scheelite Pass, then climbs a bit and makes a long traverse below Bauerman Ridge. Now the trail turns east and crosses this ridge at a large flat meadow with lots of flowers, larches, and views. From here the glorious tour rounds a lovely basin and arrives at the dark, rounded rock formation called Teapot Dome. Meadows and larches help make this prominent landmark yet another memorable location along the Boundary Trail. About 0.5 mile beyond Teapot Dome, the trail passes through a lovely semiopen meadow, where a tiny trickling creek provides welcome water. Good camps can be found among the nearby trees.

As you continue hiking east, the Boundary Trail makes an irregular traverse around Haig Mountain and drops to a forested saddle. You pass a small pond and then ascend through forest to a low rise and enter the large tundra wonderland of Horseshoe Basin. The trail leads through beautiful open terrain as it rounds aptly named Rock Mountain and soon reaches shallow Louden Lake. Flowers and larches enhance the setting of this scenic pool, although by autumn it's usually nothing more than a mud puddle. The beautiful route continues from Louden Lake through more meadows and comes to a junction in the center of Horseshoe Basin. To the northeast rise the gentle slopes of Arnold Peak, and all around are fields of stunted flowers and scattered trees. The open terrain of Horseshoe Basin invites easy side trips both on and off the trail. Worthwhile goals include tiny Smith Lake, the summit views from Arnold Peak and Armstrong Mountain (both walk-ups), and Long Draw, with its silvery forest of snags.

SMITH LAKE SIDE TRIP: For hikers who just can't pass up a trip to mountain lake, Smith Lake is a tempting body of water in proximity to Horseshoe Basin. A small campsite accommodates those wishing to make their visit an overnight stay. Abundant stands of larch trees make this area especially scenic in late autumn. The shallow lake doesn't provide any options for fishing, and the swimming is less than ideal, but it certainly adds a scenic touch to an already beautiful basin.

TIP: Horseshoe Basin is within easy reach of weekend backpackers from Iron Gate Campground. Camp here on a weekday to increase the odds of having it all to yourself.

The recommended loop turns south from Horseshoe Basin, passing through more open country to a junction near wide Sunny Pass. The most heavily traveled trail goes southeast from here on its way to Iron Gate Campground. Your route, however, turns right (southwest) and gradually descends a wide draw, where views become less frequent as trees crowd the route. Eventually you drop to a marshy meadow, hop over a small creek, and begin a forested climb. About 1 mile from the creek you'll pass a small, wet meadow on the left.

WINDY LAKE SIDE TRIP: Don't miss the short side trip from here to tiny Windy Lake. To reach it, turn left (east) at the meadow and climb off-trail for about 0.3 mile to this irregularly shaped pool with an excellent campsite on its northwest shore. Larches are abundant here, making this a glorious spot in the fall. At any season, however, this small lake would rate five stars because of the flowers, trees, and outstanding view of Windy Peak.

To complete your trip, return to the trail from the Windy Lake side trip and then climb a series of steep switchbacks to a ridgetop junction. The very hard-to-follow Basin Creek Trail bears right (west), but you continue straight (south) and ascend a few hundred more feet over the next 1.5 miles to the flank of Windy Peak and a junction with the Windy Creek Trail.

WINDY PEAK SIDE TRIP: Energetic hikers should allow time for a side trip from this junction to Windy Peak, the former site of a lookout tower. Simply leave the trail heading east and go steeply cross-country for 0.3 mile to the top. Like the view from most former lookout sites, the one from here is truly outstanding.

Turn right (southwest) onto the Windy Creek Trail and enjoy beautiful views from the top of the descent before entering the catastrophically burned basin of Windy Creek. The trail here is in remarkably good condition for being in a burned area and should make for easy downhill hiking for its 4.8-mile length back to the junction with the Cathedral Driveway Trail. Take a left (southeast) here and hike the final 0.5 mile back to the trailhead to complete this scenery-packed exploration of the eastern Pasayten Wilderness.

VARIATION

For hikers with less available time, a shorter version of this loop skips some great scenery but also eliminates about 25 miles (and three days) of hiking. To do this loop, simply turn right (south) at the junction along Boundary Trail below Wolframite Mountain, and return via the Tungsten Creek Trail to the Chewuch River.

POSSIBLE ITINERARY

	CAMP	MILES	ELEVATION GAIN
Day 1	Horseshoe Creek	6.3	400'
Day 2	Four Point Lake	6.6	2,300'
	Side trip to Remmel Mountain	3.0	1,500'
Day 3	Upper Cathedral Lake	11.1	2,300'
Day 4	Beyond Teapot Dome	12.8	1,900'
Day 5	Horseshoe Basin	6.9	600'
	Side trip to Smith Lake	1.6	150'
Day 6	Out	10.5	1,600'
	Side trip to Windy Lake	0.6	100'
	Side trip to Windy Peak	0.6	400'

BEST SHORTER ALTERNATIVE

Take the hike from Iron Gate Campground to Horseshoe Basin at the east end of this loop for a popular day hike or quick overnighter.

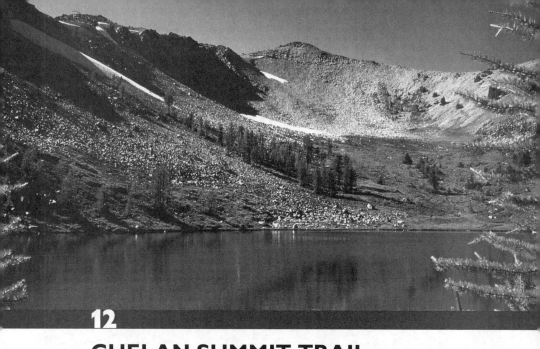

12

CHELAN SUMMIT TRAIL

RATINGS: Scenery 9   **Solitude** 6   **Difficulty** 6

MILES: 42 (47)

ELEVATION GAIN: 9,200' (11,100')

DAYS: 3–5 (4–6)

SHUTTLE MILEAGE: 29

MAPS: Green Trails *Stehekin (#82), Buttermilk Butte (#83),* and *Prince Creek (#115)*

USUALLY OPEN: July–October

BEST: Very late September–early October

PERMIT: North Cascades National Park permit required to camp at Juanita Lake. As of 2019 they are free but limited. Reservation requests should be submitted between March 15 and April 15 for the summer season. Reservation requests can only be made online; a $20 nonrefundable fee applies to reserved permits. Walk-up permits can be obtained on the first day of the trip or up to one day before. See nps.gov/noca/planyourvisit/backcountry-reservations.htm for full details. Pick up permits (whether reserved in advance or a walk-up permit) from the wilderness information center in Marblemount (if you are coming from the west) or the Chelan Ranger Station (from the east).

RULES: None

CONTACT: Okanogan-Wenatchee National Forest, Methow Valley Ranger District, 509-996-4000, fs.usda.gov/main/okawen; North Cascades National Park, 360-854-7200 ext. 515; in summer, contact the park's wilderness information center, 360-854-7245, nps.gov/noca

Above: *Tuckaway Lake*   photographed by Douglas Lorain

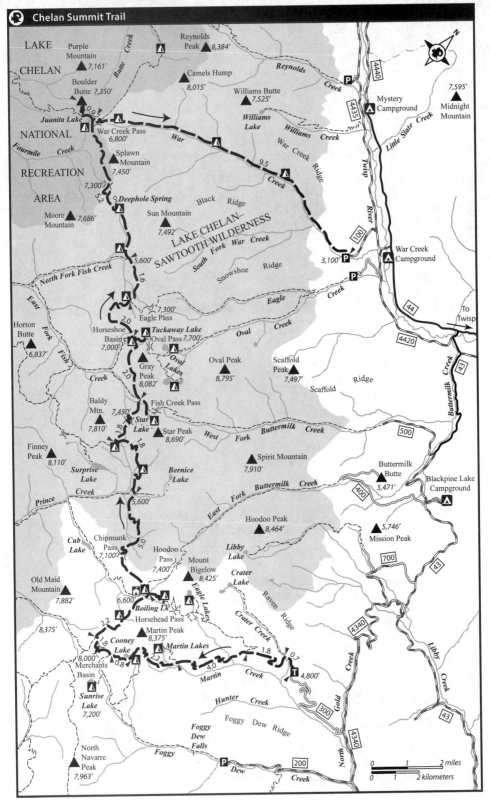

SPECIAL ATTRACTIONS

Terrific fall colors, wildflowers, extensive views, relative solitude

CHALLENGES

Motorbikes allowed on trails in southern section

HOW TO GET THERE

From the town of Twisp, drive west on Twisp River Road (County Road 1090) 10.2 miles to a junction with Buttermilk Creek Road.

To reach the north trailhead, continue straight on Twisp River Road another 3.6 miles, and turn left (southwest) at a junction just beyond War Creek Campground. Cross Twisp River, and in 0.6 mile turn left (northwest) and climb narrow gravel Forest Service Road 100 for 1.4 miles to the War Creek Trailhead.

To reach the south trailhead, turn left (south) at the Buttermilk Creek junction, veer left (east) at a fork after just 0.2 mile, and then follow one-lane paved and later gravel FS 43 for 6.4 miles. Turn left (north) to stay on FS 43 as it climbs to the turnoff to Blackpine Lake Campground. In 1 mile turn right (east), still on FS 43, and drop down into the valley of Mission Creek. In 4 miles, turn sharply right (northwest) onto FS 4340; follow this route 7.1 miles as it climbs over a saddle and goes down North Fork Gold Creek. Finally turn sharply right (west) onto FS 300 and climb 4.5 miles to the busy Crater Creek Trailhead.

NOTE: You'll need a Northwest Forest Pass to park at these trailheads.

GPS TRAILHEAD COORDINATES:

Southern (Crater Creek): N48° 13.224' W120° 16.074'
Northern (War Creek): N48° 21.508' W120° 24.982'

INTRODUCTION

East of the Lake Chelan trench rises the craggy Sawtooth Range. Although they carry the same name as the more famous mountains in Idaho, these peaks are much less crowded. Protected by the moisture-loving ranges to the west, these drier mountains feature open forests and beautiful meadows that provide endless vistas of distant peaks. Small lakes tucked beneath scenic crags compete for attention with flower-covered meadows and ridges.

In addition to those other attributes, probably the best trait of these mountains is a tree, the Lyall "alpine" larch. Throughout the summer this rather scrawny high-elevation species graces the trail with its ethereal green needles. In the last few days of September and the first week of October, however, this deciduous conifer (an oxymoron for all trees except those in the larch family) puts on arguably the best fall-color display in the state. Before shedding their needles, these trees blanket the high meadows and hillsides with gold, creating a stunning tapestry when mixed with the evergreens and reddish-brown meadows. It is truly an outstanding show, and the Chelan Summit Trail provides the best seat in the house.

The traditional southern starting point for this trail is from the Summer Blossom Trailhead off FS 8200. The problem with this approach, however, is that sane people generally prefer not to drive this narrow, steep, rutted track. The trip described here involves a little extra climbing but has a shorter car shuttle, sticks to better roads, and still includes virtually all of the Summit Trail's most scenic miles.

DESCRIPTION

From the Crater Creek Trailhead your trail starts on a dusty motorcycle expressway through typical eastside forests of ponderosa pine, Douglas fir, Engelmann spruce, and western white pine. The path climbs gently for a while and then contours to a junction beside Crater Creek. A nice hiker-only trail turns right (west) here and climbs beside this creek for 3 miles to the shores of lovely lower Crater Lake. Your route goes straight (south) as you hop across the creek and resume your long, gradual climb in semiopen woods, with occasional views to the dry hills of eastern Washington. Two long switchbacks take you to a junction with the Martin Creek Trail, where you face a decision. The shorter route turns to the right (west) and climbs gradually to the good camps and terrific scenery at the two Eagle Lakes. Larch-rimmed Upper Eagle Lake sits in a granite basin and is especially dramatic. From there you switchback up 600 feet to the fine views from Horsehead Pass and descend two long, gentle switchbacks to Boiling Lake, which has good fishing and several developed camps. From here you descend another 0.5 mile of mostly open forests to an overly developed but excellent campsite beside a creek and a junction with the Summit Trail.

A longer and perhaps more enjoyable option from the Eagle Lakes turnoff visits one of the prettiest lakes in the range. To do this, go straight (south) from the junction with the trail to Eagle Lakes, descend to a crossing of a splashing creek, and then switchback up a ridge. The trail levels off somewhat on a hillside before climbing in switchbacks to a junction with the side trail to Martin Lakes. Near this turnoff is where you first encounter alpine larches, turning the hillside a brilliant gold in the fall. The 0.6-mile side trail to Martin Lakes is blessedly closed to motorcycles and climbs to a fine campsite at lower Martin Lake.

From the Martin Lakes turnoff the main trail climbs sometimes in switchbacks gouged by wheels through increasingly open forests of subalpine fir and alpine larch. You round a lovely little basin and soon reach a poorly marked side trail near a (really) tiny creek in a sloping meadow. Turn right (south) here and gently ascend a gloriously colorful landscape of reddish-orange and gold meadows spangled with yellow larches to the open shores of Cooney Lake. Considered by many to be the "jewel of the Sawtooths," this lake has lovely camps nearby with beautiful early-morning reflections of the talus slopes and cliffs of an unnamed peak to the southwest.

Leaving the larch-rimmed shores of Cooney Lake, you travel uphill above the south shore on an obvious but rarely maintained route that steeply climbs a talus-and-meadow slope to the southwest. The route tops out on a ridge with fine views back down to Cooney Lake and across Merchants Basin to the south. You turn right (southwest) at a junction and follow a trail that traverses an open hillside to an 8,000-foot pass. From here you switchback fairly steeply down a rocky slope to a junction with the Summit Trail.

Your route goes right (north) here and gently travels up and down through an enchanting landscape of larch-dotted meadows and forests. The trail crosses a few tiny creeks (possible camps) before losing some elevation to a junction with the trail to Boiling Lake. Nearby is a well-developed camping area, including log picnic tables, fire pits, a privy, and a small U.S. Forest Service ranger cabin. The area is heavily used by people with horses and motorbikes, which greatly decreases its appeal for backpackers, but it's the last good camp for 5.5 miles.

BOILING LAKE SIDE TRIP: If you took the longer trail via Cooney Lake, you should consider making a side trip at least as far as Boiling Lake (0.5 mile) and, if possible, over Horsehead Pass to Upper Eagle Lake (3.3 miles).

From the junction below Boiling Lake, your route goes northwest on the Summit Trail, which is now closed to motorbikes, so you leave them behind in favor of God's quiet wilderness. The path climbs briefly to a junction with the Hoodoo Pass Trail, where you go straight (west). The trail now makes a brief climb, then contours to Chipmunk Pass, which, like all the other passes you will visit, has excellent views. Below you to the southwest is Cub Lake, while to the southeast is Martin Peak and the rugged Sawtooth Ridge above Boiling Lake. Dominating the view to the north is impressive Star Peak, rising majestically above the forested canyon of Prince Creek. From this grandstand the Summit Trail descends gently through meadows, talus slopes, and larches in six fairly long switchbacks, and then follows a cascading creek downstream. Eventually the path leaves the stream and goes up and down across a forested hillside to where you hop across Prince Creek. Just beyond this crossing, an unsigned boot trail takes off to the right. This unofficial path goes steeply up to Bernice Lake, in a high cirque to the east.

About 0.2 mile beyond the Bernice Lake junction is another junction, this one with the Prince Creek Trail. Continue straight (northwest) and begin climbing once again through woods and sloping meadows. At a small creek about 0.4 mile after the Prince Creek junction, you'll arrive at a leaky wooden shelter and several good tent sites on the hillside just below it.

From this camp the trail climbs steadily but not steeply with a few irregularly spaced switchbacks. The route is mostly in dense woods, but there are also a few meadow openings, where you may see deer or other wildlife. About 1.3 miles from Prince Creek Camp

Larch trees along the Summit Trail north of Tuckaway Lake
photographed by Douglas Lorain

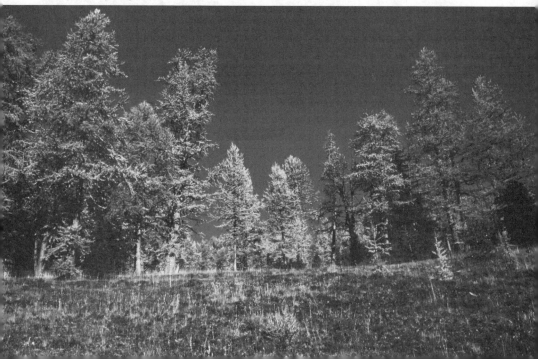

is a junction with the trail to Surprise Lake and a good but often dry camp about 100 yards to the west. The side trip from here to large Surprise Lake is especially appealing to anglers, as the fishing is usually excellent.

The main Summit Trail turns right (north) at the junction and resumes climbing over increasingly open terrain. After gaining about 800 feet, you top out at a 7,450-foot pass.

TIP: Very ambitious hikers can scramble east from this pass up steep, rocky, exposed slopes all the way to the summit of Star Peak, where you'll enjoy perhaps the best vistas of the entire trip.

From the pass the trail descends through partial forest and talus fields to an open meadow, where there is a four-way junction with the very faint Fish Creek Trail.

STAR LAKE SIDE TRIP: Don't miss the 0.5-mile side trip from this junction to Star Lake. To reach it, turn right (east) and follow the trail up the sloping, larch-dotted meadows to the east. Leave the sketchy path after about 0.3 mile and continue up more meadows to the small lake in a dramatic basin beneath the dark, towering cliffs on the northwest side of Star Peak. A superb camp can be found at this lake just above the outlet. You can make a strong case that larch-rimmed Star Lake is the prettiest spot in the entire Sawtooth Range.

As you continue north on the Summit Trail, the next 2 miles climb across the western slopes of the ridge, leading you through a mix of pine and fir forests and meadows. Eventually you switchback down a larch-covered hillside to Horseshoe Basin, where there is an excellent campsite beside a creek and a junction with the Oval Pass Trail.

TUCKAWAY LAKE SIDE TRIP: From here you can hike east to take steep side trips of varying lengths. For a short trip, you need only go as far as sublime Tuckaway Lake, in a high sloping basin. Somewhat farther and higher than Tuckaway Lake are the views from Oval Pass. If you have lots of time and energy, continue down the other side of the pass to visit one, two, or all three of the charming Oval Lakes.

The main trail continues northwest from Horseshoe Basin and gradually climbs through meadows and across larch-covered slopes that are glorious in the fall. The trail tops out on a ridge, turns right, and descends moderately steeply across a hillside. From here you will have superb views to the west, including Glacier Peak and your first good look down on Lake Chelan. The trail descends fairly steeply into yet another scenic basin with a small creek and nice camps. At the junction with the Eagle Pass Trail in this basin, your route goes straight.

Continuing north on the Summit Trail, you temporarily leave the larch zone in favor of denser forests of fir, pine, and spruce as you drop into the canyon of North Fork Fish Creek. At the bottom of the descent, your route goes straight (northwest) at a junction with a trail to Lake Chelan. About 0.1 mile beyond this junction is an unmarked boot path to the left, which leads to a nice camp in the trees beside a small creek. From here you make a moderately long uphill hike as you regain your previously lost elevation. Initially the route is in a shady forest, but it soon changes to more open woods and meadows. About halfway up this 1,800-foot climb, you'll come to a nice camp near Deephole Spring. This is where you once again begin to encounter larches. More climbing through meadows and alpine-larch forests leads to a high pass sprinkled with larch and whitebark pine. The view from here includes many of the serrated peaks of North Cascades National Park and the Glacier Peak Wilderness to the north and west. The closer tall mountain to the north is Reynolds Peak. A large wooden post here identifies your entrance into the Lake Chelan National Recreation Area.

TIP: Don't miss a quick side trip to the little knoll south of this pass, where you can spend hours picking out local landmarks like Bonanza Peak, Forbidden Peak, Goode Mountain, the Triplet Lakes, and Lake Chelan, to name only a few of the possibilities. On very clear days you can even see a small part of the top of Mount Rainier.

From the pass you descend fairly steeply for about 0.5 mile, then go up and down (mostly up) while traversing open slopes on the west side of the divide. The path comes to a junction with the Boulder Creek Trail just above the shores of shallow and rather marshy Juanita Lake. Several designated camps are on the west side of this tiny, larch-rimmed pond.

NOTE: You must have a National Park Service backcountry permit to camp here. You can obtain these from the U.S. Forest Service ranger station in Twisp before your trip. Without a permit you will have to cross over War Creek Pass and camp on the U.S. Forest Service land to the east.

BOULDER BUTTE SIDE TRIP: A fine side trip from Juanita Lake goes west on the Purple Creek Trail for 0.5 mile, then turns right (northwest) and switchbacks up a side trail to the summit of Boulder Butte. On a clear day the vistas from this high point extend all the way to Canada.

To complete the recommended trip, go east on the Boulder Creek Trail from Juanita Lake and immediately cross over the low saddle called War Creek Pass. Here you leave the national recreation area and reenter the Lake Chelan–Sawtooth Wilderness. The trail descends the east side of the pass for about 0.1 mile to a junction. Turn right (east) and regretfully leave the larches behind, as the trail drops steadily in several switchbacks to a small marshy area, where you could make a poor campsite if you don't have a permit for Juanita Lake.

You are now traveling on the historical War Creek Trail, which follows the route of an 1882 Army survey expedition led by First Lieutenant Henry Pierce. The well-engineered trail goes gradually downhill, never wasting energy on unnecessary uphills as it leads through a mix of forests and the lower edge of a burn area. About 3 miles from the pass is the first reasonably good camp. In general the route stays in the trees well above War Creek, but you cross several tributary creeks that provide ample water. About 5.5 miles down from the pass is an excellent, spacious camping area next to a sturdy log cabin near the creek. Beyond the cabin there are very few landmarks or views, but hiking this gentle trail is easy and enjoyable, so the miles go by quickly. Most of the way travels through old-growth Douglas fir forests or large avalanche meadows, where quaking aspens display shimmering yellow leaves in the fall. Occasionally the trail closely approaches the clear waters of War Creek, providing opportunities for anglers to try their luck. Gradually the path drops into the ponderosa pine belt and the forest becomes more open. The trail ends about 0.4 mile beyond where you meet the end of an old logging road.

VARIATION

As mentioned in the text, you can shorten this trip a bit by skipping the trail to Cooney Lake and taking the shortcut to Boiling Lake.

POSSIBLE ITINERARY

	CAMP	MILES	ELEVATION GAIN
Day 1	Cooney Lake	8.7	2,700'
Day 2	Prince Creek Camp	10.6	1,800'
	Side trip to Boiling Lake	1.0	400'
Day 3	Horseshoe Basin	4.8	1,950'
	Side trip to Star Lake	1.0	350'
	Side trip to Tuckaway Lake	1.1	400'
Day 4	Juanita Lake	8.8	2,450'
	Side trip to Boulder Butte	1.8	750'
Day 5	Out	9.5	300'

BEST SHORTER ALTERNATIVE

A superb one- or two-night sampling of this scenic realm follows a loop at the south end past Martin and Cooney Lakes and returns via the Eagle Lakes.

View north toward Star Peak from Chipmunk Pass
photographed by Douglas Lorain

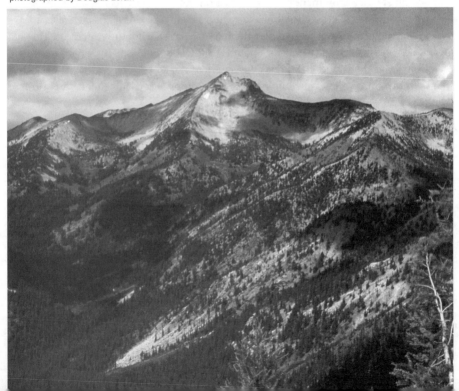

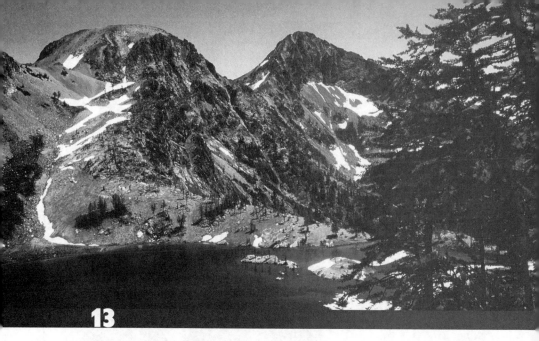

13

ENTIAT RIVER LOOP

RATINGS: Scenery 9 **Solitude** 5 **Difficulty** 6
MILES: 43 (50)
ELEVATION GAIN: 10,900' (12,800')
DAYS: 4–7 (5–7)
SHUTTLE MILEAGE: n/a
MAPS: Green Trails *Holden (#113)* and *Lucerne (#114)*
USUALLY OPEN: Mid-July–early October
BEST: Late July–mid-August
PERMIT: None required
RULES: Maximum group size of 12 people or stock; no fires near Ice Lakes; camp at least 200 feet from water
CONTACT: Okanogan-Wenatchee National Forest, Entiat Ranger District, 509-784-4700, fs.usda.gov/main/okawen

SPECIAL ATTRACTIONS •

Diverse and impressive mountain scenery, flowers, views

CHALLENGES •

Flies, chilly stream crossings, motorbikes on lower trail

Above: *Spectacle Buttes over Lower Ice Lake*
photographed by Douglas Lorain

119

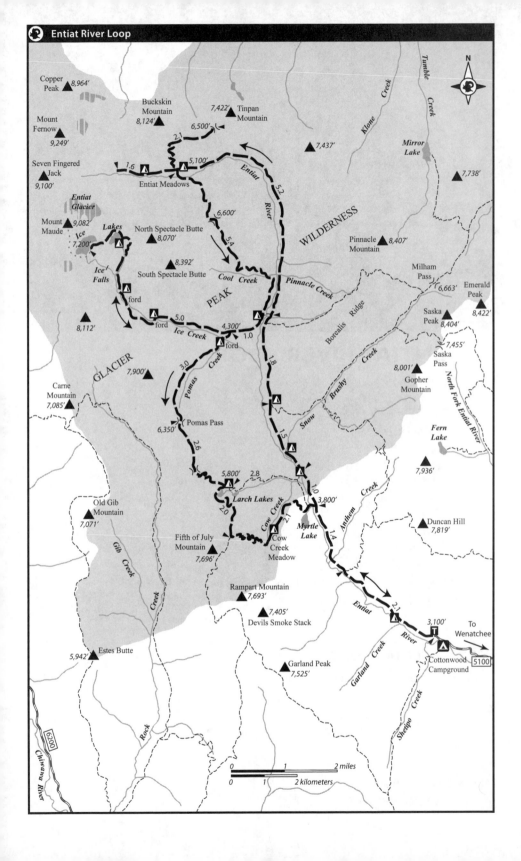

Copper Peak ▲ 8,964'

Mount Fernow ▲ 9,249'

Seven Fingered Jack ▲ 9,100'

Entiat Glacier

Mount Maude ▲ 9,082'
Ice 7,200'

Lakes

Buckskin Mountain ▲ 8,124'

Tinpan Mountain ▲ 7,422'

6,500'

2.1

5,100'

1.6

Entiat Meadows

North Spectacle Butte ▲ 8,070'

South Spectacle Butte ▲ 8,392'

Ice Falls

ford

ford 5.0

ford

Ice Creek

▲ 8,112'

Entiat River

5.2

6,600'

5.4

Cool Creek

Pinnacle Creek

PEAK

4,300'

1.0

WILDERNESS

▲ 7,437'

Mirror Lake

▲ 7,738'

Pinnacle Mountain ▲ 8,407'

Milham Pass
6,663'

Emerald Peak ▲ 8,422'

Saska Peak ▲ 8,404'

7,455'

Saska Pass

▲ 8,001'
Gopher Mountain

Klone Creek

Tumble Creek

Borealis Ridge

North Fork Entiat River

GLACIER

▲ 7,900'

Carne Mountain ▲ 7,085'

3.0

Pomas Creek

Pomas Pass
6,350'

2.6

Brushy Creek

1.8

1.5

Snow Creek

Fern Lake

▲ 7,936'

5,800' 2.8

Larch Lakes

Old Gib Mountain ▲ 7,071'

2.0

Cow Creek

2.1

1.0

3,800'

Myrtle Lake

1.4

Anthem Creek

Duncan Hill ▲ 7,819'

Fifth of July Mountain ▲ 7,696'

Cow Creek Meadow

Gib Creek

Rampart Mountain ▲ 7,693'

▲ 7,405'
Devils Smoke Stack

Entiat River

2.1

3,100'

To Wenatchee

Cottonwood Campground

5100

Estes Butte ▲ 5,942'

Garland Peak ▲ 7,525'

Garland Creek

Sherpo Creek

Rock Creek

6200

Chiwawa River

N

0   1   2 miles

0   1   2 kilometers

HOW TO GET THERE

From Wenatchee, drive north on US 97 Alternate on the west side of the Columbia River for 14.4 miles to the community of Entiat. Turn left (west) onto Entiat River Road and follow this scenic drive about 32 miles. Turn left (west) onto Forest Service Road 5100, and drive 4.8 miles, all the way to its end at the trailhead just past Cottonwood Campground.

WARNING: The upper several miles of the Entiat River Road (above Silver Falls) were closed 2014–2016 due to hazards from landslides and fires. The U.S. Forest Service reopened the road in 2017, but it may close again if the hazards return. In addition, the road closure led to no trail maintenance being done during the closure, which could mean lots of blowdown and other issues on the trail. It is, therefore, especially important that hikers check on the latest conditions before taking this trip.

NOTE: You'll need a Northwest Forest Pass to park at this trailhead.

GPS TRAILHEAD COORDINATES: N48° 01.464' W120° 39.072'

INTRODUCTION

The Glacier Peak Wilderness features so many great hikes that it was difficult to select only a few representative backpacking trips for this book. The decision to include the Entiat River Loop, however, was an easy one. With an eastside location, this area enjoys more sunshine than westside hikes, and crowds are thinner due to the longer drive from major cities. In addition, wildlife is common and the scenery features two of the grandest destinations in Washington. Set in a deep mountain basin, surrounded by 9,000-foot peaks, and carpeted with wildflowers, Entiat Meadows is one of the most beautiful mountain meadows in the state (and that's a category with plenty of competition). By contrast, the perhaps even more impressive Ice Lakes present a stark alpine setting with twisted trees, glacier-scoured rocks, and icy summits towering all around. Add to these two climaxes the many miles of lovely forests, view-packed ridges, heather meadows, and deep glacial canyons, and you have a fabulous mix of world-class splendors.

DESCRIPTION

The main price for entry here is paid in the first few miles. The "trail" here is overrun by motorcycles with their usual noise, fumes, and dust, making it more of a narrow road than a true trail. The dusty expressway climbs very gently in miniature ups and downs through forest, where occasional views through the trees provide tantalizing glimpses of the glories to come. Pleasant camps beside the river welcome those who got a late start. Keep straight (northwest) at a junction at 2.1 miles with the little-used route to Duncan Hill. Then at 3.5 miles, you reach a junction with the Cow Creek Trail, another motorcycle roadway that crosses the river on a bridge and climbs briefly to Myrtle Lake. This pool is the destination of almost all the machines. You'll come back that way on the recommended loop.

Now entering blessedly quiet forest, your trail continues straight (northwest) from the Myrtle Lake junction and soon enters official wilderness lands. You keep straight at a nice campsite beside the Larch Lakes Trail junction and reach a crossing of rushing Snow Brushy Creek, where a pleasant camp invites backpackers to drop their loads and relax.

As the trail continues north from the creek, occasional openings in the forested slopes provide long looks up the ridge to the east. Another good camp is located at the junction with the Snow Brushy Creek Trail about 0.9 mile past its namesake stream.

The trail continues its gentle up-and-down tour of the Entiat River Valley, generally staying in forests burned by large fires in 2006. Deer and porcupines are common in these charred woods, the latter sometimes making nocturnal visits to chew on sweaty pack straps. Views improve as the slope of the climb picks up, especially the scenes to the west of the Ice Creek Valley with its surrounding peaks. After going well past the mouth of this side canyon, you'll finally reach a junction with the Ice Creek Trail. Camps are a short distance down this trail near the bridgeless crossing of the Entiat River.

To continue the trip, go straight (north) at the junction and maintain your long, moderate climb. Meadows become more frequent, and views of the towering cliffs on both sides grow more enticing as you hike. In July colorful blossoms cover these meadows.

WARNING: Look for black bears in these meadows, and be sure to store your food properly at night.

As the trail and river gradually curve to the west, the climb gets steeper, the openings larger, and the views grander. Eventually, the fire scars disappear as the way levels amid the grand expanse of Entiat Meadows, a series of grassy flower gardens separated by strips of trees. At the head of the basin are peaks over 9,000 feet high supporting small glaciers. The hulking dark masses of Mount Maude on the southwest wall and Seven Fingered Jack to the west are particularly impressive. Some of the best of the many camps here are beside the stream near the start of the meadows, and more good camps are near the head of the basin.

WARNING: Like many areas in the North Cascades, Entiat Meadows is a haven for flies. Be prepared to do your share of swatting and swearing.

HOLDEN RIDGETOP VIEWPOINT SIDE TRIP: After setting up your tent, be sure to set aside some time for exploring. For a very ambitious side trip, follow a very steep, unsigned, and sometimes-sketchy path up the north wall of the canyon. The hard-to-find route starts on the west side of a long strip meadow and goes through trees and open areas that provide grand views of Entiat Meadows and its surrounding peaks. The trail ends at a pass with views north to the Holden area and Bonanza Peak.

UPPER ENTIAT MEADOWS SIDE TRIP: For an easier but still highly recommended side trip, simply follow the main trail west, up through the meadows to the rocky head of the basin beneath high cliffs and ridges.

TIP: Bring an extra-wide-angle lens; you'll need it.

The easiest way to continue this trip is to retrace your route along the pleasant Entiat River Trail to the Ice Creek Trail and turn west. A more demanding alternative, however, serves up better scenery. (Note: Be sure to check with rangers before your trip on the current conditions of this route, especially to ask if maintenance has been performed to remove dead snags in the fire-damaged areas.) To do the latter, begin by crossing the stream at lower Entiat Meadows and following the poorly marked Cool Creek Trail. The faint and irregularly maintained path initially goes left (east) along the stream, and then begins heading south on a very steep ascent of mostly forested slopes. The route follows the west side of a gully, crosses a small creek in a sloping basin, and then charges up a rocky slope to an obvious 6,600-foot pass, where you'll want to rest and enjoy the view.

From the pass the path drops through scenic, rocky meadows dotted with larch trees and then regains this lost elevation as it tops an open ridge with views west to the prominent Spectacle Buttes. The easy-to-lose path drops through heather meadows and then reenters the burn zone as it switchbacks steeply down beside cascading Cool Creek. After crossing the creek near the bottom of your descent, you turn south and hike through charred but regrowing forests above the Entiat River. Stick with this rather rugged route

Cow Creek Meadow
photographed by Douglas Lorain

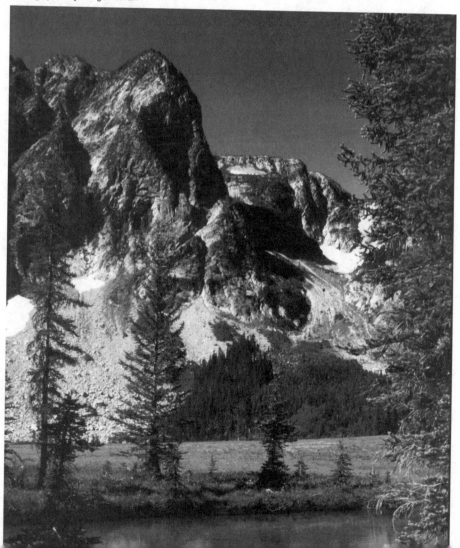

all the way to a junction with the Ice Creek Trail. The closest and best camps are a short distance to the left (east) near the unbridged crossing of the Entiat River.

SIDE TRIP TO ICE LAKES: If the weather is good, don't miss the spectacular side trip up Ice Creek to Ice Lakes. From the Entiat River go west on the Ice Creek Trail, cross a badly burned hillside (expect lots of deadfall if trail maintenance has not yet been completed), and descend to a junction with the Pomas Pass/Larch Lakes Trail. The recommended exit route of the loop goes left (southwest) here, but for now you go straight (west). Walk up the canyon, partly in burned forest, partly in brushy meadows with tantalizing glimpses of the surrounding peaks. The trail leaves the burn zone and comes to a good campsite just before it crosses Ice Creek at a potentially treacherous and always chilly ford. The route then continues upstream, mostly in meadows choked with willows, to a second, somewhat simpler ford. As it gently climbs the valley, the trail alternates its course among mixed woods, rocky areas, and meadows. Shortly after passing a nice campsite, the trail abruptly begins a tough climb along the headwall of the Ice Creek Valley. Stupendous vistas of the cliffs and spires of the surrounding peaks improve as you climb, and views back down the massive U-shaped valley are also impressive. The steep, sketchy, rocky route finally tops out on a knoll a little above Lower Ice Lake before dropping to this spectacular lake's rocky shores. The lake is set amid scattered larch trees and slabs of rock and features terrific views of the Spectacle Buttes towering to the east and Mount Maude close by to the northwest. Mountain goats are commonly found in this area, and they can be nuisances for campers. Fires are prohibited in this area.

TIP: The rocky terrain favors freestanding tents.

A little less than 1 mile to the west of Lower Ice Lake is Upper Ice Lake, reached by sketchy, boot-beaten paths.

TIP 1: It's not shown this way on maps, but the simplest way to reach the upper lake is to travel west to the outlet stream, then follow this creek upstream.

TIP 2: Be sure to carry an extra-wide-angle lens to Upper Ice Lake, as the enormous mass of Mount Maude is difficult to capture without one.

From the ridge beside Upper Ice Lake, there are superb views of the lower lake and the Ice Creek Valley.

Really ambitious hikers who are also experienced scramblers or climbers can make their way from Upper Ice Lake up the southwest ridge of Mount Maude, all the way to its 9,082-foot summit. Those with the ability and the inclination need no further instructions. Needless to say, the view from the top is terrific, one of the best in the state of Washington.

WARNING: Although not technical in nature, this climb should be contemplated only by very experienced persons and only in good weather.

Convincing yourself to leave this alpine paradise is difficult, but eventually, simply return down the Ice Creek Trail the way you came.

If you are pressed for time, you can now return to civilization the way you left it, via the Entiat River Trail. However, it would be a shame to miss taking in more scenery by hiking the Pomas Pass and Larch Lakes Trails, so return to the previously mentioned junction and turn south. You soon ford Ice Creek and begin a forested ascent of the trail up the canyon of Pomas Creek. The path generally stays on the canyon wall well above the creek, and small switchbacks keep the grade reasonable. The final push to 6,350-foot Pomas Pass is rewarded by fine views down Rock Creek Valley to the west and uncounted peaks all around.

From the pass your trail turns left (southeast) and climbs the west side of the next high point in the Entiat Mountains. Views back to Pomas Pass and the unnamed jagged summit north of the pass are excellent. The trail rambles south and east along a scenic route with almost continuous views. Small wildflowers underfoot add to the scenery and help to make the miles go by quickly. Eventually, the trail descends to a saddle and then drops several hundred feet to the sparkling waters and good camps at Upper Larch Lake.

From Upper Larch Lake hikers have a choice of several routes back to the trailhead. The shortest alternative switchbacks east down the Larch Lakes Trail to the Entiat River and follows that stream back to the trailhead. The second option, which is recommended, climbs a scenic ridge south of Larch Lakes through stunted alpine trees on the side of Fifth of July Mountain and then turns left (east) at a junction and switchbacks steeply down to lovely Cow Creek Meadow. This meadow features a nice camp, water, and a particularly impressive view of a huge rock monolith on the side of Fifth of July Mountain. From here the trail drops to Myrtle Lake and the Entiat River Trail.

The final alternative involves strenuous ups and downs but features excellent views and is especially attractive for lovers of ridge walks. For this route, simply continue south from Fifth of July Mountain and then lose and regain more than 1,000 feet before you return to the ridge crest near Devils Smoke Stack. The path then closely follows the scenic ridge past Garland Peak before returning to Cottonwood Campground via the Shetipo Creek Trail.

WARNING: While scenic, this final option is long, strenuous, and bone dry, and parts of it are open to motorcycles.

VARIATIONS

You can shorten the trip by skipping the rugged loop back from Entiat Meadows via the Cool Creek Trail. You could also skip the return along the ridge that includes Pomas Pass and the Larch Lakes.

POSSIBLE ITINERARY

	CAMP	MILES	ELEVATION GAIN
Day 1	Snow Brushy Creek	5.1	900'
Day 2	Entiat Meadows	8.0	1,350'
	Side trip to Holden ridgetop viewpoint	4.2	1,450'
	Side trip to upper Entiat Meadows	3.2	450'
Day 3	Ice Creek	6.4	1,950'
Day 4	Ice Creek		
	Day hike to Ice Lakes	10.0	3,200'
Day 5	Cow Creek Meadow	8.7	3,400'
Day 6	Out	4.5	100'

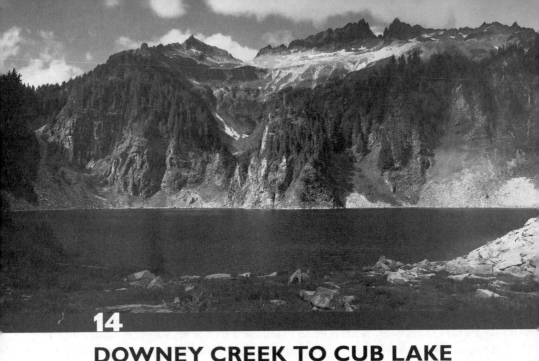

14

DOWNEY CREEK TO CUB LAKE

RATINGS: Scenery 10 **Solitude** 8 **Difficulty** 10
MILES: 24 (27)
ELEVATION GAIN: 5,600' (7,150')
DAYS: 3–4 (3–4)
SHUTTLE MILEAGE: n/a
MAPS: USFS *Darrington Ranger District* and Green Trails *Cascade Pass (#80)*
USUALLY OPEN: July–October
BEST: Late July–September
PERMIT: None required. The undeveloped trailhead does not require a Northwest Forest Pass.
RULES: Maximum group size of 12 people or stock; the usual Leave No Trace principles apply
CONTACT: Mount Baker–Snoqualmie National Forest, Darrington Ranger District, 360-436-1155, fs.usda.gov/main/mbs

SPECIAL ATTRACTIONS

Old-growth forest, mountain lakes, splendid subalpine scenery, mountain views, fishing and berries

Above: *Itswoot Lake*
photographed by Mark Wetherington

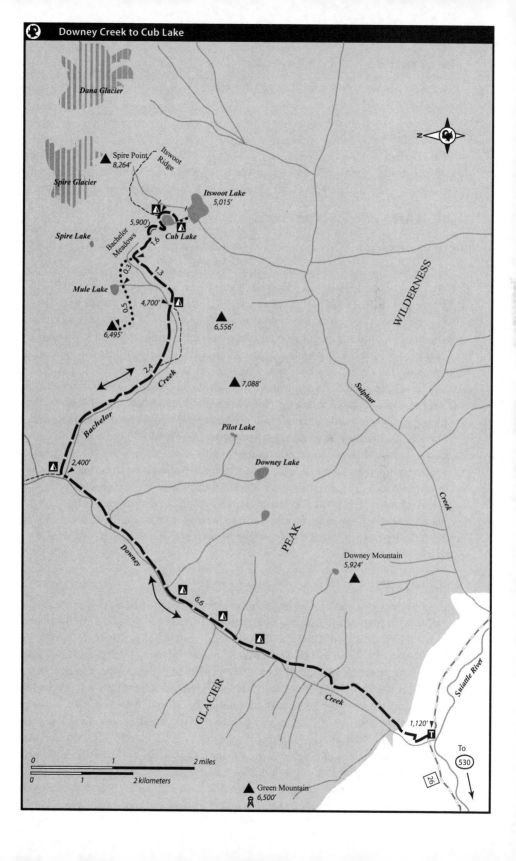

N

Dana Glacier

Spire Point
8,264'

Itswoot
Ridge

Spire Glacier

Itswoot Lake
5,015'

Spire Lake

5,900'

Bachelor
Meadows

1.6

Cub Lake

Mule Lake

0.3

1.3

0.5

4,700'

6,495'

6,556'

2.4

7,088'

Bachelor

Creek

Pilot Lake

Downey Lake

WILDERNESS

Sulphur

Creek

2,400'

Downey

PEAK

Downey Mountain
5,924'

6.6

GLACIER

Creek

Suiattle River

1,120'

To
530

26

0   1   2 miles
0   1   2 kilometers

Green Mountain
6,500'

CHALLENGES

Extremely poor tread on parts of Bachelor Creek Trail, steep climbs and descents, cross-country travel

HOW TO GET THERE

From Darrington, take WA 530 north for 7.4 miles to the junction with Forest Service Road 26. Turn right (east) onto FS 26 (Suiattle River Road) and continue approximately 20.5 miles to a parking lot on your right, just after you cross the bridge over Downey Creek.

GPS TRAILHEAD COORDINATES: N48° 15.570' W121° 13.374'

INTRODUCTION

The Glacier Peak Wilderness contains some of the most spectacular scenery in the Northern Cascades. The Ptarmigan Traverse, consistently rated as one of the most beautiful routes in North American mountaineering, crosses the high country of the wilderness, with Downey Creek being its southern terminus. While fairly well known among mountaineers, the delightful scenery of Cub and Itswoot Lakes and the adjacent high country have never made it an overly popular backpacking destination. That likely has to do with the section of trail along Bachelor Creek, which serves as a formidable gatekeeper to the lakes and stunning mountain setting and which has a somewhat exaggerated reputation as a path of almost Jurassic brutality. However, for well-conditioned backpackers, this trip offers a challenging and immersive wilderness experience that borders on the divine.

Although this hike can be done as a bare-bones out-and-back to Cub Lake, doing so is almost unfathomable given the rewards that await you on the side trips to Mule Lake, Point 6,495, and Itswoot Lake. The summit of Point 6,495 affords breathtaking views that don't require an ice ax or crampons to obtain, and shallow Mule Lake allows for a refreshing post-peak swim. Itswoot Lake and its soul-stirring blue depths are complemented by a waterfall with a jagged skyline of mountains behind it and hungry trout beneath its surface. If the berries are ripe and the weather is good, this area is as close to paradise as most backpackers can get.

DESCRIPTION

The Downey Creek Trail begins on the opposite side of the road from approximately the middle of the parking lot. A charming sign marks the trail and denotes its trail number (#768) and the fact that it's not maintained for stock. It should be noted here that up ahead the Bachelor Creek Trail (#768.1) is barely maintained for *humans,* but you'll discover that firsthand in due time. For now, enjoy the well-defined tread of the Downey Creek Trail as it climbs a few hundred feet on switchbacks before leveling out, passing a voluntary trail register, and entering the Glacier Peak Wilderness at the 0.5-mile mark.

To say that the next few miles are pleasant forest hiking would be akin to saying that Seattle has gotten to be a pretty big town over the years. Ferns, old-growth firs and other stately conifers, and a lush understory flank the trail, and a sense of timelessness permeates the air. This is a forest that calms, humbles, and inspires reverence—it truly is a work of art and deeply pleasurable to hike through. The path gently curves into the hillside and back again toward the creek several times as it gently gains elevation. Several small tributary streams are easily rock-hopped or crossed in a long-legged stride or two, except at times of unusually high water.

WARNING: The huge old-growth trees are awe-inspiring when standing but can pose significant obstacles when they fall across the trail.

The forest monopolizes the view for the majority of the hike to Bachelor Creek. However, just over 3.3 miles from the trailhead, you reach a spot where Downey Creek is within arm's reach, and you are treated to a view up the stream before returning to your sylvan immersion. For the most part, the trail is not overly difficult or overgrown, and several sections of boardwalk allow you to avoid muddy sections. The only creek crossing that will likely give you any trouble, and only at peak runoff, is located at approximately the 5-mile point and is the unnamed stream that drains Downey and Pilot Lakes. Although there are suitable campsites at 3 and 3.5 miles, as well as a nicer site tucked off the trail at 4 miles, the most logical campsite for the first night is immediately after you cross Bachelor Creek on a log bridge. Several flat spots amid the towering conifers and the lovely sounds of Bachelor Creek's descent to join Downey Creek make it an inviting place to spend the night. From here, you start the hardest part of the hike fresh the next morning.

Although the junction with the Bachelor Creek Trail (#768.1) isn't signed, it's unmistakable as it heads southeast, takes off uphill, and parallels Bachelor Creek's north bank. The initial 0.25 mile or so is easy to follow and even contains a few helpful switchbacks. Just when you think you might be able to let your guard down, you will likely begin to run into downed trees or other obstacles that require you to sidestep, if you're lucky, or exert

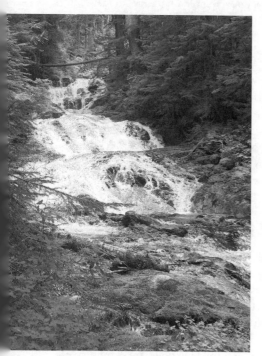

considerably more effort to move past them. The vegetation also begins to encroach on the trail in a way that is more concerning than charming. Before long, you'll find yourself in slide alder and other vegetation that ranges from seasonally benevolent (various berry bushes) to downright malicious (devil's club), but most often seems frustratingly indifferent to your attempts at making forward progress.

In the midst of the thick vegetation, and about 1.8 miles from the junction at Downey Creek, you approach a fork in the trail. The right (south) fork leads to a creek crossing and takes you through another junglelike section before emerging at a campsite. The left (east) fork, which is recommended, allows you to continue upstream another 0.5 mile through open forest before crossing the creek to the previously mentioned campsite. While this route is not perfect (the trail is faint), it does provide you with a welcome reprieve from the crowding vegetation and is certainly not any more difficult than the alternative path.

Falls on Bachelor Creek
photographed by Mark Wetherington

The creek crossing, which can be accomplished via downed logs, is shallow and benign and not any cause for concern in late summer. The spacious campsite on the other side is shaded by well-spaced evergreens, but it's awkwardly located for backpackers considering it as a base camp. If you arrive at the recommended campsite at the junction of Downey Creek Trail and Bachelor Creek Trail with energy and daylight to spare, pushing up here could be a reasonable alternative as the first night's campsite.

As you follow the trail upstream past the campsite, the views start to open up, and blooming wildflowers seem to congratulate you for making it through the thick vegetation and persevering along the challenging footpath.

Not wishing to lose its reputation for brutality, the trail soon begins an extremely steep climb. If you abide by the mantra of "If you can't say something nice, don't say anything at all," then the next 0.5 mile of trail will render you speechless. Fortunately, when you finally emerge into Bachelor Meadows, you will be rendered speechless for much more pleasant reasons. This delightful basin is situated under steep slopes crowned by exposed rock. Several small streams tumble down into the meadow, which has nice displays of wildflowers in season. Perhaps best of all, as it parallels the meadow, the trail is in remarkably good condition and allows you to actually enjoy the act of hiking.

> **SIDE TRIP TO MULE LAKE AND POINT 6,495:** If the weather is favorable, we recommend making the side trip to Mule Lake and Point 6,495 before pushing on up to Cub Lake. Begin from the top of Bachelor Meadows, where the trail begins its climb toward a pass to the east. Leave the trail here, cross the creek as it bisects the meadow, and head generally west through open forest for less than 0.3 mile to Mule Lake. A few game paths may help you find the route of least resistance, but we would be surprised if you saw a boot print in them. This shallow lake is less picturesque than Cub or Itswoot, but it's nonetheless a scenic attraction and worth the visit.
>
> From Mule Lake to Point 6,495, you make a steep, cross-country climb, but it's fairly straightforward and doesn't require traversing any particularly exposed or sketchy sections to reach its summit. The modest height of the summit doesn't limit the splendor of its views, with Glacier Peak on display to the south and numerous other peaks and ridgelines spiking the sky as you look in any direction.
>
> **TIP:** If it's a warm day, a quick dip in Mule Lake is a sublime post-summit treat.
>
> **WARNING:** If you choose to do this side trip on the exit leg of your hike, as the author did, you set yourself up to lose more than a vertical mile of elevation from the summit to the trailhead.

From the top of Bachelor Meadows, the trail makes its way up to the unnamed pass above Cub Lake. On a clear day, the scene from this pass is nothing short of magnificent. The beautiful pools of Cub Lake and (to a lesser extent) Itswoot Lake are visible below, and the rock-and-ice mass of Dome Peak dominates the horizon to the east. At this point, just a steep scramble away from great campsites, you will regret it if you only allotted a single night to spend in this paradise.

From the pass it's a steep descent to Cub Lake, and trekking poles are extremely useful. Take your time, and be sure to spread out a bit if hiking with a group, so that any domino effect can be avoided should someone be unfortunate or uncoordinated enough to lose their footing.

Once you arrive at the head of the lake, an obvious spur trail goes left (northeast), leading to a suitable camping area for a few tents. This camp, a few hundred feet from the lake, provides spectacular vistas of Spire Point and its glaciated ridge, as well as views into the basin that drains into Itswoot Lake. A small waterfall pouring into this basin is a particular highlight, but the whole area is simply astounding. If the campsites in this area are taken—most likely by mountaineers focused on summiting the nearby peaks—an equally appealing site lies on a small knoll just above the outlet of Cub Lake. It is of utmost importance that you practice Leave No Trace camping in this fragile area, especially in regard to disposing of human waste.

From your campsite, you have a plethora of options for adventure. You can continue on the increasingly steep and rugged mountaineer's path to Itswoot Ridge and its sweeping panoramas of the Glacier Peak Wilderness or carefully descend to Itswoot Lake. Both Itswoot and Cub have trout that are eager to rise for dry flies, and serious anglers would likely enjoy spending an entire day at Itswoot Lake. Sightseers will also highly approve of Itswoot Lake. Its cerulean waters and the dramatic waterfall of its inlet stream, not to mention the skyline of jagged peaks rising above it, make for a wonderful place to simply walk around and admire the grandeur.

ITSWOOT LAKE SIDE TRIP: To reach Itswoot Lake, follow the outlet of Cub Lake on a concerningly steep descent among boulders of varying size and stability. The outlet gully eventually fans out into a steep and broad talus slope. Pick your way carefully down to the lakeshore, and take exceptional care to minimize your impact when visiting this delightful and isolated subalpine treasure. There are no obvious existing campsites at Itswoot Lake, making it best suited as a day-use lake from a base camp near Cub Lake.

Because you will be retracing your steps back to the trailhead, there should be few navigational hurdles that need explaining on the return hike. However, be attentive to following the trail as you near the junction with Downey Creek Trail. It's surprisingly easy to lose the trail in this section, and if you do, we suggest that you immediately backtrack to a definitive portion of the trail. It's much better to simply cut your losses than to try a shortcut. Believe us, thrashing around in devil's club on the creek bank and spending 10 minutes to progress a mere 300 feet is *really* not recommended.

POSSIBLE ITINERARY

	CAMP	MILES	ELEVATION GAIN
Day 1	Bachelor Creek	6.6	1,300'
Day 2	Cub Lake	5.3	3,600'
	Side trip to Mule Lake and Point 6,495	1.6	1,100'
Day 3	Cub Lake		
	Day hike to Itswoot Lake	2.0	450'
Day 4	Out	11.9	700'

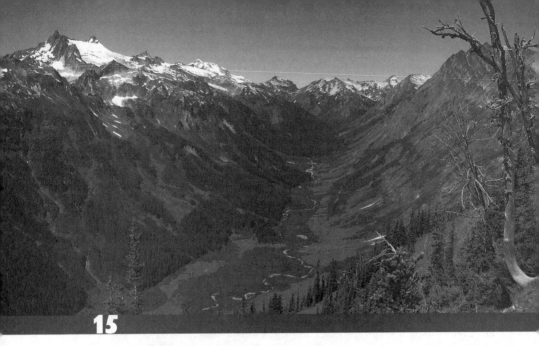

15

GLACIER PEAK LOOP

RATINGS: Scenery 10   **Solitude** 5   **Difficulty** 8

MILES: 110 (138)

ELEVATION GAIN: 23,700' (32,100')

DAYS: 9–12 (10–14)

SHUTTLE MILEAGE: 3.6 miles (or you can walk it)

MAPS: Green Trails *Benchmark Mtn. (#144), Glacier Peak (#112), Holden (#113),* and *Wenatchee Lake (#145)*

USUALLY OPEN: Very late July–early October

BEST: Mid-August

PERMIT: None required. Just sign the register at the trailhead.

RULES: Maximum group size of 12 people and/or stock; no camping or fires within 0.25 mile of Image Lake

CONTACTS: Okanogan-Wenatchee National Forest, Wenatchee River Ranger District, 509-548-2550, fs.usda.gov/main/okawen; Mount Baker–Snoqualmie National Forest, Darrington Ranger District, 360-436-1155, fs.usda.gov/main/mbs

SPECIAL ATTRACTIONS ·

Stupendous mountain scenery, abundant alpine wildflowers

Above: *Napeequa Valley from Little Giant Pass*
photographed by Douglas Lorain

CHALLENGES ••

Black bears, clouds of flies in August, frequent bridge washouts, likelihood of some bad weather, rugged trail coming out of Napeequa Valley, unbridged river crossings, very long trip with no chance to resupply

HOW TO GET THERE ••••••••••••••••••••••••••••••••••

Take US 2 to the crossroads known as Coles Corner, which is 20 miles east of Stevens Pass and 15 miles northwest of Leavenworth. Turn northeast on WA 207, following signs to Lake Wenatchee State Park, and drive 4.5 miles to a fork just after a bridge over the Wenatchee River.

If you have two cars and want to shorten the trip by leaving out the beautiful but very demanding Napeequa Valley segment, you'll want to leave one car at the White River Trailhead. To reach it, go left at the fork, still on WA 207, and proceed straight on the main paved road 6 miles to a junction. Turn right onto White River Road, which becomes Forest Service Road 64 and turns to gravel, and continue another 10.2 miles to the road-end trailhead.

To reach the recommended starting and ending point for the full loop, go right onto Chiwawa Loop Road at the fork near the Wenatchee River bridge. In 0.4 mile, turn right onto County Road 22, drive 0.8 mile, then turn left onto paved Chiwawa River Road (which becomes Forest Service Road 62). You'll reach the end of the pavement after 9.2 miles, and then continue on a narrow but decent gravel road for 10 miles to the Little Giant Trailhead on your left. This is the ending point of the loop. Be sure to get out here and walk 60 yards down the trail to check out the ford of the Chiwawa River. If it looks feasible, then you won't be turned back by this potentially difficult obstacle at the end of your adventure.

To continue to the starting point, stay on increasingly bumpy FS 62 another 3 miles, veer left at a junction, and drive a final 0.6 mile to the large Trinity Trailhead parking area on the left.

NOTE: You'll need a Northwest Forest Pass to park at these trailheads.

GPS TRAILHEAD COORDINATES:
Trinity Trailhead: N48° 04.345' W120° 51.017'
Little Giant Trailhead: N48° 01.535' W120° 49.681'
White River Trailhead: N47° 57.767' W120° 56.692'

INTRODUCTION ••••••••••••••••••••••••••••••••••••••

Like most of the taller mountains in the Cascade Range, Glacier Peak is a massive stratovolcano, now covered with glaciers and offering stupendous views and scenery. To the south, other major Cascade peaks rise above a relatively nondescript landscape of forested hills and ridges. This mountain, however, lies in the higher and more rugged North Cascades region, and as a result it's surrounded by tall, jagged peaks and ridges covered with glaciers of their own, presenting scenery that, even without the major peak, would be worthy of a place in this book.

continued on page 136

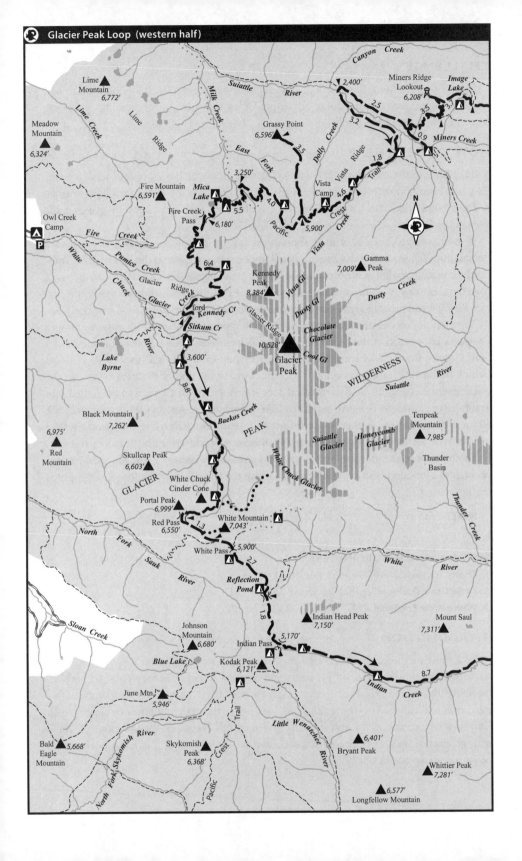

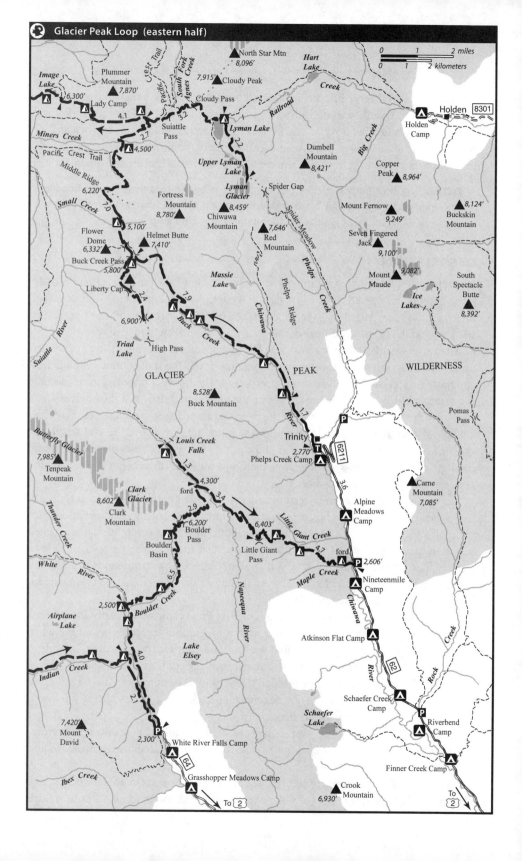

0   1   2 miles
0   1   2 kilometers

Image Lake 6,300'
Plummer Mountain 7,870'
Lady Camp 4.1
North Star Mtn 8,096'
Hart Lake
7,915' Cloudy Peak
Cloudy Pass
Holden 8301
Holden Camp
Miners Creek
Pacific Crest Trail
2.7
Suiattle Pass
Lyman Lake
2.2
Railroad
Creek
Big Creek
Pacific Crest Trail
4,500'
Upper Lyman Lake
2.2
Lyman Glacier
Dumbell Mountain 8,421'
Copper Peak 8,964'
Middle Ridge 6,220'
Fortress Mountain 8,780'
Spider Gap
Mount Fernow 9,249'
8,124' Buckskin Mountain
Small Creek
7.0
Helmet Butte 7,410'
Chiwawa Mountain 8,459'
7,646' Red Mountain
Seven Fingered Jack 9,100'
Flower Dome 6,332'
5,100'
Buck Creek Pass 5,800'
Massie Lake
Spider Meadow
Phelps Ridge
Phelps Creek
Mount Maude 9,082'
Ice Lakes
South Spectacle Butte 8,392'
Liberty Cap
2.4
6,900'
7.9
Buck Creek
Chiwawa River
Triad Lake
High Pass
GLACIER
8,528' Buck Mountain
PEAK
WILDERNESS
Pomas Pass
Butterfly Glacier
7,985' Tenpeak Mountain
Louis Creek Falls
1.7
River
Trinity 2,770'
6211
Phelps Creek Camp
Carne Mountain 7,085'
Clark Glacier
8,602' Clark Mountain
1.3
4,300' ford
2.9
3.4
6,403'
3.6
Alpine Meadows Camp
Thunder Creek
6,200' Boulder Pass
Little Giant Creek
White River
Boulder Basin
6.5
Napeequa River
Little Giant Pass
4.7 ford
2,606'
Nineteenmile Camp
Maple Creek
Airplane Lake
2,500'
Boulder Creek
Lake Elsey
Atkinson Flat Camp
Chiwawa River
4.0
Indian Creek
62
Rock Creek
2.1
Schaefer Creek Camp
Riverbend Camp
7,420' Mount David
2,300'
64
White River Falls Camp
Schaefer Lake
Finner Creek Camp
Ibex Creek
Grasshopper Meadows Camp
To 2
Crook Mountain 6,930'
To 2

continued from page 133

Taking in all of this remarkable landscape, however, requires a long and rugged adventure that will necessarily start off with a very heavy pack, and that will potentially deal with days of poor weather. But if you are up for the challenge, this could be the trip of a lifetime. In the opinion of this writer, this hike is at least the equal (and perhaps even surpasses) the much more famous and hard-to-get-a-permit-for Wonderland Trail around Mount Rainier.

NOTE: The final portion of this trip climbing out of the Napeequa Valley is quite challenging and should only be attempted by strong and experienced hikers. With a reasonable car shuttle, it is possible to skip this part of the loop.

DESCRIPTION

The trail begins beside a signboard on the west side of the parking lot and rambles north through an open forest of Douglas fir, western hemlock, western white pine, and Engelmann spruce. After just 70 yards, you take a bridge over rushing Phelps Creek, then wind around the private buildings of the small mining settlement of Trinity.

After a very gentle 1.7 miles, you bear left (northwest) at a fork and soon pass a fair campsite that is well suited for those who got a late start. The trail continues uphill, now at a more noticeable but still far from steep grade. The forest and undergrowth become increasingly lush as you go upstream beside the unseen but easily heard Chiwawa River. Views are limited to a few glimpses of the nearby craggy ridges, but these are more than enough to encourage you to keep going. The route takes you over several small and unnamed side creeks, none of which should do more than get the soles of your boots wet. At about 3 miles you cross a bridge over the Chiwawa River, then climb 80 yards up the opposite bank to a spacious campsite.

The trail now begins a long, steady, moderately graded uphill with frequent, irregularly spaced switchbacks. As the forest gradually thins, a few brushy meadows afford nice views of very rugged Buck Mountain to the south, as well as several unnamed jagged peaks around High Pass to the west. It's obvious that many of these sloping meadows were created by large avalanches, which regularly knock down thousands of trees and create significant headaches for trail crews. If you see any of these hard-working crews, please be sure to thank them for their efforts.

At 6.7, 7.0, and 7.4 miles, you pass large and very good campsites. Shortly after the last of these sites, you complete a switchback with a long uphill leg, probably all the while cursing the clouds of annoying flies that buzz around your face as you climb. In mid- to late August, a much more welcome swarm arrives: flocks of noisy and colorfully yellow evening grosbeaks, which migrate through this area in large numbers. Also welcome are the views to the northwest of the obvious notch of Buck Creek Pass, which is still over a mile away, as the evening grosbeak flies.

At around 9.1 miles you hop over a small creek, then continue gradually uphill, crossing open wildflower-covered slopes for 0.5 mile to a junction just above the meadows and tree islands of Buck Creek Pass.

The main trail goes straight, but if you need a campsite or want to do the wildly scenic side trip to High Pass, turn left (southwest) at the junction and descend 0.1 mile to Buck

Creek Pass with its terrific views looking west to Glacier Peak. A tiny but reliable spring feeds a creek that provides water for several excellent campsites in this area. August weekends are often very busy, however, so be prepared for company.

> **HIGH PASS SIDE TRIP:** Beyond Buck Creek Pass, the High Pass Trail goes south, switchbacking up the north slope of pointed Liberty Cap, then contouring across the west side of this peak in sloping meadows. In addition to world-class vistas to the west of aptly named Glacier Peak, these open slopes have outstanding displays of August-blooming lupine, pasqueflower, partridge foot, bistort, yarrow, lousewort, valerian, aster, arnica, false hellebore, alpine buttercup, both pink and white heather, paintbrush, Cusick's speedwell, and countless other wildflowers. At the south end of these glorious meadows is a saddle, where a faint boot path turns back to the north as it follows a ridge to the top of Liberty Cap, where you can enjoy magnificent panoramas.
>
> The main path continues south, climbing to a second saddle, where you switch to the northeast side of the ridge. After a short uphill traverse, you hit the ridgetop again just above another saddle where the official trail ends. From this point you'll enjoy the best views of all, down Buck Creek's canyon to the east, over to Fortress Mountain to the northeast, south to heavily glaciated Clark Mountain, and southwest to Triad Lake and the rugged ridge that encloses this ice-bound pool. Filling the sky to the west is ever-present Glacier Peak. Beyond this saddle, the route to High Pass becomes a difficult scramble over rocks and icy snowfields. You may need an ice ax to safely travel this section, especially if the snow is hard. Most hikers simply turn around at the last viewpoint, well satisfied with their adventure.

Back at the junction just above Buck Creek Pass, you turn northwest and walk 0.25 mile to a saddle and an unsigned but obvious junction with a boot trail that goes west up Flower Dome. Although not in a class with the route to High Pass, the short climb to the top of Flower Dome is worth your time. The main trail goes straight (north), descends a series of switchbacks, then makes a downhill traverse through forest to the bridgeless but easy crossing of Small Creek. On the other side is a campsite, although most of the best tent spots have been obliterated by fallen trees.

The trail now makes a fairly steep ascent, gaining 1,100 feet in a little less than 2 miles to the top of Middle Ridge. A use trail goes right (southeast) here, climbing the ridge to some excellent overlooks of Glacier Peak, Fortress Mountain, Plummer Mountain, Bonanza Peak, and other landmarks. Your trail goes straight at the unsigned Middle Ridge junction, descends across scenic meadows, then reenters forest and follows a small creek. At the bottom of the 1,700-foot descent is a junction with the Pacific Crest Trail (PCT).

You turn right (northeast), and after 0.4 mile you come to some very good campsites about 80 yards before a bridge over slightly silty Miners Creek. From here the trail climbs gradually but steadily away from Miners Creek as it makes occasional switchbacks on a heavily forested slope. About 1.7 miles up from the creek, a fine viewpoint presents an excellent perspective of Fortress and Chiwawa Mountains. The former summit features a small glacier that feeds Miners Creek. After another 0.6 mile, you reach a junction. Turn left (west), almost immediately hop over a small creek, and 100 yards later reach a very good campsite near an old mine site and a well-maintained (but locked) cabin.

LYMAN LAKE AND LYMAN GLACIER SIDE TRIP: From a base camp at this convenient location, you can make an extremely scenic day hike. First, return to the northbound PCT, then climb to the east, gathering nice views looking southwest to Glacier Peak and south to Fortress Mountain. After about 1.1 miles, and just 0.2 mile or so before you reach Suiattle Pass, a possibly unsigned trail forks to the right (east). The PCT goes left (north) on its way to Suiattle Pass.

Take the right fork as it climbs around a ridge a bit above Suiattle Pass, then makes a rough up-and-down traverse of the north side of an unnamed butte. The rugged trail is rocky and often icy until late summer as it crosses this shady slope. After about 1 mile you intersect a trail coming up from a junction with the PCT in the valley below.

Go right (northeast) and climb a series of switchbacks to high and often windy Cloudy Pass, from which an obvious and not-too-difficult climber's route heads northeast to the tremendous viewpoints atop Cloudy Peak and North Star Mountain. The main trail goes straight at Cloudy Pass and winds down mostly forested and relatively gentle slopes to Lyman Lake.

The views from any side of this large, turquoise-colored lake are superb, and several excellent campsites are in the vicinity.

WARNING: Black bears are a big problem in this area. If you camp here, be especially careful to guard your food, and don't be surprised if you have to get up in the middle of the night to bang pots in an effort to scare away the thieving bruins.

A dead-end trail goes along the west side of Lyman Lake to a pretty waterfall. A better exploring option crosses the lake's outlet creek and climbs a ridge to the east of the lake. This wildly scenic path goes over a little rise, then travels above timberline as it passes a series of shallow meltwater lakes amid the bouldery wasteland below receding-but-still-active Lyman Glacier. This impressive ice sheet sits in a dramatic bowl beneath Chiwawa Mountain.

Back at the campsite below Suiattle Pass, you head almost due west as the trail contours across the slopes on the south side of Plummer Mountain. After 1.6 miles you pass a broken-down log cabin that used to be part of the long-defunct Glacier Peak mines, and then come to a junction. Go right (uphill and northwest), following signs to Image Lake, and climb eight switchbacks on a brushy and partly forested slope. At the top of the switchbacks is a tiny creek and Lady Camp, one of the places where visitors to busy Image Lake are encouraged to camp.

The trail's grade now eases as it goes very gradually uphill across open slopes sprinkled with alpine wildflowers. More memorable than the flowers, however, are the nearly continuous picture-postcard views of shining Glacier Peak rising over the deep, forested chasm of the Suiattle River. It's truly breathtaking! After about 1.5 miles of happily striding along through this wonderland, you come to a junction. The trail to the right (north) goes to distant Canyon Lake. You go straight (west) and descend into the meadowy basin holding gorgeous Image Lake. The view from the meadows on the northeast side of Image Lake across to Glacier Peak are so outstanding that they're often depicted in national calendars, despite the considerable effort required by photographers to get here. To protect against damage from too many boots, the lake is strictly a day-use area, and horses are not allowed in the basin. A designated backpacker camping area is located well below Image Lake.

Once you've had your fill of Image Lake, continue west on the trail, which follows a high ridge 0.8 mile to a junction. The recommended main loop goes left, downhill (south), here.

> **SIDE TRIP TO MINERS RIDGE LOOKOUT:** Having come this far, you may as well first continue straight (west) on a trail that goes another 0.2 mile to Miners Ridge Lookout, a staffed facility with a view to die for.

Having had your fill of the scenery, backtrack 0.2 mile from the lookout and turn south at the junction onto a trail that begins a seemingly endless series of switchbacks down a mostly forested slope. Occasional breaks in the tree cover offer excellent views looking southwest to Glacier Peak. After 2.6 miles you reach a junction, where you keep right (west) and continue the long switchbacking descent. Just as it seems the downhill will never end, you'll hear the Suiattle River below you and finally come to a junction with the PCT. If you're in need of a campsite, the best in this area can be found about 0.9 mile to the left (upstream and east) at the trail crossing of Miners Creek.

Unless you've heard reports from other hikers of a convenient nearby log spanning the raging Suiattle River (don't count on it), you now must take a long detour. The former PCT bridge was about 1 mile upstream from here, but that washed out in one of the infamous floods that are so common in this area. The new bridge is now miles downstream, so turn right (west) and follow the trail along the river, sometimes near its banks but more often in the wet forest environment a little up the hillside. After 2.5 miles on a mostly gentle downhill path and past some magnificent old cedars, you come to a point where the PCT forks to the left (south). Turn that way, and a few minutes later reach the impressive (and hopefully permanent) new trail bridge over the river. As you look up the river, take in the nice views to the nearby forested ridges, with glimpses of the high peaks at the river's headwaters. After the crossing, you turn back upstream (east) and follow a new section of trail through old-growth forests for 3.2 mostly viewless miles to a junction beside somewhat silty Vista Creek. You can cross the creek here (a log is usually available) to a fine campsite on the south side.

The PCT keeps right (southwest) at the junction and begins an extended climb. You will gain 3,100 feet in the next 9.5 miles, so settle in for a long, tiring slog. Numerous irregularly spaced switchbacks keep the grade relatively gentle, but they also add mileage, so it seems to go on forever. About 1.8 miles into the climb, you cross a tiny, clear tributary creek just before a small but serviceable campsite near rushing Vista Creek. The trail then switchbacks up a hillside covered with brush and dense forest, although a couple of openings along the way offer very nice views of Glacier Peak if the clouds have parted and the notorious North Cascades weather is cooperating. Finally, as you approach the top of Vista Ridge, the forest gradually peters out, and you find yourself switchbacking up beautiful wildflower-covered hillsides. On a clear day the vistas extend to countless rugged North Cascades peaks to the east and north. You pass very scenic, but usually dry, Vista Camp, then gain another 500 feet before topping out at just over 5,900 feet.

Shortly after you make a quick descent, you'll come to a switchback and see an unsigned trail going off to the right (north).

> **GRASSY POINT SIDE TRIP:** The trail that goes to the right here is the Grassy Point Trail, and it's well worth a side trip if the weather is sunny and you have the

time. The view of the hulking north face of Glacier Peak from the end of this 3.5-mile dead-end trail is outstanding.

The main PCT keeps left (southwest) at the Grassy Point turnoff and contours across the upper part of a sloping basin at the head of East Fork Milk Creek. Along the way you hop over several small creeks and pass side trails leading down to a couple of exposed but extremely scenic campsites. Finally you cross a ridge and enjoy fine views to the west of rugged Lime Ridge rising over the deep canyon of Milk Creek.

The trail drops into that canyon, switchbacking 36 times as it descends. Without regular maintenance, this section of trail quickly becomes overgrown with head-high brush, and especially after it rains, it can be soggy and rather miserable. At the bottom of this 1,600-foot descent is a possibly unsigned junction with a section of the PCT that was closed due to yet another bridge washout. You go straight on a new trail, descend eight more switchbacks, and come to a junction with the Milk Creek Trail. This once-popular trail has gone unmaintained for several years due to flood damage and a destroyed bridge across the Suiattle River at the trail's lower end.

You go sharply left (south) at the Milk Creek junction and climb 0.3 mile to a new bridge across Milk Creek. History shows that bridges across this (and any other) large stream in this wilderness often don't live up to their "permanent" expectations, but hopefully the wooden span will be there when you hike through because Milk Creek is swift, cold, and silty and wouldn't be much fun (or possibly even safe) to ford. The new section of PCT now ascends a series of nine well-graded switchbacks to an unmarked junction with the old and abandoned PCT. From here you go right (southwest) and keep steadily but gradually climbing countless switchbacks, sometimes on older tread and sometimes on newer trail that was built to avoid some severe landslides and washouts. You briefly break out of the forest to cross a rocky creek before resuming the woodsy and rather monotonous uphill route. A little more than halfway up this second set of switchbacks, you reach a grassy bench, with a small, clear creek and good campsites.

TIP: These sites are better and more sheltered than those at nearby Mica Lake, another 0.5 mile ahead.

More uphill switchbacks over open terrain take you to the rocky shores of deep

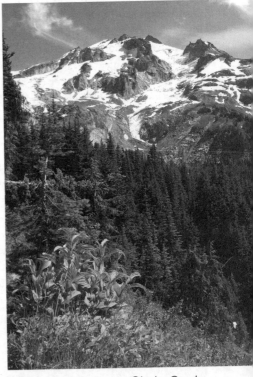

Glacier Peak from near Glacier Creek
photographed by Douglas Lorain

and often ice-bound Mica Lake. Camping here is rather stark but also very scenic. In addition to the many charms of the lake itself, the views to the northeast of Dome Peak peeking over the shoulder of Grassy Point are superb. Another 900 feet of circuitous uphill through rocky areas and heather meadows take you to Fire Creek Pass. Not surprisingly, the views from here are terrific and encompass a portion of the top of Glacier Peak to the southeast, nearby Fire Mountain to the west-northwest, and long vistas to the southwest including distinctive Sloan Peak.

The trail winds its way slowly down from the pass through meadows then partial forest to a basin with a possible campsite at the head of Fire Creek. It then climbs around a little ridge before making a long up-and-down traverse to good campsites near Pumice Creek. From the PCT crossings of the two ridges on either side of Pumice Creek, the views of massive Glacier Peak are positively overwhelming.

From Pumice Creek you cross Glacier Ridge, then make your way over to small, clear Glacier Creek before beginning a long, toe-jamming descent along a narrow, forested ridge. About 1.5 miles from Glacier Creek, you go left (east) at a junction and descend to silt-laden Kennedy Creek. The log bridge that used to be here is now broken and unusable, so expect to have to make a ford or tricky rock-hop to get across.

The trail briefly follows Kennedy Creek downstream, then turns south and climbs to the top of a minor ridge, where there is a junction with the new trail to White Chuck River and Lost Creek Ridge. You go left (south), still on the PCT, and descend briefly to an easy rock-hop crossing of Sitkum Creek. Just after this crossing is a spacious campsite. The PCT then gradually descends 0.7 mile to a junction with an old and now abandoned section of the White Chuck River Trail. You keep left (southeast) and walk 0.3 mile to a campsite just before a log bridge over a small, unnamed creek.

The PCT gives tired hikers a break for the next couple of miles as it leads you on a gentle stroll through old-growth hemlock and cedar forest to a campsite just before the bridge over rushing Baekos Creek. An intermittent climb for the next mile takes you to a new "permanent" bridge over the milky White Chuck River. Unless they have been recently washed away, twisted remains of the last "permanent" bridge can still be seen in a rocky chasm just upstream.

After this crossing the uphill grade becomes steadier as you ascend a set of 12 switchbacks, then come to a nice one-tent campsite beside a small, clear creek. From here the trail follows the creek upstream through gradually thinning forest and eventually up to the high basin at the head of the White Chuck River. Flowers, views, campsites, and fine scenery abound here.

WHITE CHUCK GLACIER SIDE TRIP: For an excellent side trip, make your way off-trail to the east toward an obvious waterfall on White Chuck River. Once there, follow a sketchy boot path that climbs steeply up the right side of the falls to a nearly flat upper basin. The faint path then ascends two more levels of increasingly steep, rocky terrain to a glacial lake that usually has floating icebergs even in late summer. Old maps show this lake at the base of White Chuck Glacier, but the ice has receded considerably since then. With some rock scrambling over moraine, you can still visit the glacier, and the stark but impressive scenery makes this worthwhile.

Meanwhile the main PCT slowly winds its way up and away from the rolling mead-owlands of the White Chuck Basin, passes the dark volcanic landmark of White Chuck Cinder Cone, and switchbacks up to rocky Red Pass. From here you'll catch a glimpse of Glacier Peak, which is mostly blocked by nearby Portal Peak, and can look west to Sloan Peak and the jagged Monte Cristo Range.

The southbound trail curves east and makes a rugged, mostly downhill traverse of an open, flower-sprinkled hillside. Views here, especially southeast to Indian Head Peak and south to nearby Johnson Mountain, are outstanding. On very clear days you can even see distant Mount Rainier.

WHITE MOUNTAIN SIDE TRIP: For an even better view, scramble up to the ridgeline on your left (east), and follow it all the way to the top of White Mountain. This grandstand offers simply stupendous vistas of pyramid-shaped Glacier Peak.

You go straight (southeast) where the North Fork Sauk Trail angles up from the right, and soon reach White Pass. Here an unsigned trail goes east, providing access to the tech-nically demanding "high" route to Thunder Basin. Another much shorter path heads west down to good camps on a nearby meadow-covered bench.

The PCT rambles south, going up and down along a lovely open ridge with excellent views. Hoary marmots are nearly constant companions here and often make loud alarm "whistles" at the approach of hikers. About 2 miles from White Pass is tiny Reflection Pond, with (yes) good reflections of Indian Head Peak, as well as a couple of nice camp-sites amid the mountain hemlocks and subalpine firs on the pond's west shore.

In a saddle about 0.2 mile south of Reflection Pond is a junction with White River Trail. A glance at the map leads to the conclusion that this trail is the shortest, easiest way to com-plete the loop around Glacier Peak. Unfortunately, a fire swept through White River Canyon some years ago, leaving many dead snags and enormous problems with deadfall on the trail. The U.S. Forest Service hasn't cleared the route for several years, so for now it's a slow and difficult trail. Check with the U.S. Forest Service for current conditions before you leave.

For now, travelers are advised to take the trail down Indian Creek instead, which is 6 miles longer for those doing the full loop. To reach it, continue south on the PCT from the junction with the White River Trail. For 1.8 miles this route traverses the west side of the Cascade Divide, where you gain lovely views of Johnson Mountain, Sloan Peak, and the North Sauk River Canyon. At the end of the traverse, a short downhill leads to a junction amid the large meadows around Indian Pass. Numerous nice campsites are in this area, although finding nearby water can be a problem in late summer.

You turn left (east) at the Indian Pass junction and begin a gradual descent, sometimes in lush meadows and sometimes in dense forest. After 1 mile you reach a small but rea-sonably good campsite on your right about 150 yards before the trail crosses a small creek in the first of several long, sloping meadows. The route, which steeply descends a series of these meadows, often has lots of brush, so be prepared to get soaked if it has rained recently. Indian Creek is sometimes heard on your right (south), but it's rarely seen. At nearly 3 miles from Indian Pass, you reach another good campsite.

Beyond this second campsite along Indian Creek, the trail becomes much gentler, with only minor ups and downs. The only difficulty comes from the miles of brush you must hike through, which often overhangs the trail. In fairness to the U.S. Forest Service, plants grow so quickly in the North Cascades that keeping trails clear of brush is a Herculean and very expensive task. So just accept it as part of the hiking experience in this part of the world, and if you have a choice, try not to hike through shortly after a rainstorm.

Near the bottom of the canyon, after playing hide-and-seek with elusive and slow-moving Indian Creek for several miles, you pass a good campsite, and a little over 1 mile later you make eight downhill switchbacks to a bridge over Indian Creek. A good campsite is on your left immediately before the bridge.

The trail turns downstream (south), following the initially unseen White River, which so recently added the waters of Indian Creek to its own. On the other side of this large stream is the continuation of the loop trail, but fording the river is usually too dangerous, so an extended downstream detour is required. That downstream section, however, is very easy and enjoyable, as the trail wanders gently downhill under the shady canopy of an old-growth forest. Adding beauty to the scene, the river is a lovely turquoise color from glacial runoff at its headwaters. After 2.1 miles you keep left (southeast) at the signed junction with Mount David Trail, and 20 yards later you cross a substantial bridge over the White River. Immediately on the other side of this crossing is the parking lot and trailhead at the end of Forest Service Road 64. If you left a second car here and plan to skip the upcoming section to the Napeequa Valley, then your hike is now complete.

Those intrepid, experienced, and athletic types who have the time and energy to complete the entire loop only briefly touch this evidence of civilization before turning left (north) at the parking lot onto White River Trail. This trail is gentle and fun as it goes upstream and travels through attractive forested terrain. About 3.7 miles up the White River Trail is a log crossing of Boulder Creek and some mediocre campsites. Just 0.3 mile later is a junction near a cluster of much better campsites.

You turn right (east) onto Boulder Pass Trail and almost immediately begin what will turn out to be a long and exhausting climb. You start with 18 switchbacks that gain about 1,100 feet on a mostly forested hillside. From there you duck into the canyon of Boulder Creek, climb past a nice trailside campsite, then 0.4 mile later make a simple rock-hop crossing of the stream. The trail keeps charging uphill, traversing a very brushy slope, where you'll enjoy excellent views of Boulder Basin and imposing Clark Mountain. As you approach the lower portion of Boulder Basin, the trail abruptly pulls away from the creek and ascends six switchbacks to upper Boulder Basin. Here you'll find lots of wildflowers and numerous very good campsites set under the cliffs on the southeast side of Clark Mountain.

The trail isn't finished climbing yet, however, so after a nice rest or overnight, wind your way up dozens of sometimes rocky but well-graded switchbacks to 6,200-foot Boulder Pass. The views here are worth all the sweat, especially those views looking seemingly straight down into the depths of the Napeequa River Valley, almost 2,000 feet below.

Reaching those depths is your next challenge. It's a long way down, but 68 switchbacks and a brushy traverse later, you finally reach the banks of the Napeequa River and another challenge. There is no bridge, and the slightly milky waters of this major mountain stream can be waist deep in early August. By late August, however, just over knee-deep is the norm, so while the crossing will be cold and a bit tricky, it *should* be reasonable for late-summer hikers. Check with the U.S. Forest Service about the latest conditions before you leave, but note that the information may not be updated and accurate. The other hazard that must be noted is the uncountable *billions* of flies that buzz around and are famously found throughout the Napeequa River Valley. Fortunately, once the sun goes down, the *?&*! flies disappear.

Once across the river and through a tangle of thick willows and alders, it's only about 100 yards up the opposite bank to a signed junction.

> **LOUIS CREEK FALLS SIDE TRIP:** The Little Giant Trail, which is the return route of the loop, goes to the right (southeast). Before heading that way, however, it's well worth taking a side trip up the Napeequa Trail, which goes left (northwest). This trail is no longer maintained by the U.S. Forest Service, but despite being brushy in places, it is easy to follow. As this path goes uphill across a slope above the river, there are fine views to the southwest of massive Clark Glacier on the slopes of the mountain of the same name. After a little over 1.2 miles you pass an inviting campsite just before the trail passes below the long, sliding cascade of Louis Creek Falls. A sketchy and very brushy trail continues up the valley, but this falls is the logical turnaround point for the side trip.

The rough and poorly maintained Little Giant Trail goes down the valley from the junction near the river ford and leads you on a difficult 1.5-mile journey through muddy slop, thick brush, tall grasses, and dense thickets of willow and alder at the bottom of the valley. Even though the path slowly loses elevation, the hiking is quite tiring. Fortunately, once it finally pulls away from the valley and begins to climb the canyon walls, the trail is somewhat less overgrown. It is, however, very narrow, badly sloping, and completely open to the sun and flies, so it's *tough* going. In addition, despite numerous irregularly spaced switchbacks, the route is often ridiculously steep. All of these factors make the trail not only difficult but occasionally even dangerous, so this is *strictly for strong and experienced hikers*. But, oh my goodness, the VIEWS! With every step, the scenes back down the classic U-shaped Napeequa River Valley and up to its surrounding jagged peaks just get better and better. The winding, turquoise-colored river at the bottom adds considerably to the setting.

The crowning glory comes when you (*finally!*) top out at Little Giant Pass. From this high point Glacier Peak makes its appearance above the head of the long Napeequa River Valley. You can also look east into the Chiwawa River Valley, but as nice as that is, it doesn't remotely compare to the glories to the north and west. Although you may have never heard of this spot before, in good weather, this is one of the finest and most photogenic views in North America. I am fortunate enough to have visited many of the leading contenders, and, believe me, that is *not* an exaggeration.

The trail, now maintained to a somewhat higher standard, switchbacks down the open slope east of Little Giant Pass, where there are good views of the Chiwawa River Valley and its flanking ridges. Although unrelentingly steep and badly eroded in places, this trail is still easier and safer than the route climbing to Little Giant Pass from the west. About 0.9 mile from the pass is a small but nice campsite beside a tiny trickling creek. Another 0.5 mile takes you to an exposed and rocky rib, where you must look for small cairns in order to stay on the trail. About 2.3 miles down from the pass, you come to a large tributary of Little Giant Creek with reliable water and a small but good campsite.

From here the trail steeply gains a little more than 200 feet to cross a minor ridge, then resumes its downhill trek. Fortunately, most of the remaining descent is much easier on the knees, as a series of relatively gentle switchbacks takes you down to some possible campsites near an easy hop-over crossing of Maple Creek. In another 0.2 mile of nearly level walking, you arrive at the banks of the clear Chiwawa River. There is no bridge and only occasionally will you find a logjam, so expect to ford. In early summer this can be a difficult business, but by mid-August the water is usually only a little more than knee-deep and not overly swift. In late August and September you may see spawning salmon in the river's clear waters. About 60 yards up the other side of the crossing is the Little Giant Trailhead. To reach your car, turn left (north) and make the easy 3.6-mile walk up FS 62.

VARIATIONS

As mentioned previously, with a car shuttle, it is possible to shorten this trip by ending it at the White River Trailhead. If you have limited time and the ability to do sometimes long and tedious car shuttles, the full loop could also be done as three section hikes, utilizing trailheads on the Suiattle River and the White River.

POSSIBLE ITINERARY

	CAMP	MILES	ELEVATION GAIN
Day 1	Buck Creek Pass	9.6	3,200'
Day 2	Junction below Suiattle Pass	9.7	2,150'
	Side trip to High Pass (morning)	4.8	1,200'
Day 3	Junction below Suiattle Pass		
	Day hike to Lyman Lake and Glacier	10.8	3,150'
Day 4	Miners Creek	12.2	1,200'
	Side trip to Miners Ridge Lookout	0.4	150'
Day 5	Camp along Vista Creek	8.4	700'
Day 6	Vista Ridge	5.6	2,750'
	Side trip to Grassy Point	7.0	1,600'
Day 7	Fire Creek	10.5	3,200'
Day 8	Upper White Chuck Basin	12.0	2,000'
	Side trip to White Chuck Glacier	4.4	1,300'
Day 9	Reflection Pond	5.0	1,250'
	Side trip to White Mountain	1.2	1,000'
Day 10	Near mouth of Indian Creek	10.5	250'
Day 11	Boulder Basin	11.1	2,500'
Day 12	Louis Creek Falls	5.8	2,100'
Day 13	Out	9.4	2,400'
	(plus a road walk of 3.6 miles)		

BEST SHORTER ALTERNATIVES

Highlights on either end of this long loop at Buck Creek Pass and Little Giant Pass can be reached by either very long day hikes or (much better) one-night backpacking trips. For a shorter loop, try a 36-mile hike to Buck Creek Pass, Suiattle Pass, and Lyman Lake; then exit via Spider Gap (beware of lingering snow, which may require an ice ax) and Phelps Creek.

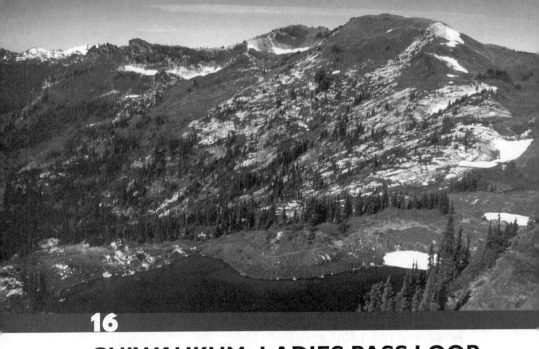

16

CHIWAUKUM–LADIES PASS LOOP

RATINGS: Scenery 8   **Solitude** 4   **Difficulty** 6

MILES: 38 (55)

ELEVATION GAIN: 10,000' (13,700')

DAYS: 4–6 (4–7)

SHUTTLE MILEAGE: 4

MAP: Green Trails *Chiwaukum Mtns. (#177)*

USUALLY OPEN: Late July–October

BEST: Late July–mid-August

PERMIT: Required. Free and available at the trailhead.

RULES: Maximum group size of 12 people and/or stock; no fires above 5,000 feet (which includes all the lakes on this trip); camp only at designated sites at Lake Mary and Upper Florence Lake

CONTACT: Okanogan-Wenatchee National Forest, Wenatchee River Ranger District, 509-548-2550, fs.usda.gov/main/okawen

SPECIAL ATTRACTIONS •

Gorgeous ridgetop gardens, good views

CHALLENGES •

Rattlesnakes along lower Chiwaukum Creek, crowded in places

Above: *Looking down on Upper Florence Lake*
photographed by Douglas Lorain

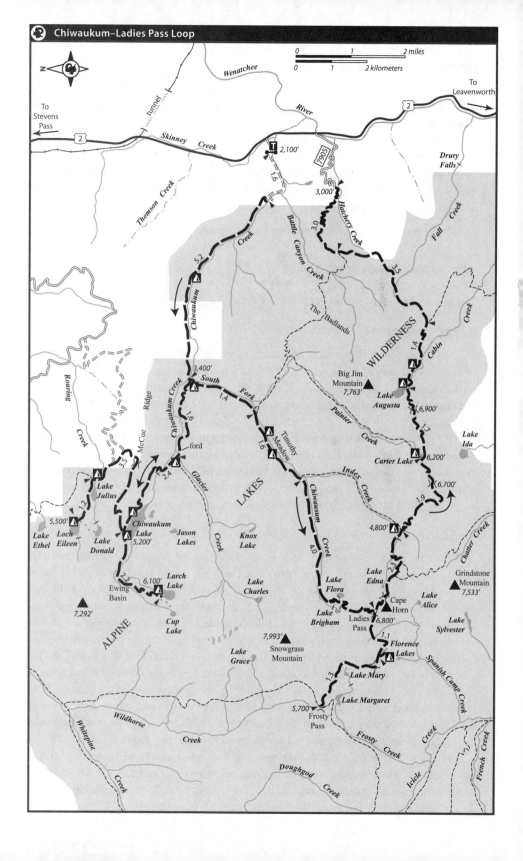

To Stevens Pass

To Leavenworth

2

Wenatchee

River

2

Skinney Creek

Thomson Creek

tunnel

Drury Falls

Fall Creek

2,100'

7905

1.6

3,000'

3.0

Hatchery Creek

3.5

Battle Canyon Creek

Chiwaukum Creek

5.2

3,400'

South Fork

1.4

1.6

The Badlands

WILDERNESS

1.4

Cabin Creek

Big Jim Mountain 7,763'

Lake Augusta

6,900'

Painter Creek

Lake Ida

1.7

Roaring Creek

McCue Ridge

3.5

ford

2.4

Glacier Creek

Chiwaukum Creek 5,200'

1.6

Timothy Meadow

1.6

Carter Lake

6,200'

6,700'

Index Creek

1.9

LAKES

1.2

Lake Julius

5,500'

Lake Ethel

Loch Eileen

Lake Donald

Jason Lakes

Knox Lake

Chiwaukum Creek

4.0

4,800'

Lake Edna

2.3

Grindstone Mountain 7,533'

Lake Alice

Lake Charles

2.2

6,100'

Larch Lake

Ewing Basin

7,292'

ALPINE

Cup Lake

Lake Grace

Snowgrass Mountain 7,993'

Lake Flora

Lake Brigham

Ladies Pass

Cape Horn

6,800'

1.1

Florence Lakes

Lake Sylvester

Spanish Camp Creek

Chatter Creek

1.3

Lake Mary

Lake Margaret

5,700'

Frosty Pass

Frosty Creek

Creek

Wildhorse

Creek

Whitepine Creek

Doughgod Creek

Icicle Creek

French Creek

HOW TO GET THERE ●

From Leavenworth, drive west on US 2 for about 10 miles, and then turn left onto Chiwaukum Creek Road (Forest Service Road 7908). Follow this gravel route 0.2 mile to a gate and the trailhead.

If you have two cars, leave the second car at the Hatchery Creek Trailhead. To reach it from the Chiwaukum Creek Trailhead, head south on US 2 E for 0.8 mile, and turn right (west) onto FS 7905, just north of the Wenatchee River bridge. Follow this narrow gravel road 2.2 miles, and turn right to remain on FS 7905. Continue another 0.3 mile to the marked trailhead parking area on the right.

NOTE: You'll need a Northwest Forest Pass to park at these trailheads.

GPS TRAILHEAD COORDINATES:
Northern (Chiwaukum Creek): N47° 41.334′ W120° 44.448′
Southern (Hatchery Creek): N47° 40.273′ W120° 45.287′

INTRODUCTION ●

The Alpine Lakes Wilderness has many supremely beautiful areas and a diversity of charms. This attractive loop trip gives you a nice sampling of what this part of the wilderness has to offer, with a minimum of regulatory hassles, especially in contrast to the nearby Enchantment Lakes country. You don't need reservations or special permits to hike here, and despite the fine scenery, the crowds are small enough that the U.S. Forest Service has managed to keep the regulations to a minimum. This hike takes you to spectacular high lakes, through larch-studded alpine meadows, along view-packed ridges, through deep canyons, and past high waterfalls. Along the way you'll travel on some trails that are fairly crowded, as well as others that are so rarely traveled, they're easily lost amid the greenery of meadows.

DESCRIPTION ●

From the Chiwaukum Creek Trailhead you hike past the gate on the closed road as it heads upstream (west) across private property. The public has an easement to pass through here, but you must stay on the road. The forests are typical for this elevation on the east side of the Cascades and are mostly composed of grand and Douglas fir with some ponderosa pine and western red cedar. In addition, big-leaf and vine maple display nice colors in October. After 1.6 miles, just beyond a fork in the road and a bridge on the left, the trail leaves the road and veers off to the right (northwest). You climb four short switchbacks, enter the wilderness, and begin a long but gentle ascent beside the creek. The trail is dusty from fairly heavy horse use but never steep, and it generally stays close to the clear, rushing waters of Chiwaukum Creek. Fires in 2013 hit this area pretty hard, clearing out some of the brush but negatively impacting the scenery for most hikers. Still, in August you should be able to snack on thimbleberries, which look and taste like tart raspberries.

Just shy of the 4-mile point, you pass the first good creekside campsite. Farther upstream you travel through an area that was selectively logged in the 1970s and then cross North Fork Chiwaukum Creek on a footlog. About 0.1 mile beyond the crossing is a decent campsite and a junction. The loop trail goes left (south) here.

First, however, you really must visit Chiwaukum and Larch Lakes. To do so, turn right (west) and make a moderately steep and often quite brushy climb through a recently burned forest. The ascent levels out as you skirt the edge of an overgrown marshy area and continue to Glacier Creek.

WARNING: The bridge that once spanned this creek is now gone, and the U.S. Forest Service does not plan to replace it. Logs may be available but cannot be relied upon, so be prepared to make a cold and potentially tricky ford, especially before midsummer.

About 100 yards beyond the crossing is a junction with the Glacier Creek Trail and a spacious campsite. Stock is not allowed on the trail above this point.

Go straight (northwest) at the junction, and after 0.2 mile cross North Fork Chiwaukum Creek at a sliding cascade. There is no bridge here, but you can usually find a log to shimmy across just downstream. From this point the easy hiking is over because the trail charges steeply uphill over mostly open terrain, gaining 1,400 feet in about 1.6 miles.

WARNING: This south-facing hillside can be uncomfortably hot on sunny afternoons. Start with a full water bottle and make frequent rest stops.

Lake Edna
photographed by Douglas Lorain

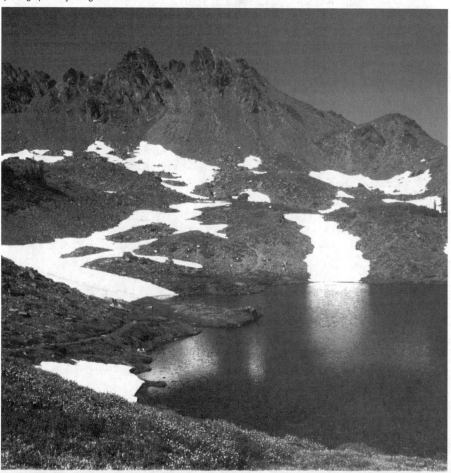

As you gain elevation, there are good views up the narrow canyon of Glacier Creek and back down the wider valley of Chiwaukum Creek.

The climb tops out on a hillside about 100 feet above large and very deep Chiwaukum Lake. You descend to the lake and then go up and down along the scenic north shore past a few decent camps. At the west end of the lake you'll come to a very good camp beside a junction. This is a fine spot to set up camp and do some exploring.

LOCH EILEEN SIDE TRIP: For a full day side trip from your camp at Chiwaukum Lake, leave the northwest end of the lake and follow the McCue Ridge Trail up a forested hillside to a ridgetop with decent views both north and south.

TIP: The side trip this far makes a fairly easy morning stroll.

The trail now drops partway down the other side of the ridge to a confusing junction near the end of a jeep track (not shown on most maps). Turn left (northwest) here, following signs to Lake Julius, and continue downhill. Next you come to a remote trailhead on a primitive road sometimes used as a shortcut approach by those with motorbikes but closed to other vehicles. Veer left (northwest) here, drop to a very good camp beside the clear waters of Roaring Creek, cross the creek on small logs, and turn left (west) at a junction a few hundred yards later. After passing pleasant Lake Julius, you steeply climb across open slopes to dramatic Loch Eileen. This lake sits in a cliff-walled cirque with a cascading waterfall feeding into it. The lake has good camps just above the outlet.

TIP: If you still have plenty of energy, use it to scramble up a very faint trail that climbs over steep rock slabs on the ridge south of Loch Eileen to Lake Donald, another beauty.

LARCH LAKE SIDE TRIP: A shorter recommended side trip is also spectacular. Follow the gradually diminishing North Fork Chiwaukum Creek Trail through a marshy meadow with lots of flowers, then curve south and cross the creek on a log. From here you climb moderately steeply through beautiful creekside meadows to Ewing Basin and a rock-hop crossing of the now-fairly-small creek. From here you ascend this view-packed mountain valley through flowery meadows and over switchbacks in open forests to Larch Lake, 2.2 miles and 900 feet up from Chiwaukum Lake. Larch Lake is everything an alpine lake should be: It has fish; flowery meadows, talus slopes, and scattered firs and alpine larches border the shores; and all of these features are surrounded by several picturesque serrated peaks. You can camp in this paradise if you choose, but rules require that you do so at least 200 feet from shore. Also be aware that the camps here are quite exposed and not recommended in bad weather. From Larch Lake adventurous hikers can scramble up a scree slope southwest of the lake to austere Cup Lake in a snowy, cliff-walled basin.

To continue your tour, return to Chiwaukum Lake and retrace your route back down to the junction near the confluence of the South and North Forks of Chiwaukum Creek. Turn right (south) and climb through forests and across rocky slopes above cascading South Fork Chiwaukum Creek.

WARNING: Unless trail crews have been through recently, this stretch of trail can get extremely brushy. Wear long pants to protect your legs from abuse.

After 1.4 miles you pass a frothing waterfall and immediately above it reach a junction with the Painter Creek Trail. Go straight (southwest) and climb exposed, often hot slopes with scattered quaking aspens and wildflowers, including fireweed and goldenrod. Shortly after the path levels off at inviting Timothy Meadow, you'll find nice, shady camps set aside separately for horses and hikers, both to the left of the trail. If these don't suit you, several more good sites appear over the next 0.3 mile in the various openings that comprise Timothy Meadow.

The trail now climbs steadily but not steeply through strips of trees made up primarily of Engelmann spruce and true firs. The majority of the route, however, traverses large, sloping meadows and avalanche chutes covered with tall grasses and wildflowers. A particularly abundant flower here is monkshood. This generally rather uncommon plant has 4-foot-tall stalks, each boasting several unusually shaped blue flowers.

NOTE: The Index Creek Trail goes left (south) in this area and is shown on most maps, but it is usually unsigned and is very faint. You probably won't even notice it.

As you continue to gain elevation, there are ever-improving views of Snowgrass Mountain and the imposing cliffs and waterfalls at the head of this canyon. It looks, in fact, as if the trail would have a hard time getting up there. Rest assured that it does, but the climb won't be easy.

Lake Augusta
photographed by Douglas Lorain

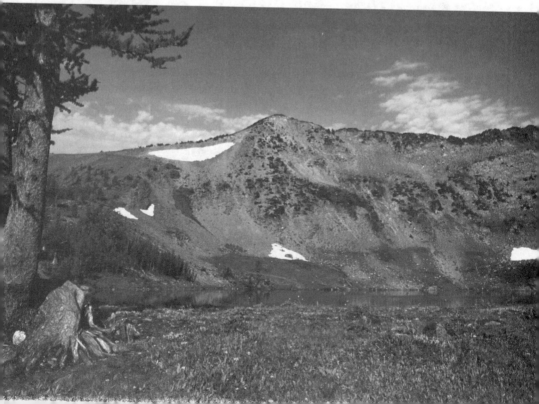

You make a sometimes-tricky rock-hop over the creek and follow the canyon as it curves south and approaches a tall, veil-like waterfall on the left. The knowledge that you must climb not only to the top of this high falls but well above it is a little discouraging (c'mon legs, you can do it!), but the scenery is terrific and keeps you going. A dozen switchbacks lead you to the trees above the falls, where a poorly signed but obvious path goes left (east) to Lake Flora, the first of many small lakes with feminine names in the Ladies Pass area. From here you go up to a small meadow with a designated horse camp, where you switchback to the right and continue your long uphill trek. Larches, flowers, views, and hoary marmots all abound in this lovely high meadowland. You pass an unsigned and faint way trail that veers off to the right (west) toward Lake Brigham, as your tour continues ever higher through this glorious high country. More switchbacks over heather, scree slopes, and possibly some snowfields finally take you to 6,800-foot Ladies Pass.

Not that you will need any prompting, but drop your pack here and enjoy the vista. Back to the north is the South Fork Chiwaukum Creek Canyon, from which you came. To the immediate east is the pinnacle of Cape Horn. To the south is ruggedly beautiful Grindstone Mountain. Directly below you to the south is the green basin at the head of Spanish Camp Creek, and below that is the deep, green valley of Icicle Creek. Farther south you can see Mount Daniel, the countless icy summits of the Alpine Lakes country, and even a small part of Mount Rainier. If the scenery before was terrific, then I can think of no adequate word to describe what it's like here.

There is a junction with the Icicle Ridge Trail at Ladies Pass. The direct route to continue your loop turns left (east), but to miss out on the side trip to the right (west) would be foolish.

FROSTY PASS SIDE TRIP: So take your lunch and a camera, and wander west around a basin and up to a ridgeline. From here you continue to the side trail that drops to exposed but lovely Upper Florence Lake, where there are good camps (you are required to use designated sites). Beyond this lake you continue west to another small ridge with still more terrific views. Added to the previous views are Mount Stuart and more of Mount Rainier to the south; Glacier Peak, Mount Baker, and numerous lesser summits to the north; and even part of the Olympic Mountains in the distance to the west. If all this doesn't satisfy you, then continue down to Lake Mary and forest-rimmed Lake Margaret. From here it's only a short distance to Frosty Pass and sketchy trails leading to Lake Grace or the distant Doelle Lakes. All in all, you'll find more than enough to fill many happy hours.

To continue with your loop trip, go east from Ladies Pass, climb steeply across the north side of Cape Horn, and then go through a saddle and drop to tiny Lake Edna. The few available camps here are too fragile and exposed for comfort, so spend the night elsewhere.

Your route now drops fairly steeply to a junction, with the popular hiker's trail going south to Chatter Creek. You turn left (southeast) and descend to a second junction with a spur of the same trail. Go straight (east) and follow a sometimes faint and almost always steep trail as it crosses a small creek twice and switchbacks down into the next canyon. The trail bottoms out at a point where you hop across Index Creek to a trail junction. The faint remnants of the Index Creek Trail go to the left (north).

TIP: If you need a campsite, a couple of fair ones are about 50 yards downstream.

Your trail goes straight (southeast) at the Index Creek junction and makes an unrelenting 1,900-foot climb. The now-familiar pattern takes you first through dense forest, then to heather meadows, and finally up to scattered larches amid slopes covered with flowers to a windswept pass with panoramas. The sketchy trail then drops a short way to tiny Carter Lake, which is ringed by meadows and larches and has good camps.

TIP: The shallow waters of Carter Lake warm up much more than other, deeper lakes in this wilderness. Don't miss the opportunity to take a swim here in late summer.

Immediately beyond Carter Lake you bear right (east) at a junction with the Painter Creek Trail, then climb through a couple of wet meadows where the trail is easily lost (look for cairns). Beyond these meadows you make an extremely steep climb to the last high pass of the trip, from which you can look west to the many scenic peaks you've been traveling among over the last few days. From the pass you descend steeply to the scenic basin holding Lake Augusta. This high lake features excellent, if somewhat exposed, camps.

TIP: If the lake is too crowded, good camps are also in the meadows below.

The heavily used trail leading away from Lake Augusta drops through a lovely larch-studded basin, and then contours for a while and climbs in four switchbacks over the ridge on your left. You veer left (northeast) at a ridgetop junction, staying on the much more heavily used Hatchery Creek Trail. This dusty path gradually winds down through attractive open forests and wildflower glades for about 1.5 miles before passing through a small part of the blackened landscape left behind by the Hatchery Fire in 1994. Appropriately, fireweed has colonized this area, adding its pink blossoms to the otherwise rather bleak landscape.

The trail tops a low, meadowy ridge and then descends through unburned forest to a junction with the Badlands Trail. You go straight (north) and switchback down 2,300 feet in three well-graded but very dusty miles to the Hatchery Creek Trailhead. For those with just one car, it's an easy 4.5-mile road walk back to the Chiwaukum Creek Trailhead.

POSSIBLE ITINERARY

	CAMP	MILES	ELEVATION GAIN
Day 1	Chiwaukum Lake	10.8	2,400'
Day 2	Chiwaukum Lake		
	Day hike to Loch Eileen	9.4	1,700'
Day 3	Timothy Meadow	6.2	600'
	Side trip to Larch Lake (morning)	4.4	900'
Day 4	Upper Florence Lake	6.0	3,100'
	Side trip to Frosty Pass	2.8	1,100'
Day 5	Lake Augusta	7.1	3,400'
Day 6	Out	7.9	500'
	(plus 4.5-mile road walk)		

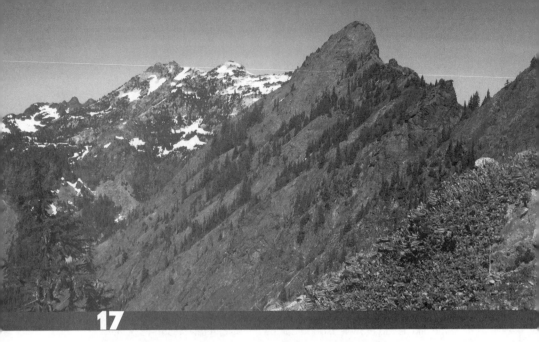

ALPINE LAKES TRAVERSE

RATINGS: Scenery 8   **Solitude** 4   **Difficulty** 6

MILES: 66–76 (85–95)

ELEVATION GAIN: 12,050'–14,750' (15,700'–18,400')

DAYS: 5–9 (6–10)

SHUTTLE MILEAGE: 135

MAP: Trails Illustrated *Alpine Lakes Wilderness (#825)*

USUALLY OPEN: Late July–early October

BEST: Very late July–August

PERMIT: Required. Free and available at the trailhead.

RULES: Maximum group size of 12 people and/or stock; campsites must be at least 200 feet from any lake or stream; fires prohibited above 4,000 feet west of the Cascade Divide and above 5,000 feet east of the divide; fires prohibited within 0.5 mile of Lake Ivanhoe, as well as Deep, Glacier, Hope, Mig, Spectacle, and Upper Park Lakes; designated campsites must be used at Gravel Lake; livestock prohibited within 0.5 mile of Spectacle Lake

CONTACTS: Mount Baker–Snoqualmie National Forest: Snoqualmie Ranger District, 425-888-1421; Skykomish Ranger District, 306-677-2414; fs.usda.gov/main/mbs. Okanogan-Wenatchee National Forest: Cle Elum Ranger District, 509-852-1100; Wenatchee River Ranger District, 509-548-2550; fs.usda.gov/main/okawen

Above: *Red Mountain from the trail up to Kendall Katwalk*
photographed by Douglas Lorain

SPECIAL ATTRACTIONS

Excellent mountain scenery, dozens of beautiful lakes

CHALLENGES

Snow and ice across the trail until midsummer, potentially tricky stream crossings in early summer, relatively crowded

HOW TO GET THERE

Public transportation was formerly available to both ends of this hike. Seattle Transit buses, however, no longer access Snoqualmie Pass, so you'll either need to drive or make other arrangements. One quite reasonable alternative, especially for those flying in from out of town who don't want to rent a car, is to hire a cab at the airport. The drive is fairly short and on the freeway, so the cost is rather reasonable (about $160 one-way plus tip as of 2019). You can also save some money and take the transit bus as far as North Bend (less than $5 as of 2019), then a cab from there to the pass (about $80 as of 2019).

From the ending trailhead at Stevens Pass, you can return to Seattle using Northwestern Trailways (northwesterntrailways.com). There is regular service from the pass to the Seattle bus depot, but reservations are required. As of 2019, the fare was $32 one way from Stevens Pass to Seattle. If you have to change your scheduled day or time, a $20 additional fee applies. Depending on the size of your backpack, you may have to check it as baggage and pay a small fee. Visit the website for more information.

If you are driving yourself, reach the southern (starting) trailhead from Seattle by heading east on I-90 to Snoqualmie Pass and taking Exit 52 for West Summit. Turn left onto WA 906, which takes you under the freeway, and 150 yards later turn right at a small trailhead sign. Drive 0.1 mile and then fork right into the large Pacific Crest Trail hiker's parking lot.

To leave a car at either of the possible northern (ending) trailheads, drive 27 miles north of Seattle on I-5 to Everett. Take Exit 194 and head east on US 2. Drive 58.2 miles, or about 10 miles past the turnoff to Skykomish, to a somewhat obscure junction just past the Iron Goat interpretive site. If you are making the shorter trip that ends at Scenic, then turn right (south) here, drive over a set of railroad tracks, then immediately turn right and proceed 0.3 mile on a rough dirt-and-gravel road to the Surprise Creek Trailhead.

If you plan to do the longer route, continue driving another 6 miles on US 2 to Stevens Pass, where a large parking area lies on the south side of the highway.

NOTE: You'll need a Northwest Forest Pass to park at these trailheads.

GPS TRAILHEAD COORDINATES:

Southern (Snoqualmie Pass): N47° 25.668' W121° 24.810'
Northern (Stevens Pass): N47° 44.772' W121° 05.160'
Alternate (Surprise Creek): N47° 42.468' W121° 09.402'

continued on page 160

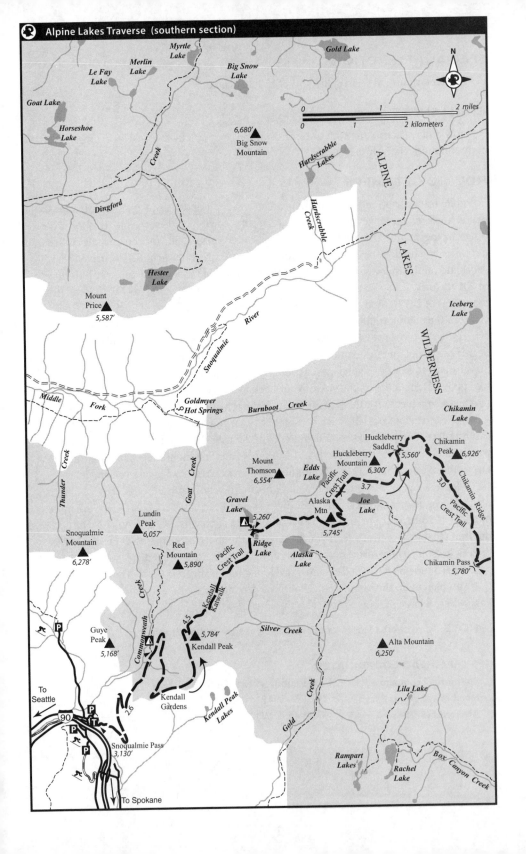

N

0   1   2 miles
0   1   2 kilometers

Le Fay
Lake

Merlin
Lake

Myrtle
Lake

Big Snow
Lake

Gold Lake

Goat Lake

Horseshoe
Lake

Creek

6,680'
Big Snow
Mountain

Hardscrabble
Lakes

ALPINE

Dingford

Hardscrabble
Creek

Hester
Lake

LAKES

Iceberg
Lake

Mount
Price
5,587'

River

Snoqualmie

WILDERNESS

Middle   Fork

Goldmyer
Hot Springs

Burnboot   Creek

Chikamin
Lake

Thunder   Creek

Goat   Creek

Mount
Thomson
6,554'

Edds
Lake

Huckleberry
Mountain
6,300'

Huckleberry
Saddle
5,560'

Chikamin
Peak 6,926'

Lundin
Peak
6,057'

Gravel
Lake
5,260'

Pacific
Crest Trail

3.7

Alaska
Mtn

Joe
Lake

Chikamin
Ridge

Pacific
Crest
Trail

3.0

Snoqualmie
Mountain
6,278'

Red
Mountain
5,890'

Pacific
Crest
Trail

Ridge
Lake

5,745'

Alaska
Lake

Chikamin Pass
5,780'

Commonwealth

Creek

Kendall
Katwalk

.45

5,784'
Kendall Peak

Silver   Creek

Alta Mountain
6,250'

Lila Lake

To
Seattle

Guye
Peak
5,168'

Kendall
Gardens

Kendall Peak
Lakes

Gold   Creek

2.6

90

Snoqualmie Pass
3,130'

Rampart
Lakes

Rachel
Lake

Box Canyon Creek

To Spokane

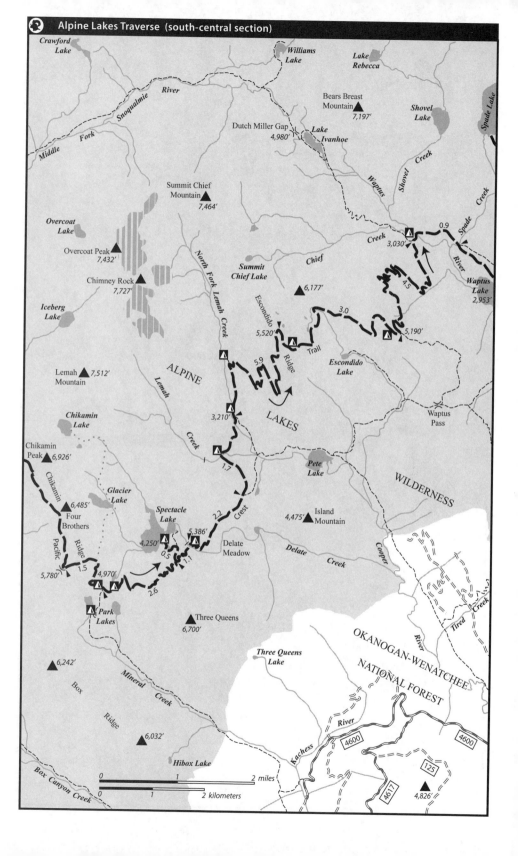

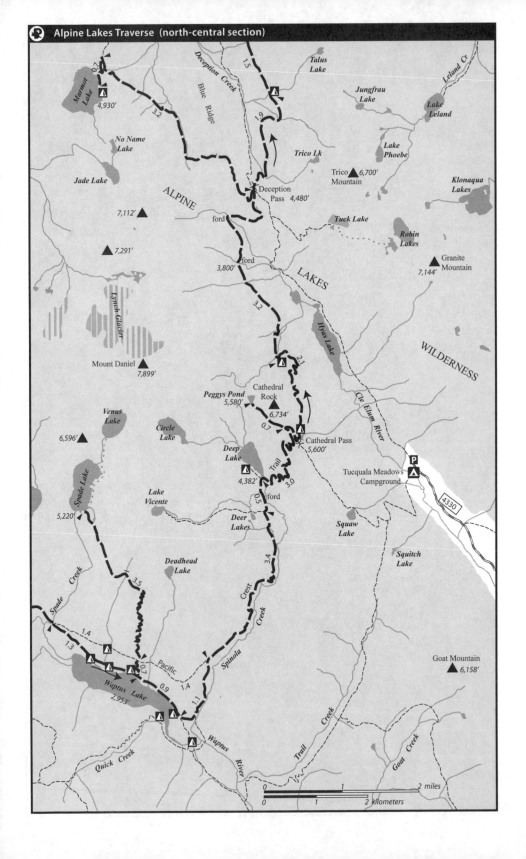

Marmot Lake 4,930'

No Name Lake

Jade Lake

Deception Creek

Blue Ridge

ALPINE

7,112'

7,291'

Lynch Glacier

Mount Daniel 7,899'

Venus Lake

6,596'

Circle Lake

Peggys Pond 5,580'

Deep Lake 4,382'

Lake Vicente

Spade Lake

5,220'

Deadhead Lake

Spade Creek

3.5

1.4

1.3

Pacific

Waptus Lake 2,953'

Quick Creek

Waptus River

Talus Lake

Jungfrau Lake

Leland Cr

Lake Leland

Trico Lk

Lake Phoebe

Deception Pass 4,480'

ford

ford 3,800'

3.2

Trico Mountain 6,700'

Klonaqua Lakes

Tuck Lake

Robin Lakes

Granite Mountain 7,144'

LAKES

Hyas Lake

WILDERNESS

Cathedral Rock 6,734'

0.7

Cathedral Pass 5,600'

Cle Elum River

Tucquala Meadows Campground

P

4330

Trail

3.0

0.5 ford

Deer Lakes

Squaw Lake

Squitch Lake

Crest

Spinola Creek

3.4

Goat Mountain 6,158'

0.9

1.4

1.1

0.7

Waptus

Trail Creek

Goat Creek

0   1   2 miles

0   1   2 kilometers

1.5

1.9

0.7

3.2

2.1

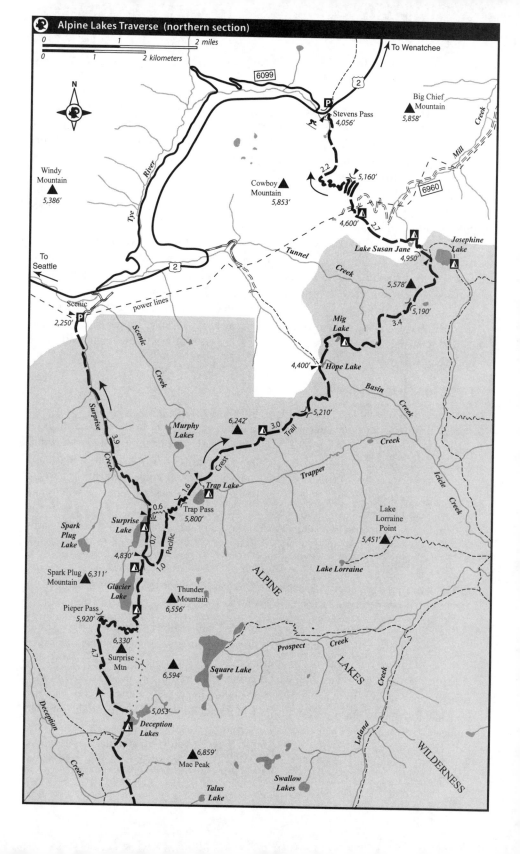

0   1   2 miles
0   1   2 kilometers

N

To Wenatchee

2

6099

P
Stevens Pass
4,056'

Big Chief
Mountain
5,858'

Mill

Creek

Windy
Mountain
5,386'

Cowboy
Mountain
5,853'

2.2

5,160'

6960

4,600'
2.7

Lake Susan Jane
4,950'

Josephine
Lake

Creek

5,578'

5,190'

To
Seattle

2

Scenic
2,250'
P

power lines

Tunnel

Mig
Lake

3.4

Scenic

Creek

4,400'
Hope Lake

Basin

Creek

Surprise

3.9

Murphy
Lakes

6,242'

3.0
5,210'

Trail

Creek

Creek

Trapper

Crest

Spark
Plug
Lake

Surprise
Lake

0.6

1.6
Trap Lake

Trap Pass
5,800'

Lake
Lorraine
Point
5,451'

4,830'

0.7

Pacific

1.0

Spark Plug   6,311'
Mountain

Glacier
Lake

Thunder
Mountain
6,556'

ALPINE

Lake Lorraine

Pieper Pass
5,920'

4.7

6,330'
Surprise
Mtn

6,594'

Square Lake

Prospect   Creek

LAKES

Creek

Deception

5,053'
Deception
Lakes

6,859'
Mac Peak

Talus
Lake

Swallow
Lakes

Leland

Creek

WILDERNESS

Creek

continued from page 155

INTRODUCTION

The large and exceptionally rugged Alpine Lakes Wilderness fills a wide swath of land in the central Washington Cascades and serves as a transition zone between the gentler terrain to the south and the icy crags of the North Cascades. This is a land of heavily forested canyons, ice-sculpted peaks, and enough lakes to make even residents of Minnesota, with its famous 10,000 lakes, envious.

The Pacific Crest Trail (PCT) cuts through the heart of this wilderness, visiting along the way many of the best beauty spots and providing side trips to many more. Close proximity to Seattle and easy access to both the north and south trailheads (you can even do it with public transportation) make this an exceptionally convenient extended backpacking trip, in addition to being an exceptionally beautiful one. The trail isn't easy, with thousands of switchbacks along the way that constantly take you up and over ridges and down into deep valleys, but it's well worth every drop (or gallon) of sweat.

If you are doing this as a car shuttle rather than using the bus for transportation, a shorter alternate ending point is at the old railroad stop of Scenic. This saves at least a full day of hiking on a marginal section of the PCT, and it's pretty in its own right, with some of the best old-growth forests in this part of Washington.

DESCRIPTION

Starting just behind the kiosk at the southeast end of the parking lot, the trail passes a picnic table and 50 yards later reaches a T-junction. The trail to the left (north) is an equestrian spur to the stock trailhead. Go right (east) and begin a well-graded uphill under the shade of old-growth forests composed mainly of tall Douglas firs and droopy western hemlocks. You ascend three long and generally well-graded switchbacks, where many large trees were blown down in a 2011 storm, then make a gentle downhill hike across a talus field, where you'll gather decent views over the Snoqualmie Pass area to the west and north. You cross a small creek just below a pretty waterfall and about 250 yards later come to a signed junction. The Red Mountain Trail, which heads for Commonwealth Basin, veers to the left (north).

> **TIP:** If you got a late start and need a place to camp, you can follow this trail about 0.1 mile to some fair campsites along Commonwealth Creek.

The PCT goes right (northeast) at the junction and begins a moderately steep climb. You soon switchback to the south and reenter dense forest, although you get occasional glimpses of the surrounding rugged country. After another long switchback (get used to switchbacks; you'll encounter thousands on this trip), you break out of the old-growth forest and can really start to appreciate your surroundings. Particularly picturesque vistas highlight the charms of rugged Snoqualmie Mountain to the northwest and the rounded pinnacle of descriptively named Red Mountain to the north. In the distance to the south is the bulky summit of ice-covered Mount Rainier. At your feet, abundant midsummer wildflowers, including lupine, valerian, paintbrush, phlox, penstemon, and columbine, give this area the local nickname of the Kendall Gardens.

The tread narrows as you continue uphill, and you often have to navigate dangerous snowfields that can stick around into August. A final fairly steep uphill takes you over the divide just north of Kendall Peak, where you gain new vistas across the deep valley of Gold Creek to Alta Mountain and Chikamin Peak, among other impressive summits.

Now you head north on the Kendall Katwalk, a narrow section of trail that the builders simply blasted into a steep hillside. The route is airy and spectacularly scenic but not suitable for those with a fear of heights. It *is* suitable for lovers of great views, however, as they are here in abundance. Throughout this exposed section, the path maintains a northerly heading, staying high and not far below the rugged ridgeline on your left. You round a minor ridge, from which you can look down to large Alaska Lake, then drop slightly to a saddle at 7.1 miles between small Ridge Lake on the right (south) and narrow Gravel Lake on the left (north). Camping is prohibited at Ridge Lake, but there are good sites at Gravel Lake, where you are required to set up your tent at designated locations.

The northbound PCT traverses rocky slopes, making a long loop high above Alaska Lake, then climbs to go around the narrow eastern ridge of Alaska Mountain. From here a set of rather steep switchbacks descends a north-facing slope that often holds snow well into August. At the bottom of this descent, you go through a forested saddle above deep and oblong-shaped Joe Lake. The trail turns east to cross the steep, open slope above Joe Lake, then rounds a ridge and takes you through a lovely meadow-covered glen with wildflowers, a small creek, views galore, and a couple of small ponds. Camping is prohibited in this vicinity to protect the fragile environment.

Just past this grassy paradise, you walk through wide Huckleberry Saddle, then ascend mini switchbacks to a high viewpoint before turning southeast and making an extended and very scenic traverse across the slopes above the headwaters of Gold Creek. Marmots whistle at your approach, and your head will be on a swivel, taking in all the views of the many nearby rugged peaks and the distant dome of Mount Rainier. The jagged line of Chikamin Ridge rises on your left (east). Near the end of this traverse, a minor uphill leads to the gap at Chikamin Pass, from which you'll have fine views looking east across the basin holding the Park Lakes to cliff-edged Three Queens and the distant and distinctive spires of Mount Stuart.

You cross a steep slope, then come to a relatively flat area, where you may see a faint boot route going left (north) on its way to Glacier Lake and stark Chikamin Lake (a great side trip for experienced hikers, but only in good weather). The PCT then makes a few lazy switchbacks down to some no-fire campsites (the first since Gravel Lake) and a junction with Mineral Creek Trail, which goes right (south) and drops to campsites at the Park Lakes.

Your route stays left (east) on the PCT and soon passes a spur trail to more no-fire campsites near Upper Park Lake on your left (north). From here you ascend a couple of switchbacks, taking you well above the shimmering Park Lakes; pass a pair of shallow ponds; then top a ridge radiating to the northwest from Three Queens. Looking to the north, you can see the irregular shape of Spectacle Lake far below, with the almost unbelievably contorted pinnacles, cliffs, and glaciers of Lemah Mountain in the background.

Brace your knees because next up is a toe-jamming festival of short switchbacks leading down to the basin of Spectacle Lake and Delate Creek. After about 1.6 miles of this tedious and tiring downhill, you reach a junction.

SPECTACLE LAKE SIDE TRIP: A must-see side trip goes left (northwest) here and, a short distance later, presents you with a wide vista across the glorious basin of Spectacle Lake. It's easy to see how this huge mountain gem got its name, as the spectacle looking across the waters to the dramatic sharp summit of Lemah Mountain to the northwest and the more rounded but no less beautiful views of Chikamin Peak to the west is superb. Several waterfalls tumble down to the lake from the heights above. The trail steeply drops some 200 feet in 0.4 mile over roots and rocks to the shoreline, where a maze of social trails leads to hidden nooks and crannies for private viewing. Much of the shoreline is rather steep, limiting the best campsites to those on a peninsula that juts far out into the lake from the southeast shore.

From the Spectacle Lake turnoff, the PCT goes down 17 more switchbacks, then crosses a wooden bridge over Delate Creek in the middle of a thunderous and very photogenic waterfall. You then pass a campsite and descend another dozen gentle switchbacks before finally concluding the infernal zigzagging. You then make a gradual downhill trek through woods burned in a 2009 fire to a junction with the Pete Lake Trail. Keep left (north) on the PCT, and go around the base of a small, forested knoll to a bridge over rampaging Lemah Creek. A nice campsite beckons on the north side of this crossing.

A mostly level traverse through forest leads to a bridged crossing of North Fork Lemah Creek and a junction where you stay left (north).

As you have undoubtedly noticed by now, this is a trail with lots of big ups and downs, so I hope you're ready for another up because here it comes. It starts gently as you pass a very good campsite along North Fork Lemah Creek, then gradually veer away from this stream. At the first major switchback, an unofficial use trail goes straight (north) and drops to another nice campsite on the creek.

The PCT soon returns to its obsession with switchbacks as you climb irregularly spaced turns up the southwest flanks of Escondido Ridge. The mostly well-graded climb is usually dry and can be hot, so it's best to tackle this in the cool of the morning. As you gain elevation, the views of Lemah Mountain, Chimney Rock, and other scenic peaks grow ever more impressive. As you near the top, the forest thins and the wildflowers and views become outstanding, especially looking east to towering Mount Stuart and west to the cliffs and glaciers of Lemah Mountain. From here you drop briefly from a high point to a small pond, where camping is prohibited. Fortunately, tired hikers have a nearby option because, only about 0.3 mile farther, you reach some designated campsites on a partly forested hillside.

The trail rounds a point, then comes to a second basin, this time with a string of beautiful alpine tarns and scenic rock outcrops. Camping is not allowed here, in order to protect the fragile ecosystem. After an extended traverse, you reach a basin with water shortly before you come to the edge of a ridgeline and a junction with the Waptus Burn Trail. Your route continues north.

Now it's back to switchbacks as you soak in the outstanding views looking northeast to the glacier-covered summits of distant Mounts Daniel and Hinman. Closer at hand, just across the deep abyss filled by Waptus River and Waptus Lake, rises the sharp pinnacle of Bears Breast Mountain. The downhill, often on brushy slopes, seems to go on forever, as a total of 24 well-graded turns lead toward the valley floor. As you near the bottom, a switchback opens up to a view of a nice little waterfall just west of the trail. Once on flatter ground near the valley floor, you go through brushy areas overhung by enormous bracken ferns, then hop over a seasonal creek and come to a nice campsite beside a junction. The trail to the left (northwest) climbs to popular and attractive Lake Ivanhoe.

Keep straight (north) on the PCT and 0.1 mile later reach a bridge over the rampaging Waptus River. From here a lazy stroll through forest for 0.8 mile leads to a bridge across Spade Creek and immediately thereafter a junction.

The PCT veers left (northeast), staying on a forested hillside well above Waptus Lake. But having come this far, you'll surely want to at least visit and probably camp near this huge and very beautiful wilderness lake, so bear right (southeast) and make a gentle downhill hike to reach the shoreline. The path follows the northern shore of this almost 2-mile-long lake and passes the side trip option to Spade Lake (described below) and several nice campsites along the way. Camps are usually located where an inlet creek drops down the wooded hillside on your left. The most scenic (and popular) campsites are at the lake's east end near the outlet. From this spot you'll wake up to terrific views looking down the length of huge Waptus Lake to the pointed summits of Bears Breast and Summit Chief Mountains.

SPADE LAKE SIDE TRIP: A little more than halfway down the shore of Waptus Lake, or 0.9 mile up from the east-end campsites, is a signed junction. To visit outstandingly beautiful Spade Lake, turn uphill (north) here and begin a wickedly steep ascent on a hiker-only trail. Old-growth western hemlocks and Douglas firs shade the early part of this punishing route. That shade is a blessing because you'll sweat gallons as you push your way uphill on interminable switchbacks. After just 0.7 mile, you cross the PCT and keep climbing, as the trail eventually curves to the northwest. You cross a small creek just below an impressive little waterfall, and finally level out as you traverse an open hillside with tremendous views looking west to the spire of Bears Breast Mountain. You walk past a small pond and finally come to the rocky shores of Spade Lake. You're to be forgiven for wondering if this would all be worth it while you were hiking up that trail, but such doubts are immediately forgotten at the destination. This large and quite deep mountain gem is surrounded by granite mounds, snowy peaks, and talus slopes, and picturesque peninsulas jut into its clear waters. On a scale of scenic beauty, precious few lakes in the Pacific Northwest are in the same class as Spade Lake. Camping here is not recommended, mostly because sane people would rather not haul their heavy packs up that trail. If you want to see more of this remarkable terrain, and you somehow still have extra energy, then circle around the east side of Spade Lake and scramble up to austere Venus Lake, which sits directly beneath the cliffs and snowfields of Mount Daniel.

About 0.2 mile beyond the camps at the east end of Waptus Lake is a junction with Spinola Creek Trail. Bear left (east then north) on this route, and hike 1.1 miles up the trail's namesake creek to a reunion with the PCT. From here it's a steady climb with scattered switchbacks as you make your way up the long valley of Spinola Creek. The terrain consists of a pleasant mix of meadows, forest, and rocky slopes, and there are nice views up to the ridges enclosing this narrow canyon. After 3.1 miles, you cross a small tributary creek amid subalpine meadowland, then go straight (north) where the faint Lake Vicente

Trail branches to the left (west). Soon after this junction, you pass a campsite, then come to a cold ford of the outlet creek for Lake Vicente. Just beyond this ford is Deep Lake. A rocky butte southeast of Mount Daniel towers over this teardrop-shaped lake, making for excellent scenery. If you are looking to spend the night (no fires allowed), the best campsites are along a dead-end side trail that goes up the lake's southwest shore.

You make an ankle-deep wade across Spinola Creek where it pours out of Deep Lake, then begin a long climb on well-graded switchbacks. Views improve as the tree cover lessens, giving you nice perspectives of the east side of tall Mount Daniel. After gaining 1,200 feet, you reach a junction at a switchback.

> **PEGGYS POND SIDE TRIP:** For a scenic break from all that climbing, turn left (northwest) at this junction. Take a narrow and rugged trail that first contours under the towering cliffs of Cathedral Rock, then goes up a little valley on open slopes to Peggys Pond. I don't have any idea who Peggy was, but she must have won beauty contests because her pond is spectacular. Perky subalpine firs and mountain hemlocks dot the steep shoreline, which displays abundant wildflowers in midsummer and outstanding fall colors in October. Towering over the entire scene is the huge blocky mass of andesite that is Cathedral Rock, an unmistakable landmark in this part of the Alpine Lakes Wilderness. The whole package makes Peggys Pond an ideal lunch spot.

From the Peggys Pond junction, the PCT makes its way out to a final switchback to reach a junction at Cathedral Pass, where there are great views up to the monster rock formation of Cathedral Rock to the northwest. Looking southeast, you can see the tall pyramid of

Kendall Katwalk
photographed by Douglas Lorain

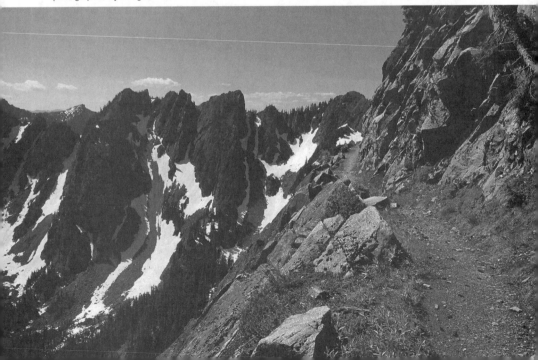

distant Mount Stuart. You go left (north) and drop briefly to a meadow-covered bench with a couple of seasonal ponds and a larger more reliable pond, which has scenic campsites.

The northbound PCT now traverses the east side of Cathedral Rock, tops a little ridge, and then begins going steadily downhill, first in a series of very short switchbacks, then in two longer turns to reach a meadow-covered basin. A couple of good campsites are located at this pleasant location. Still losing elevation, the trail takes you down forested slopes to a pair of creek crossings, the second of which can be wet and difficult in high water. This marks the low point of this section; from here you gain elevation, crossing avalanche chutes and traveling through dense conifer forests. After an easy ford of the headwaters of Cle Elum River, you ascend through a forest of large subalpine firs to reach a five-way junction at Deception Pass.

> **MARMOT LAKE SIDE TRIP:** A lengthy but commensurately rewarding side trip from Deception Pass takes you to Marmot Lake. To reach it, turn sharply left (southwest) at the pass onto the Lake Clarice Trail and descend 1.3 miles to a meadow-covered cirque basin with a small pond and nice views up to Mount Daniel. From there you descend through forest, then make a gentle climb over slopes with lots of huckleberries. These plants offer tasty treats in late summer and acres of red fall foliage in October. At 3.2 miles from Deception Pass is a junction. Turn left (south) and climb a set of switchbacks to reach large Marmot Lake, which has campsites, a forested shoreline, fine fishing and swimming, and partially obstructed views of Mount Daniel.

Continuing your northerly trip on the PCT (go north-northeast from the junction), you descend around a little butte to cross the headwaters of Deception Creek in a badly eroded ditch, then contour across a hillside with nice views to the southwest of Lynch Glacier shimmering on the side of the long, bumpy ridge of Mount Daniel. After rounding a ridge, you hop over a creek, then hike another 0.3 mile to a campsite beside the small stream feeding down from Talus Lake.

From here an extended slightly uphill traverse takes you across a slope, still recovering from an old forest fire, to a junction with a spur trail coming up from Deception Creek. Keep right (northeast), soon cross a creek, and then reach the lowest of the three Deception Lakes. Although not wildly scenic, this lovely basin with its large marshy lakes is very attractive, with nice campsites and views up to the rounded summit of Surprise Mountain and a second unnamed butte to the north. The beauty and relatively easy access to these lakes make them quite popular, so expect plenty of company and overused campsites.

Still not finished with your steady climb of the mostly forested hillside above the Deception Creek Valley, you leave the Deception Lakes and ascend in long traverses and scattered switchbacks to Pieper Pass, with its nice views looking west to Three Fingers, Baring Mountain, and the heavily clear-cut valley of Tye River. In the basin to the northeast lies Glacier Lake. On very clear days you can see the snowy pinnacle of Glacier Peak far to the north.

Knee-rattling switchbacks lead down from Pieper Pass and take you past a couple of pretty little benches before finally reaching a campsite just before the crossing of a tiny creek high above the southeast shore of Glacier Lake. The trail stays above this large lake, crosses a talus slope, and reaches an unsigned junction with a steep use trail that drops to a campsite on the northeast shore of Glacier Lake. Even if you don't need to set up your tent for the night, it's worth the short side trip to visit this spot because this lake is very scenic, with the talus slopes of Spark Plug Mountain rising above the west shore and pointed Surprise Mountain visible to the south. No fires are allowed in this basin.

Just beyond Glacier Lake the PCT passes a shallow tarn on the right (east) and comes to a junction.

The remainder of the PCT north to Stevens Pass is pleasant but generally lacks the dramatic scenery you have enjoyed for the last several days. If you're using the bus for transportation, then you will have to hike that way because bus service is only available at that location. If you are using a car shuttle, however, it saves 9 miles of hiking on the PCT if you leave the northbound route at the junction below Glacier Lake and exit via the Surprise Creek Trail instead.

EXIT VIA SURPRISE CREEK TRAIL: For the shorter alternative, keep left (downhill and north) at the junction, and descend along the top of a little ridgecrest for 0.7 mile to the designated campsites beside lovely Surprise Lake. You soon cross a creek and pass a small marshy area, then go straight (north) at a junction and steeply descend on a poorly engineered trail with lots of roots and rocks. You travel through forest and over talus slopes to the banks of Surprise Creek, after which things get much easier and more pleasant as the trail takes you along this tumbling stream. The river music is nice, but an even better feature of this trail is the magnificent cathedral forests of old-growth western hemlocks and western red cedars. These are the most impressive trees along this trip and some of the last great trees still standing in this part of Washington. About 2.7 miles below Surprise Lake, you cross Surprise Creek on a log, and finish the route on easy trail to the trailhead at Scenic.

Those taking the longer exit route to Stevens Pass should go right (southeast) at the junction near Glacier Lake and loop around the headwaters of a small creek. You then make an uphill traverse, with good views down to Surprise Lake far below, and reach a junction with the Trap Pass Trail. Turn right (east) and climb a series of mostly short, steep switchbacks to the Cascade Divide at 5,800-foot Trap Pass.

Below and to the east of this pass sits Trap Lake, a sparkling oasis. The trail skirts around the lake in a series of switchbacks and traverses high on the walls above the water. You pass a very steep and unofficial access trail that drops to the north shore of the lake, but you keep straight (northeast) on the PCT and cross partly forested slopes and open areas with plenty of midsummer wildflowers. You come to a little basin with a possible campsite, then go up and down for a couple of attractive but uneventful miles before dropping to a junction beside small Hope Lake. Fires are prohibited near this heavily used lake. Continue northeast. Just 0.7 mile later the PCT reaches Mig Lake, where fires are also off-limits, but you'll find good campsites and fine places to take a swim.

From Mig Lake the PCT takes you past a shallow pond before ascending rather steeply to a forested saddle. You then contour around an eastward-trending ridge and drop to a junction on a bench with lots of tiny tarns. Circular Josephine Lake fills the basin on your right. If you turn right (northeast) at this junction, you'll gradually descend view-packed slopes to the shores of this pretty lake, where you'll find several good campsites.

TIP: These campsites are more plentiful and generally nicer than the ones at Lake Susan Jane, not far ahead on the PCT.

The PCT keeps left (northwest) at the junction above Josephine Lake and takes you through a woodsy saddle before descending to small Lake Susan Jane, which sits in a rocky cirque.

The remainder of the trip lacks scenic appeal as you contour across open slopes above the headwaters of Mill Creek and cross a rough dirt road under a set of power lines. From here you climb long switchbacks to a high ridge, then descend in twists and turns past ski runs and under ski lifts to the Stevens Pass Trailhead.

VARIATION

As mentioned previously, you can shorten this route by exiting via the Surprise Creek Trail.

POSSIBLE ITINERARY

	CAMP	MILES	ELEVATION GAIN
Day 1	Gravel Lake	7.1	2,800'
Day 2	Spectacle Lake	11.3	1,350'
Day 3	Basin north of Escondido Ridge	11.7	2,800'
Day 4	East end of Waptus Lake	10.1	200'
Day 5	East end of Waptus Lake		
	Day hike to Spade Lake	9.8	2,400'
Day 6	Basin north of Cathedral Rock	10.3	2,700'
	Side trip to Peggys Pond	1.4	150'
Day 7	Talus Lake outlet creek	5.1	450'
	Side trip to Marmot Lake	7.8	1,100'
	via Shorter Route:		
Day 8	Out to Surprise Creek Trailhead	10.8	1,750'
	via Longer Route:		
Day 8	Mig Lake	12.5	3,250'
Day 9	Out to Stevens Pass	7.6	1,200'

BEST SHORTER ALTERNATIVES

At the start of this hike, the popular trail to Kendall Katwalk is a rewarding day hike sampler. For a shorter backpacking trip, try hiking in to Waptus Lake along trails from the east. Set up a base camp here and take day hikes to great destinations like Spade Lake, Deep Lake, and Lake Ivanhoe.

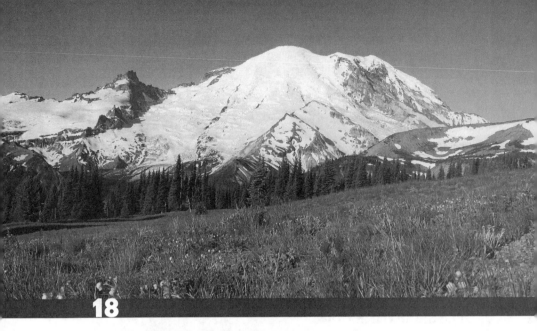

18

NORTHERN MOUNT RAINIER LOOP

RATINGS: Scenery 8 **Solitude** 3 **Difficulty** 5
MILES: 36 (49)
ELEVATION GAIN: 9,300' (13,050')
DAYS: 3–5 (4–6)
SHUTTLE MILEAGE: n/a
MAP: Earthwalk Press *Hiking Map & Guide: Mount Rainier National Park*
USUALLY OPEN: Mid-July–October
BEST: Late July–September
PERMIT: Required. Approximately 70% of permits are available for reserva-
tion, with the rest given out on a first-come, first-served basis. Reservation
requests for the summer hiking season can only be made online, beginning
March 15; a $20 nonrefundable fee applies to reserved permits. Walk-up
permits can be obtained on the first day of the trip or up to one day before.
See nps.gov/mora/planyourvisit/wilderness-permit.htm for full details.
Pick up permits (whether reserved in advance or a walk-up permit) from a
wilderness information center or ranger station.
RULES: Trailside camping is allowed only at designated sites; dogs are prohib-
ited; maximum of 5 people per campsite; fires prohibited
CONTACT: Mount Rainier National Park, White River Wilderness Information
Center, 360-569-6670, nps.gov/mora

Above: *Mount Rainier from the trail just north of Sunrise Day Lodge*
photographed by Douglas Lorain

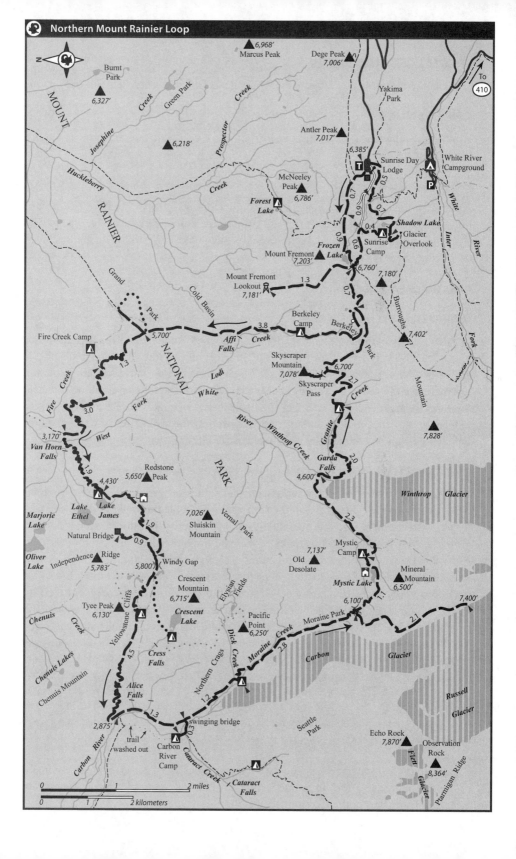

N

MOUNT

RAINIER

NATIONAL

PARK

To
410

Burnt
Park
6,327'

Green Park

Marcus Peak
6,968'

Dege Peak
7,006'

Yakima
Park

6,218'

Antler Peak
7,017'

6,385'

Sunrise Day
Lodge

White River
Campground

Josephine

Huckleberry

Prospector Creek

Green Park Creek

Creek

McNeeley
Peak
6,786'

*Forest
Lake*

0.7

0.5

0.9

0.7

Shadow Lake
Glacier
Overlook

White

*Frozen
Lake*

0.9

0.6

0.4

Sunrise
Camp

Inter

River

Mount Fremont
7,203'

Grand

Park

Cold Basin

Affi
Falls

Creek

Lodi

White

Fork

River

Winthrop Creek

Berkeley

0.9

6,760'

7,180'

0.7

Mount Fremont
Lookout
7,181'

1.3

Berkeley
Camp

3.8

Burroughs

7,402'

Fork

Mountain

7,828'

Fire Creek Camp

1.3

3.0

Fire Creek

West

*Van Horn
Falls*

3,170'

1.9

4,430'

Redstone
Peak
5,650'

Skyscraper
Mountain
7,078'

6,700'

Skyscraper
Pass

2.7

Granite Creek

*Garda
Falls*
4,600'

2.0

2.3

Winthrop Glacier

*Marjorie
Lake*

Lake
Ethel

Lake
James

1.9

Natural Bridge

0.9

7,026'
Sluiskin
Mountain

Vernal Park

7,137'
Old
Desolate

Mystic
Camp

Mystic Lake

Mineral
Mountain
6,500'

7,400'

*Oliver
Lake*

Independence Ridge
5,783'

Windy Gap
5,800'

Crescent
Mountain
6,715'

Elysian
Fields

6,100'

1.1

*Chenuis
Creek*

Tyee Peak
6,130'

Yellowstone Cliffs

*Crescent
Lake*

4.5

*Cress
Falls*

Pacific
Point
6,250'

Moraine Creek

Moraine Park

2.8

Carbon

2.1

Glacier

*Russell
Glacier*

Chenuis Lakes

Chenuis Mountain

*Alice
Falls*

Northern Crags

Dick Creek

1.2

Seattle
Park

Echo Rock
7,870'

Observation
Rock
8,364'

Flett Glacier

2,875'

trail
washed out

1.3

swinging bridge

0.3

Carbon River
Camp

Carbon River

Cataract Creek

*Cataract
Falls*

Ptarmigan Ridge

0   1   2 miles

0   1   2 kilometers

SPECIAL ATTRACTIONS

A scenic but shorter alternative to the Wonderland Trail, many excellent side trip options

CHALLENGES

Snagging a permit for this trip can be difficult; black bears and mosquitoes require the usual precautions

HOW TO GET THERE

From Sumner head east on WA 410, and go about 50 miles to the northeast part of Mount Rainier National Park. Turn right (southwest) onto White River Road, following signs to Sunrise, and proceed 15.5 miles to the huge road-end parking lot and trailhead next to Sunrise Day Lodge.

GPS TRAILHEAD COORDINATES: N46° 54.852′ W121° 38.538′

INTRODUCTION

Pairing an exceptionally scenic section of the famous Wonderland Trail with the lesser known but also very scenic Northern Loop Trail, this hike makes a fun loop in the northern part of Mount Rainier National Park. It's an excellent alternative for hikers looking to experience the mountain's many charms but who lack the time or ambition to tackle the entire Wonderland Trail (see Trip 19). The shorter overall distance also allows hikers more time to check out the many superb side trips along the way, visiting several of Mount Rainier's outstanding but usually overlooked backcountry gems.

DESCRIPTION

From the northwest end of the parking lot, pick up a heavily traveled trail that heads up the slope toward the ridge to the north. After about 0.15 mile this trail splits and you take the left (west) branch, soon reaching the ridgetop and another junction. Go left again, following the view-packed ridgeline to the west as you travel through sloping meadows filled with wildflowers and around a small promontory along the ridge. At 0.7 mile you go straight (west) at a junction, and then contour along the south side of the ridge to Frozen Lake. This stark body of water, fenced off from public access, is used as a water source for Sunrise Day Lodge. A short walk across open alpine slopes leads to a five-way junction at a pass. The recommended return route to Sunrise at the end of the loop goes downhill to the left (east).

> **MOUNT FREMONT LOOKOUT SIDE TRIP:** For a particularly impressive view of Mount Rainier, turn right (north) at the junction onto the trail to Mount Fremont Lookout. This path climbs a bit, then follows a high, up-and-down ridgeline to the north. After 1.3 miles you reach the staffed lookout facility on a ridge north of Mount Fremont. The location offers superb vistas southwest over the rolling expanse of Berkeley Park to the massive bulk of ice-covered Mount Rainier.

Back at the five-way junction, go west on the Wonderland Trail as this path gradually descends 0.7 mile to a fork in the upper parts of the rolling meadowlands of Berkeley Park. This is the start of the recommended loop.

BERKELEY PARK POND SIDE TRIP: For a quick break, drop your heavy pack here and wander across the trailless tundra to the north about 200 yards to an unnamed pond. Looking across this shallow body of water, you'll enjoy fine reflections of the top third of Mount Rainier.

For a counterclockwise loop, bear right (north) on the Northern Loop Trail, and continue descending through wildflower-covered meadows, making a long switchback toward the defile holding Lodi Creek. The trail goes downstream beside this clear creek as you enter increasingly forested terrain and reach attractive Berkeley Camp. This is a pleasant place to spend the night near a small meadow and beneath the crags of Skyscraper Mountain to the west.

The trail continues along Lodi Creek another 0.6 mile, then climbs away from the water just above unseen and hard-to-reach Affi Falls. A little more intermittent uphill takes you to the spectacular meadowy expanse of Grand Park. This large and remarkably flat meadow is unusual in a region where nearly all of the landscape is dramatically up and down. The reason for this is that the meadow sits atop an old basalt flow, whose sides have not yet eroded away into the steep slopes and canyons found elsewhere in the park. The trail skirts the southwest side of Grand Park and comes to a junction.

GRAND PARK SIDE TRIP: The trail to the right (northeast) crosses Grand Park on its way to remote Lake Eleanor. Although that lake is pretty, going that far really isn't necessary. What you will definitely want to do, however, is to wander north about 0.5 mile, then explore off-trail through the expansive grassy wonderland of Grand Park. For photographers, a particular feature to look for is a tiny shallow pond near the south end of the park that offers postcard-perfect reflections of Mount Rainier.

The Northern Loop Trail goes left (northwest) at Grand Park, climbs briefly over a knoll, and then reenters forest. About 0.3 mile from the junction, things open up at a stunning viewpoint of Mount Rainier and jagged Sluiskin Mountain rising majestically over the depths of West Fork White River Canyon. Past this viewpoint it's all downhill and all in forest, as 13 moderately steep switchbacks take you to the junction with the 0.35-mile spur trail to Fire Creek Camp. This camp is not particularly scenic, but it is shady and has reliable water from a trickling creek.

The main trail keeps heading downhill in forest, utilizing 22 irregularly spaced switchbacks along its moderately steep, winding course. Eventually you reach a point just above the West Fork White River, and then parallel that river downstream 0.5 mile to a junction with a long-abandoned trail. Go left (west) and soon hike through a boulder-strewn floodplain, crossing the river's silt-laden flow on a log bridge. Just across the log bridge is pretty Van Horn Falls, which you can reach with a bit of scrambling through thickets of thorn-covered devils club plants.

As you might expect, now an extended uphill begins. There are no views, but the forest provides welcome shade, as approximately 25 mostly short and generally quite steep switchbacks take you up to a junction with the short side trail to Lake James Camp. The camps here are comfortable. For a better view across the water, continue straight on the

Northern Loop Trail another 150 yards, cross a bridge over the lake's inlet creek, and come to an unmarked side trail. This path goes to an attractive spot on the shore of the lake, although no camping is allowed here. The shallow lake, surrounded by forested ridges, has no views of Mount Rainier, but it is tranquil and very pretty.

The Northern Loop Trail quickly pulls away from Lake James, ascending four switchbacks in 0.4 mile to a junction with the 0.2-mile spur trail to the Lake James Ranger Cabin. Go straight, and continue zigzagging uphill. Once the switchbacks end, you leave the forest and ascend a lovely rolling meadowland with excellent views of nearby Sluiskin and Crescent Mountains. This area has some of the densest concentrations of huckleberries in the park, so be prepared for a feast from mid-August to mid-September.

WARNING: All those berries also attract black bears, which are often encountered here during the same period.

About 0.15 mile before you finally top out at Windy Gap, you will reach a junction.

NATURAL BRIDGE SIDE TRIP: To visit one of Mount Rainier's more interesting backcountry highlights, turn right (northeast) at the junction and hike mostly downhill through meadows. The gentle section eventually ends with 10 short switchbacks taking you to an overlook just above a large rock arch. It's hard to photograph this geologic landmark, but the view past the arch down to clear Lake James and greenish Lake Ethel is very nice.

Back on the Northern Loop Trail, you soon top out at Windy Gap, where there are several ponds and a particularly pretty shallow lakelet reflecting the bulky ramparts of Crescent Mountain. At the west end of this lakelet, an unsigned boot path goes left (west-southwest).

CRESCENT LAKE SIDE TRIP: To visit large and quite scenic Crescent Lake, bear left on the unofficial boot path. This sometimes-sketchy route takes you around a ridge, then drops to the western shore of deep Crescent Lake. With an off-trail camping permit, you can spend the night at a little-used campsite here. Only the most experienced cross-country hikers should consider going beyond Crescent Lake, but those up for a very tough challenge can scramble over a ridge south of Crescent Lake. From there you go south and very steeply downhill (be extremely careful) to the scenic and remote marshy flat (a haven for millions of frogs) called Elysian Fields. In addition to its wonderful views, this is a great place to listen to bugling elk in September. For an additional goal, you can keep going on a short, rocky climb west to Pacific Point, which features one of the best but least-visited views of Mount Rainier in the park.

Heading west from Windy Gap, the Northern Loop Trail descends a dozen switchbacks through gorgeous meadows to Yellowstone Cliffs Camp. This spot offers excellent views to the north of the line of impressive cliffs and spires forming the Yellowstone Cliffs. The remarkably diverse and interesting vegetation in this meadow includes such attractive flora as bear grass, huckleberries, heather, and numerous wildflowers.

The loop continues west, gradually descending through a series of small meadows, then plunging down 21 waterless and moderately steep switchbacks that take you down the southern slopes of Chenuis Mountain. The knee-jarring but shady descent ends at the bottom of the Carbon River Canyon and a junction. To the right (southwest) a short trail takes you to a seasonal log bridge over the silty Carbon River and a junction with the Wonderland Trail. Until recent years, the official Wonderland Trail went left (south) and followed the west side of the Carbon River up to Carbon River Camp. That section of the Wonderland Trail has been repeatedly washed out, however, and the National Park Service has now officially closed this route.

Instead, go straight (south) at the junction with the trail across the Carbon River, and follow a maintained path that crosses the hillside east of the river. This route is mostly forested, but it does offer a few decent views of the river and the nearby ridges. After 1.3 miles you come to a junction beside a swinging suspension bridge over the Carbon River. If you are spending the night at Carbon River Camp, you'll have to cross (one hiker at a time, please) this very narrow, bouncing, and rather frightening bridge and then walk approximately 0.2 mile west to a junction. Turn right (north), almost immediately cross Cataract Creek, and walk down the old Wonderland Trail 0.1 mile to Carbon River Camp. As mentioned previously, the trail north of this camp is abandoned.

To continue the loop, go straight (south) at the junction just before the Carbon River bridge and settle in for a long, steep climb. It begins easily enough with a pleasant stroll through forest, but you soon leave this welcome shade and climb a very steep and rocky tread on the slopes immediately adjoining the Carbon Glacier. As always, stay off the unstable ice, which is covered with rocks and full of crevasses and other hazards. Above the ice, the trail ascends a slope fully exposed to the hot afternoon sun, so try to hike this section in the cool of the morning. A pair of new and relatively gentle switchbacks detours around a washed-out area, then it's back to the steep climb on the rocky, open slope. You finally catch a break when you cross a log bridge over rushing Dick Creek and reach small but scenic Dick Creek Camp, located on a rock outcrop directly overlooking the ice of Carbon Glacier.

After the camp, 11 more steep switchbacks take you up to pretty Moraine Creek and a gentler section of trail for 0.5 mile along this stream's banks. The terrain starts to open up as you pass through a series of

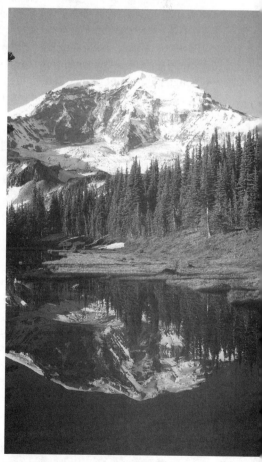

Mount Rainier and a pond above Mystic Lake
photographed by Douglas Lorain

lovely subalpine meadows, carpeted with numerous types of wildflowers in midsummer. Another set of four switchbacks and you finally reach Moraine Park, a rolling meadowland with lots of whistling hoary marmots and fine views looking southwest to Observation Rock and Ptarmigan Ridge. Leaving Moraine Park, the long uphill finishes as you huff your way up 10 more switchbacks to a 6,100-foot pass.

> **TIP:** A shallow pond on the west side of the trail provides the ideal foreground for tremendously photogenic views of Mount Rainier, with the towering face of enormous Willis Wall filling your camera's viewfinder.

> **WILLIS WALL VIEWPOINT SIDE TRIP:** Adventurous hikers won't want to pass up a side trip to a close-up look at Willis Wall. To do this, pick up an unofficial but easy-to-follow use trail that circles the pond then climbs to the south. You pass the first excellent viewpoint after only 0.8 mile, but keep going because, another 1.3 miles of rocky travel later, you'll come to an even better spot directly above Carbon Glacier. The only downside is that two of your body parts may be jeopardized here: the views up to Willis Wall are both neck-craning and jaw-dropping.

Back at the pass, the Wonderland Trail rapidly descends five switchbacks to a little valley, and then goes over a small ridge to reach the shores of meadow-rimmed Mystic Lake. Although glimpses of Mount Rainier are blocked by nearby Mineral Mountain, there are good views looking north across the water to Old Desolate. This lake makes a lovely spot to rest or eat lunch.

After rounding the south side of Mystic Lake, you keep straight where a side trail goes left to the Mystic Patrol Cabin. Just 0.2 mile later is the turnoff to Mystic Camp. This spot is popular with both backpackers and black bears, so don't expect much privacy, and be careful with your food. Mosquitoes are also abundant until about mid-August, so you may have to deal with them as well.

About 0.2 mile beyond Mystic Camp, you cross West Fork White River on a log, then turn downstream, following this clear and cascading creek. After another 0.2 mile you jog to the right, cross another creek in a rocky gully, and then go gradually downhill through forest before breaking out into a rocky wasteland left behind by the rapidly retreating Winthrop Glacier. Small pioneering trees are starting to take hold in this recently icy area, which offers good views to the east of feathery Garda Falls and the rugged pinnacles of Burroughs Mountain. Looking south, you are also treated to impressive looks at the wide icy mass of Mount Rainier. After completing your descent, you cross the glacial flow of Winthrop Creek on a log bridge.

A brief climb above the bridge takes you to a log spanning Granite Creek immediately below the lower portion of Garda Falls. On a warm afternoon, the cooling spray from this cartwheeling waterfall is quite refreshing.

After Garda Falls the route ascends beside rushing, silt-laden Winthrop Creek, then steeply climbs several switchbacks on a rocky tread above the ice- and rock-covered expanse of Winthrop Glacier. As usual, towering over the entire scene is the impressive mass of Mount Rainier. After a rest stop at a particularly good viewpoint atop a rocky promontory, you charge up another set of very steep switchbacks on a brushy slope for about 0.8 mile. At the top, things get easier as you wander gently up and down in forest for about 0.3 mile to a log bridge over Granite Creek and come to Granite Creek Camp, a viewless but comfortable spot to spend the night.

Four long and moderately graded switchbacks take you above the camp, and your long ascent comes to an end as you top out on a ridge just above Skyscraper Pass. The views of Mount Rainier filling the sky to the south are outstanding.

> **SKYSCRAPER MOUNTAIN SIDE TRIP:** For an even better view, take an obvious use trail north, briefly descending to the saddle of Skyscraper Pass. From there the path steeply climbs a ridge to the summit of Skyscraper Mountain. As expected, the views of Mount Rainier will take your breath away, but you can also look north and east to Grand Park, the rugged peaks of the Alpine Lakes Wilderness, and even very distant Glacier Peak. Look for mountain goats on the slopes of Skyscraper Mountain.

After rounding the ridge above Skyscraper Pass, the Wonderland Trail makes a downhill traverse to the open, rolling meadowlands of Berkeley Park and returns to the junction at the start of the loop. Keep straight (east) and gradually ascend 0.7 mile back to the five-way junction at the pass near Frozen Lake.

For a different way back to Sunrise Day Lodge, stick with the Wonderland Trail, which goes slightly right (southeast) and steeply descends on a rocky tread for 0.6 mile to a junction at the end of a gravel road. You could go straight here and follow the road back to Sunrise, but for a more scenic course, turn right (south) and wander through pleasant meadows for 0.4 mile to the turnoff for Sunrise Camp, an attractive overnight spot a little above the shores of pretty Shadow Lake. Just south of this turnoff is a junction with the Sunrise Rim Trail.

Sunrise Day Lodge
photographed by Douglas Lorain

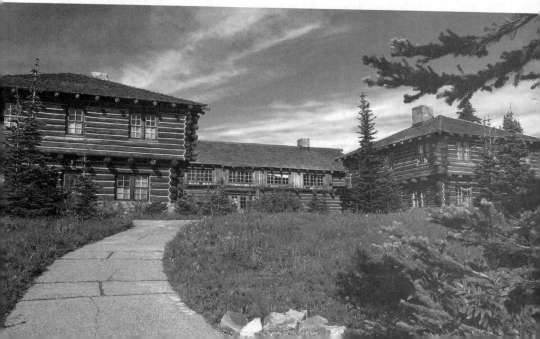

GLACIER OVERLOOK SIDE TRIP: Before turning left (east) on the Wonderland Trail, it's worth a few minutes for a short side trip to an awesome viewpoint. So go right (west) and make an uphill traverse for 0.2 mile to Glacier Overlook, a stone-lined turnaround from which you'll enjoy breathtaking views of Mount Rainier and sprawling Emmons Glacier.

To finish the trip, you turn left (east) at the junction near Sunrise Camp and soon pass an unsigned side path to Shadow Lake on your left. Keep right (east) and follow a gentle trail that goes over a small creek and through open forests of subalpine firs past a series of fine viewpoints looking southwest to Mount Rainier. At 0.7 mile from Shadow Lake, you keep straight (east) where the Wonderland Trail goes downhill to the right (south). Climb gradually through forest for 0.4 mile to a junction. On your right is a popular overlook, while just 0.1 mile to the left (north) is the Sunrise parking lot and the end of your trip.

POSSIBLE ITINERARY

	CAMP	MILES	ELEVATION GAIN
Day 1	Berkeley Park Camp	3.8	550'
	Side trip to Mount Fremont Lookout	2.6	1,000'
	Side trip to Berkeley Park Pond	0.2	50'
Day 2	Lake James	8.5	1,500'
	Side trip through Grand Park	1.2	100'
Day 3	Carbon River Camp	8.0	1,750'
	Side trip to Natural Bridge	1.8	400'
	Side trip to Crescent Lake	1.8	200'
Day 4	Mystic Camp	5.4	3,100'
	Side trip to Willis Wall Viewpoint	4.2	1,450'
Day 5	Out	9.9	2,400'
	Side trip to Skyscraper Mountain	0.7	400'
	Side trip to Glacier Overlook	0.4	150'

BEST SHORTER ALTERNATIVE

A day hike to either Grand Park or Skyscraper Mountain is fun and offers excellent scenery.

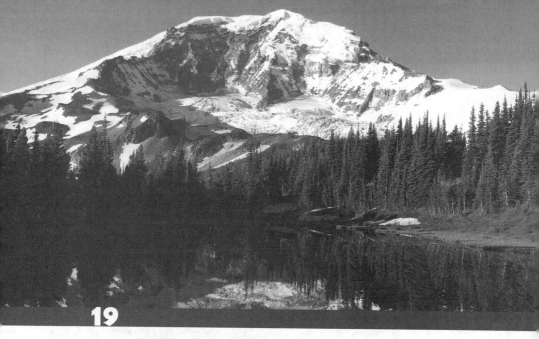

19

MOUNT RAINIER: WONDERLAND TRAIL LOOP

RATINGS: Scenery 10   **Solitude** 2   **Difficulty** 8
MILES: 91 (98)
ELEVATION GAIN: 25,150' (26,400')
DAYS: 8–13 (9–14)
SHUTTLE MILEAGE: n/a
MAPS: Green Trails *Mt. Rainier West (#269)* and *Mt. Rainier East (#270)*
USUALLY OPEN: Mid-July–October
BEST: August
PERMIT: Required. Approximately 70% of permits are available for reservation, with the rest given out on a first-come, first-served basis.

NOTE: For all intents and purposes, it's impossible to just show up and obtain a first-come, first-served permit to do the entire Wonderland Trail. Get a reservation, or plan to go elsewhere.

Reservation requests for the summer hiking season can only be made online, beginning March 15; a $20 nonrefundable fee applies to reserved permits. Walk-up permits can be obtained on the first day of the trip or up to one day before. See nps.gov/mora/planyourvisit/wilderness-permit.htm for full

continued on page 180

Above: *Mount Rainier reflected in a pond at a pass above Mystic Lake*
photographed by Douglas Lorain

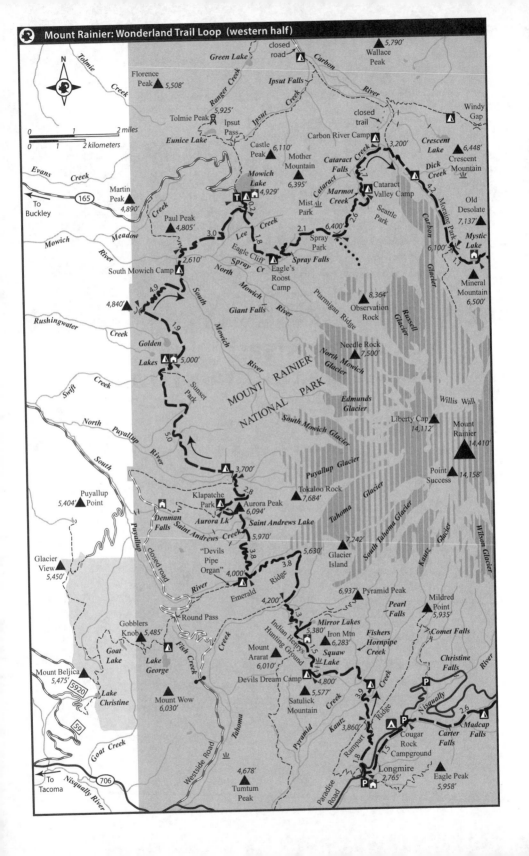

N

0   1   2 miles
0   1   2 kilometers

Tolmie Creek

Florence Peak ▲ 5,508'

Green Lake

closed road

Wallace Peak ▲ 5,790'

Ranger Creek

Ipsut Falls

Carbon River

Ipsut Creek

closed trail

Windy Gap

Tolmie Peak 🛰 5,925'

Ipsut Pass

Carbon River Camp ▲ 3,200'

Crescent Lake

Crescent Mountain ▲ 6,448'

Eunice Lake

Castle Peak ▲ 6,110'

Cataract Creek

Cataract Falls

Dick Creek

4.2

Evans Creek

Mowich Lake

Mother Mountain ▲ 6,395'

Cataract Creek

Cataract Valley Camp

Old Desolate ▲ 7,137'

To Buckley 165

Martin Peak ▲ 4,890'

0.3

4,929'

Mist Park

Marmot Creek

Seattle Park

Moraine Park

6,100'

Mystic Lake 1.1

Paul Peak ▲ 4,805'

3.0

Lee Creek

1.8

2.1

6,400'

2.6

Mowich River

Meadow Creek

Eagle Cliff

Spray Falls

Spray Park

Mineral Mountain ▲ 6,500'

Rushingwater Creek

South Mowich Camp ▲ 2,610'

North Mowich River

Spray Cr

Eagle's Roost Camp

Ptarmigan Ridge

Observation Rock ▲ 8,364'

Russell Glacier

Carbon Glacier

4.9

Giant Falls

South Mowich River

4,840' ▲

1.9

Golden Lakes ▲ 5,000'

Needle Rock ▲ 7,500'

North Mowich Glacier

Willis Wall

Swift Creek

Sunset Park

MOUNT RAINIER

Edmunds Glacier

North Puyallup River

NATIONAL PARK

South Mowich Glacier

Liberty Cap ▲ 14,112'

Mount Rainier ▲ 14,410'

South Puyallup River

5.0

▲ 3,700'

Puyallup Glacier

Tahoma Glacier

Point Success ▲ 14,158'

Puyallup Point ▲ 5,404'

2.8

Klapatche Park

Aurora Peak ▲ 6,094'

Tokaloo Rock ▲ 7,684'

Denman Falls

Aurora Lk

Saint Andrews Creek

Saint Andrews Lake 5,970'

▲ 7,242'

Glacier Island

South Tahoma Glacier

Kautz Glacier

Wilson Glacier

Glacier View ▲ 5,450'

"Devils Pipe Organ"

3.8

5,630'

3.8

Puyallup River

closed road

4,000'

Ridge

Pyramid Peak ▲ 6,937'

Pearl Falls

Mildred Point ▲ 5,935'

Emerald Ridge

4,200'

Round Pass

1.3

Mirror Lakes

Fishers Hornpipe Creek

Comet Falls

Gobblers Knob ▲ 5,485'

Fish Creek

Indian Henrys Hunting Ground 5,380'

Iron Mtn ▲ 6,283'

Christine Falls

Goat Lake

Lake George ▲

Mount Ararat ▲ 6,010'

Squaw Lake

1.5

Christine River

Mount Beljica ▲ 5,475'

5920

Lake Christine

Devils Dream Camp ▲ 4,800'

Carter Falls

Madcap Falls 2.6

59

Mount Wow 6,030'

Satulick Mountain ▲ 5,577'

3.9

Cougar Rock Campground

P

P

Westside Road

Kautz Creek

Rampart Ridge 3,860'

1.5

To Tacoma

706

Nisqually River

Tahoma Creek

4,678'

Tumtum Peak

Pyramid Creek

1.8

Paradise Road

Longmire ▲ 2,765'

Eagle Peak ▲ 5,958'

P

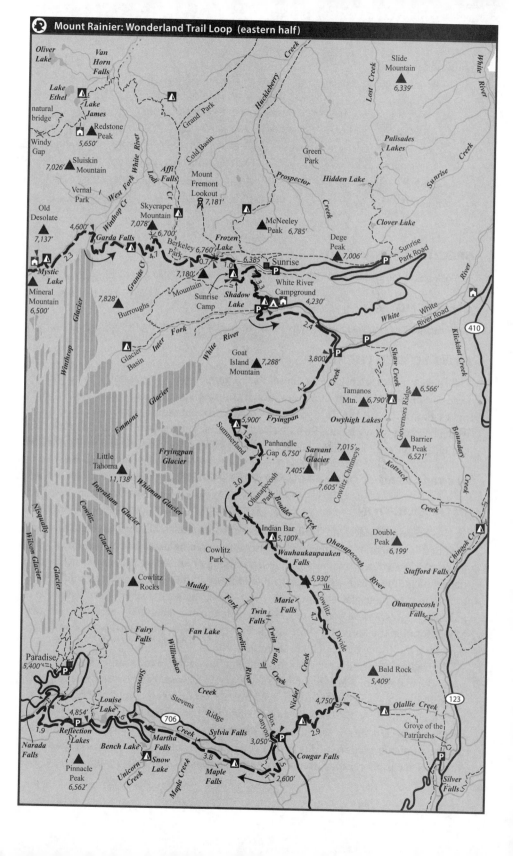

continued from page 177

details. Pick up permits (whether reserved in advance or a walk-up permit) from a wilderness information center or ranger station.

RULES: Trailside camping is allowed only at a restricted number of designated sites; Wonderland Trail loop hikers must use trailside camps (no off-trail permits are given out); maximum of 5 people per campsite; fires prohibited

CONTACT: Mount Rainier National Park, Longmire Wilderness Information Center, 360-569-6650, nps.gov/mora

SPECIAL ATTRACTIONS

Wonderful mountain views, wildflowers, wildlife, waterfalls

CHALLENGES

Campsite restrictions; long, rugged trail; difficulty in obtaining permits

HOW TO GET THERE

To reach the Mowich Lake trailhead, the recommended starting point, from Sumner, head east on WA 410 about 11.5 miles to an intersection at the south end of Buckley. Turn right (south) here on WA 165, go 1.6 miles, and turn left (south) to remain on WA 165, which becomes Mowich Lake Road. Drive 25.3 miles. The road turns to rough gravel as it climbs into the park and then ends at the Mowich Lake Campground and trailhead.

GPS TRAILHEAD COORDINATES: N46° 55.983' W121° 51.851'

INTRODUCTION

The famous Wonderland Trail, which completely circles Mount Rainier, is not only the finest long hike in Washington; it's also considered by many to be one of the best in the world. The route provides a generous sampling of all the attractions in the Cascade Range, including meadows choked with wildflowers, abundant and varied wildlife, old-growth forests, huge glaciers, impressive waterfalls, and scenic lakes. What will leave an indelible impression on your mind, however, are the ever-changing spectacular views of Mount Rainier, the Monarch of the Cascades. This monster volcano with its mantle of ice presents a multitude of faces, all of them beautiful.

The traditional starting point for this loop is at Longmire in the southwest corner of the park. The majority of hikers begin here and travel clockwise. We, however, recommend a different itinerary, starting from Mowich Lake in the northwest corner of the park. If you start at Longmire, you will face the most exhausting part of the hike in the first few days, when your pack is heavy with food and supplies. By starting at Mowich Lake, you save the most difficult section for the end of your trip. The only real drawback of starting at Mowich Lake is poorer road access, but most hikers are accustomed to that.

NOTE: Given the length of this trip, most hikers prefer to send food caches ahead rather than carrying all of their calorie needs from the start. Fortunately, the National Park Service has a very convenient program for doing this, allowing you to mail or drop off supplies at ranger stations along the way. Food caching is allowed at Mowich Lake, Sunrise, White River Campground, and Longmire. See nps.gov/mora for the latest procedures and details.

DESCRIPTION

From Mowich Lake you are immediately faced with a choice of trails. The official Wonderland Trail goes north around the west shore of the lake, climbs a bit to Ipsut Pass, and then drops down the pleasant but mostly viewless Ipsut Creek Valley to a junction about 0.3 mile above the end of the old Carbon River Road, which is now permanently closed to vehicles. From here you turn upstream (south), detouring to cross the river to avoid a washed-out and now-closed portion of trail, to a swinging bridge about 0.3 mile northeast of Carbon River Camp and a junction with the trail coming down from Spray Park. If the weather is bad or the high country is still buried in snow, this route from Mowich Lake is shorter, easier, and a better alternative than the high route.

The other option from Mowich Lake is more popular, higher in altitude, and much more scenic than the official Wonderland Trail, but it also gains 500 feet more in elevation. If the weather is good, this alternative is the superior choice due to the wildflowers and outstanding scenery.

From the Mowich Lake trailhead you cross the lake's outlet creek and follow the southbound (counterclockwise) course of the Wonderland Trail. This path makes a series of downhill switchbacks to a junction with Spray Park Trail at 0.2 mile. Here you veer left (south), leaving the Wonderland, and follow an up-and-down sidehill route through the trees. The trail, usually crowded with day hikers, makes a bridged crossing of small Lee Creek and then continues its uneven traverse of the wooded hillside. About 2 miles from Mowich Lake, the relatively easy hiking ends, as your route turns left (east) and climbs steadily in the trees along the top of Eagle Cliff. Views remain limited until you come to a short dead-end side trail that goes down about 40 yards to Eagle Cliff Viewpoint. This side trip is worthwhile because from here you have a terrific view of Eagle Cliff, the Spray Creek Valley, and snowy Mount Rainier.

TIP: Afternoons provide better lighting for photographs.

The main trail now traverses a hillside, passes Eagle's Roost Camp, and then comes to the 0.3-mile side trail to Spray Falls.

SPRAY FALLS SIDE TRIP: Don't miss the opportunity to visit this monster waterfall, where Spray Creek fans out over a long rock face. It's difficult to get a good look at the entire falls, but generally the best views are from the south bank of the creek.

WARNING: You should expect to get wet from this aptly named falls.

Beyond the Spray Falls turnoff, the main trail climbs a series of short, moderately steep switchbacks beside a small creek. As the trees start to thin and the country opens up, you cross the creek and climb gradually through the lower reaches of Spray Park. This huge, uneven, sloping meadow is justly famous for its flowers and fine scenery. Small ponds and picturesque clumps of trees add to the area's beauty. Topping it all off is Mount Rainier, which from this angle has a relatively slender profile and is almost unrecognizable as the same bulky peak observed from other directions. Observation Rock, a large ridge, partially obstructs the lower part of the peak.

Your trail makes a long, uneven climb through ever-higher terrain, eventually leaving the trees behind and ascending over rocks and snowfields to a windy, 6,400-foot-high point on the side of a ridge.

> **SIDE TRIP TO UPPER SPRAY PARK:** A terrific exploring opportunity awaits for those willing to wander off the trail from this pass southeast up to the rock gardens and great views in Upper Spray Park.

From this high pass the trail wanders down over snowfields and talus back into friendlier meadows. The large meadow below you to the left (west) is Mist Park, with remote and craggy Mother Mountain behind it. The trail continues its often-steep downhill along a small ridge, switchbacks to the right, and then descends over rocky meadows and through thin forests to small Marmot Creek. The path follows this creek downstream through gorgeous flower gardens, then steeply descends a badly eroded section of trail that is slippery with mud and fine gravel. After losing about 1,600 feet from the pass, you'll reach the short side trail to pleasant Cataract Valley Camp, a good place to set up your tent and reflect on the beauties of day one.

From Cataract Valley Camp the trail drops through heavy forest in a series of short switchbacks into the canyon of Cataract Creek. Cascading Cataract Falls provides a welcome diversion near the bottom of the switchbacks. Good views of the falls are hard to obtain, but what you can see is pretty impressive. The trail here gets less maintenance than some other park trails, so early-season hikers often have to scramble over downed trees and push through brushy areas. The trail completes its descent along a forested hillside down to a junction with a spur trail that crosses Cataract Creek to large Carbon River Camp. The trail north of this camp used to be the Wonderland Trail, but it's now closed.

From the junction near Carbon River Camp, you turn upstream (east) and make a short, gentle ascent through willows and other riparian vegetation to a memorable crossing of Carbon River on a long and very narrow swinging bridge. Hikers accustomed to the solid footing of Mother Earth may be disconcerted by the seeming instability of this structure as it bounces up and down and swings back and forth with every step. Handrails help to steady your nerves.

Once on the east bank of the Carbon River, you meet up with the newly rerouted Wonderland Trail, which turns right (southeast) and begins a long climb above the wasteland that abuts Carbon Glacier. Despite retreating in recent years, this massive ice sheet is still the lowest-elevation glacier in the Lower 48, reaching down to about 3,700 feet. Along the edge of the ice is the usual ugly moonscape of rocks associated with retreating glaciers. The transition where the rocks end and the glacier begins is hard to make out, as the ice is covered with so much debris.

WARNING: Do not venture onto or even near the ice, as it is very unstable and dangerous.

The trail beside the glacier is steep, rocky, and exposed to the sun, so despite such close proximity to all that ice, it can be quite hot.

TIP: The morning offers cooler temperatures and shade, making this section generally more comfortable, and also provides better lighting for photographs.

The route makes a pair of switchbacks around a washed-out area, then climbs above and away from the glacier to a crossing of Dick Creek just before you reach tiny Dick Creek Camp, on a bench south of the creek. The tent sites at this camp are rocky and don't accept tent stakes very well, but the scene from this high overlook is wonderful, providing particularly exciting views at sunset. Beyond Dick Creek the terrain is more pleasant, as the trail climbs in welcome shade up a hillside away from the glacier. The trail steadily ascends, following splashing Moraine Creek through a narrow meadow and then traversing a gully to the lower end of beautiful Moraine Park. This large, flat meadow has lots of flowers and terrific views of Russell Glacier and Ptarmigan Ridge to the southwest. To the south are massive Willis Wall and the summit of Mount Rainier.

Although Moraine Park is a full 2,500 feet up from the swinging bridge over the Carbon River, the ascent is not quite complete, as you still must climb another 400 feet of forested switchbacks beyond Moraine Park to reach a 6,100-foot pass. Once you arrive at the pass, it's time to drop your pack and soak in the wonderful views. A small pond on the west side of the trail perfectly reflects massive Mount Rainier. Adventurous hikers, irresistibly drawn to the great mountain, can follow boot paths into the wonderland

The snout of Carbon Glacier
photographed by Douglas Lorain

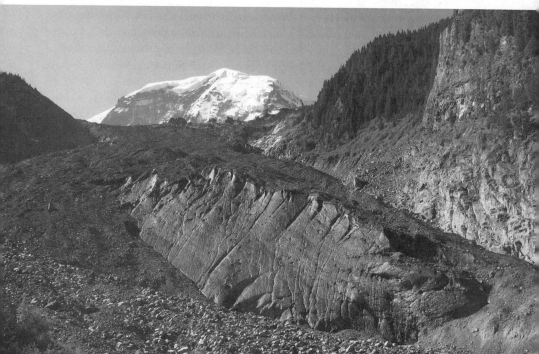

to the south. Although the explorations are superb and highly rewarding, Mount Rainier is so huge that it's actually better viewed and photographed from along the trail, farther back from the peak.

From the pass the trail makes an uneven but gorgeous descent through trees and small meadows to the shores of Mystic Lake. A small high point called Mineral Mountain sits above the south shore of this lake, blocking the view of Mount Rainier, but to the north rise the barren slopes of Old Desolate, which provide more than enough scenery to warrant an extended stay. The trail rounds the meadowy south shore of Mystic Lake, passing a spur trail to a ranger cabin, and then reenters forest and drops about 0.2 mile to a junction with a short spur trail to Mystic Camp.

From Mystic Camp the Wonderland Trail steadily descends the valley of West Fork White River, sometimes in evergreens, sometimes in deciduous creekside vegetation.

WARNING: In early summer the path here may be overrun by high water. You should expect to do a bit of wading or bushwhacking.

The route veers away from the creek and then crosses a short, rugged stretch of boulders and glacial outwash to a bridged crossing of Winthrop Creek, a boisterous stream flowing from the nearby ice and gravel of Winthrop Glacier.

Just above the crossing, Granite Creek tumbles over good-size Garda Falls, worth a look, though it's difficult to photograph from the trail. Beyond the falls the route continues climbing above the moraine of nearby Winthrop Glacier, then turns away and begins a steep switchbacking ascent to the east. Trees limit the views, but you'll enjoy occasional glimpses of massive Winthrop Glacier and the surrounding ridges. Your route continues to steadily gain elevation, rounds a small ridge, and then climbs beside the splashing waters of Granite Creek. About 2 miles from Garda Falls, you cross the creek on a flat-topped log and immediately reach Granite Creek Camp, a good place for a rest or a quiet night in the wilderness.

Beyond Granite Creek the trail climbs in long switchbacks toward Skyscraper Pass. Along the way the trees gradually thin out and eventually disappear altogether, replaced by alpine meadows and rocky slopes. From the often-windy 6,700-foot pass, superb vistas include most of the northern part of the national park. A careful observer should even be able to spot the Mount Fremont Lookout cabin to the northeast.

From the pass your trail makes a long, looping descent over talus slopes and lingering snowfields into Berkeley Park. This large, gently sloping mountain meadow sits beneath the talus slopes of Burroughs Mountain and features wildflowers, tree islands, and generally lovely mountain scenery, although intervening peaks block any view of Mount Rainier. From a trail junction at the east end of Berkeley Park, a path leads north to Berkeley Camp and spectacular Grand Park—well worth a side trip if you have an extra day.

Your trail continues east from the junction in Berkeley Park and climbs a gentle meadow to a broad saddle just south of Frozen Lake, where there is a major five-way junction. To the left, a 1.3-mile trail climbs north to the Mount Fremont Lookout, a good place to see mountain goats, while to the right a trail goes southwest to Burroughs Mountain. Your route goes slightly right and descends a moderately steep gully to the southeast for 0.6 mile to a junction with a closed road heavily traveled by day-hiking tourists.

SIDE TRIP TO SUNRISE DAY LODGE: The source of all these tourists is Sunrise, which you can reach by an easy 0.9-mile stroll along the closed road to the left (east). Here you can pick up any food you sent ahead, or indulge in such backpacking luxuries as a cheeseburger and fries. You can also throw away your garbage to lighten the load a bit.

Back at the Wonderland Trail junction with the closed road, west of Sunrise, your tour turns south and travels a virtually level 0.4 mile to Sunrise Camp, where you can set up your tent for the night, a little above tiny Shadow Lake. A short and crowded side trip follows a trail south up the slope west of Sunrise Camp for 0.2 mile to spectacular Glacier Overlook, which features great views of Emmons Glacier, the White River Valley, and ever-present Mount Rainier.

TIP: Do this side trip in the early morning, when photos are better and before the crowds of day hikers have arrived.

From Sunrise Camp the Wonderland Trail heads east, crosses the outlet of Shadow Lake, and then goes through a mix of attractive meadows and forests. You'll reach a junction after 0.7 mile, where you turn right (southeast) and follow the Wonderland Trail as it drops into the White River Valley. This switchbacking route initially has some views, but it soon enters dense forest as it makes a 2,000-foot descent to the backpacker's camping area and car campground at White River. Walk west through the campground and then pick up the Wonderland Trail again where a sign directs you south over a trail bridge spanning the raging river. From here a relatively new section of trail goes east (downstream), generally staying in the forest not far above the banks of the river for 1.5 miles to a junction with a short spur trail that leads east to the paved White River Road. You stay on the Wonderland Trail, which goes up and down on a forested hillside above the road for 0.9 mile, then comes to a junction with an access trail from the highway.

From this junction some hikers prefer to take a lower-elevation alternative to the Wonderland Trail that avoids the sometimes-dangerous snowfields and exposed terrain around Panhandle Gap. Although less scenic, it may be a superior choice, particularly during bad weather. The alternate route follows the highway east for 0.6 mile to the Owyhigh Lakes Trail, and then turns south, climbs past these attractive lakes, and descends the other side of a pass into heavily forested Chinook Creek Valley. You then hike south on the pleasant Eastside Trail, past waterfalls along Chinook Creek and the Ohanapecosh River to the massive old-growth stand called Grove of the Patriarchs. From here you follow Stevens Canyon Road to the west, and then climb the shady but viewless Olallie Creek Trail north, back to a reunion with the Wonderland Trail along Cowlitz Divide.

Unless the weather has really turned sour, most hikers opt for the wildly scenic Wonderland Trail route over Panhandle Gap rather than the lower-elevation alternative just described. From the junction with the spur trail above White River Road, the wide trail turns southwest and climbs gently through deep forests above Fryingpan Creek. The going is easy and enjoyable through this lowland valley, although views are nonexistent. You cross two side creeks and begin to climb steadily on a small, forested ridge beside Fryingpan Creek. A few switchbacks break up the grade, but views remain limited until the trail enters a lovely meadow choked with tall wildflowers.

The trail crosses the creek, goes uphill through an attractive mix of meadows and forest, and then begins a spirited climb in a series of short switchbacks across an open, meadowy slope. The climb tops out at Summerland, an absolutely gorgeous meadow carpeted with colorful wildflowers. An intervening ridge blocks a full view of Mount Rainier, but with scattered trees, small creeks, and lots of flowers, this is a magical spot. A large designated camping area, complete with an old stone shelter, lies in the trees on the left shortly after you enter the meadow.

Upon leaving Summerland you quickly climb above timberline and enter an austere alpine world of snow and rocks.

WARNING: The trail is easy to lose here, so navigate carefully.

TIP: As you climb, keep an eye out for mountain goats. This area is one of the most reliable locations in the park for spotting these agile mountain dwellers.

The path makes a sometimes-tricky stream crossing, passes a lovely snowmelt pond, and gains nearly 900 feet from Summerland to 6,750-foot Panhandle Gap. Vistas both north and south from this rocky pass are superb, but a ridge blocks the view west to Mount Rainier. To solve this problem, you can scramble up a steep boot path to a rocky high point east of the pass, where you'll be able to see about half of the mountain, including the prominent pinnacle called Little Tahoma on the eastern slopes of Mount Rainier.

From Panhandle Gap the trail goes southwest across talus slopes and large semipermanent snowfields to a gentle alpine bench.

WARNING: In foggy conditions the route is very easy to lose, especially over the featureless snowfields.

If the way is totally snow covered, do not be fooled into dropping east into Ohanapecosh Park. The correct route stays high on the bench above this park, following an up-and-down course, and then drops down a ridge above the southwest side of Ohanapecosh Park. If you lost the trail under the snow, you should be able to relocate it on this ridge, where you can look west to the cliffs and waterfalls in the basin above Indian Bar.

Your trail descends a series of short switchbacks along this ridge, as the route reenters stunted alpine forests and meadows and then descends through somewhat larger trees. The superb scenery includes lots of wildflowers, waterfalls, snowy ridges, and glaciers. Eventually the path descends steep switchbacks to the flat meadow called Indian Bar, one of the park's legendary beauty spots. Wildflowers

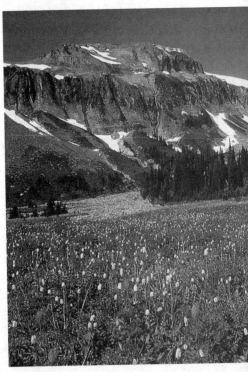

Indian Bar
photographed by Douglas Lorain

carpet the valley floor, and dozens of waterfalls cascade down the surrounding cliffs. Marmots whistle alarm calls, and in the fall you will probably hear elk bugling. At the southeast end of this paradise, the trail crosses the creek near a stone shelter. The designated backpacker camps are on the east side of the creek, a little above the crossing. Just below the bridge is thunderous Wauhaukaupauken Falls, which is almost as difficult to get a view of as it is to pronounce.

Reluctantly, you must leave Indian Bar and climb moderately steeply over a series of meadowy benches, gaining some 900 feet to a 5,930-foot knoll with simply outstanding views. (Actually, I'd prefer to use a stronger adjective, but nothing in my thesaurus seems to do this place justice.) Drop your pack and soak in the scenery for a while as you look northeast to the rugged Cowlitz Chimneys, south to distant Mount Adams, north to Indian Bar and Panhandle Gap, and, best of all, northwest to the shining summit of Mount Rainier. Trees frame superb photographs of the peak, and flowers add color to the foreground. There might not be a better lunch spot in North America.

From this knoll the Wonderland Trail makes an uneven descent along scenic Cowlitz Divide through partial forest and meadows. Black bears are common in this area, as are elk and other wildlife. The views here don't rival those from the knoll above Indian Bar, but the hiking is very enjoyable. You drop to a saddle, and then make a sidehill climb mostly in forest to another grassy knoll and more views. From here the path leaves the views behind as it reenters forest and drops to a junction in a wooded pass. The trail to the left (east) is the Olallie Creek Trail, the end of the alternate lower-elevation route described earlier.

The Wonderland Trail turns right (west) at this junction and makes a long, switchbacking descent through dense forests to a designated camping area and, just beyond, a bridge over Nickel Creek. After crossing Nickel Creek, the trail climbs a bit, and then loses elevation to reach a trailhead on Stevens Canyon Road (WA 706).

TIP: A short side trip to the road parking lot allows you to throw away any accumulated garbage.

The Wonderland Trail avoids this road by turning right (north) at a junction and following the deep and very narrow gorge called Box Canyon for 0.2 mile to a bridged crossing. You then climb a hillside above the road and cross the highway where it goes through a tunnel.

After crossing the busy highway, the trail enters wilder terrain, rounds a ridge, and makes an uneven descent through forests to a junction near the crossing of Stevens Creek. Turn left (west), cross the creek, and climb very slowly up woodsy Stevens Canyon. About 0.8 mile after crossing Stevens Creek, you'll reach the log crossing of pleasant Maple Creek. A designated camping area on your left is just before Maple Creek.

TIP: In August the brushy flat east of this camp has lots of delicious blackberries. These make a wonderful natural after-dinner treat.

From Maple Creek the trail leads northwest up the south side of Stevens Canyon, generally staying in the forests well away from the creek. On the opposite side of the canyon lies busy Stevens Canyon Road, from which you can sometimes hear the sounds of traffic. The trail passes joyous Sylvia Falls on the main stream, then continues its steady climb, alternating along the way between forests and brushy slopes. You cross Unicorn Creek just downstream from Martha Falls, a beautiful cascade that demands several photographs.

Beyond this landmark the trail steadily climbs increasingly open slopes to a crossing of Stevens Canyon Road, and then continues its ascent through open forests and briefly on the road's shoulder to Louise Lake. This quiet lake sits in a pretty basin beside the highway, but views there are limited. For better views continue uphill another 0.5 mile, turn left (south) at a junction, and reach gorgeous Reflection Lakes (not surprisingly, the reflection is of Mount Rainier). Hordes of car-bound tourists share the view here, so solitude-seeking backpackers should stop only long enough to snap a few photographs.

The trail follows the road shoulder about 0.4 mile, then veers to the right (northwest), passes a junction (continue west), and crosses the road again about 0.2 mile west of the marshy lake. The trail then travels through forest as it rounds a ridge and switchbacks down a heavily forested hillside to a junction about 1.3 miles from Reflection Lakes.

> **NARADA FALLS SIDE TRIP:** A mandatory 0.1-mile side trip to the right (northeast) goes to beautiful Narada Falls on the Paradise River, which is also accessible by a short walk from the road, so don't expect to be lonesome.

From the Narada Falls turnoff, the Wonderland Trail heads southwest and begins a long, viewless, but highly enjoyable descent of the woodsy canyons of the Paradise and Nisqually Rivers. The going is moderately steep but not too bad on the knees. You'll reach a reasonably good camp a little before the bridged crossing of Paradise River, and then continue through increasingly lush forests of Douglas fir, western yew, western hemlock, and western red cedar with an interesting mix of understory species. For variety, the trail passes Madcap and Carter Falls, both partly hidden by trees but still worth a look. The Wonderland Trail levels out as it enters the valley of the Nisqually River and follows a wide path to the crossing of this large glacial stream on a narrow log. On the opposite bank the trail comes to a highway parking area and turns downstream (south). You skirt the busy car campground at Cougar Rock as you follow a pipeline and old roadbed (now trail) through the forests along the Nisqually River.

Eventually you will come to a junction on a low and heavily forested hillside. If you don't need to resupply at Longmire, the quickest way to continue your trip is to turn right (north) here, hike about 0.1 mile to a road crossing, and pick up the well-marked Wonderland Trail on the other side.

> **LONGMIRE SIDE TRIP:** Hikers who want to visit the historic lodge and park facilities at Longmire or who need supplies should turn left (south) at the junction and descend 0.2 mile to the crowds and bustle of Longmire. In addition to lots of parking and people, this facility has a wilderness information center, a small museum, a hotel, and a restaurant.

To return to the quiet of the wilderness, retrace your route to the Wonderland Trail junction 0.2 mile north of Longmire, cross the highway, and begin hiking on trail once more. The popular route makes one quick switchback and then leaves the road behind as it wanders through lovely old forests. The easy travel ends after about 0.5 mile, where the trail begins a lengthy ascent of Rampart Ridge on numerous short switchbacks. At the top of this climb are two nearby junctions. You keep straight (north) at each, travel on a gentle up-and-down path with limited views, and then descend briefly but sharply to a bridged crossing of the glacial waters of Kautz Creek.

> **NOTE:** The placement of this seasonal bridge changes as the location of the stream moves about in the rocky floodplain. You may need to scout around a bit to find the current crossing site.

Now you climb through the valley of Kautz Creek, cross the much clearer waters of Pyramid Creek (designated camps nearby), and begin climbing once again. The trail switchbacks up a ridge, crosses splashing Fishers Hornpipe Creek, and then makes a side-hill ascent to another creek crossing. Shortly beyond this crossing, large and heavily used Devils Dream Camp offers designated sites, which are spread out so well across this forested hillside that the crowding is barely noticeable.

Beyond Devils Dream Camp the trail resumes climbing a short distance, and then begins to ease as the path breaks out of the solid forest and enters more open country. After passing marshy Squaw Lake, you climb a bit more before entering the wonderful flowery expanse of Indian Henrys Hunting Ground. Lots of wildflowers, small tarns, and superb views of Mount Rainier make this spot one of the highlights of the trip. A picturesque National Park Service patrol cabin here is usually staffed by a ranger, who is fortunate enough to spend many days amid this paradise.

The Wonderland Trail goes straight (northwest) at a junction with the Kautz Creek Trail and continues through more flower gardens for a short distance to a second junction, this one with the dead-end spur trail to Mirror Lake.

> **MIRROR LAKE SIDE TRIP:** This 0.7-mile side trip is well worth your time, as it leads northeast through a flowery vale up to a well-known view of Mount Rainier over tiny Mirror Lake. Here, Asahel Curtis photographed a famous scene for a postage stamp commemorating the national park in 1934. Adventurous hikers can continue on an obvious use trail above Mirror Lake to some outstanding close-up views of Mount Rainier from atop Pyramid Peak.

Beyond the Mirror Lake turnoff, the Wonderland Trail makes an uneven descent north through a mix of meadows and forests down to a rocky area above Tahoma Creek. A narrow swinging bridge spans the deep chasm of this boisterous stream. The bridge isn't as long as the one over Carbon River, but it's still enough to put a chill through hikers who are afraid of heights. On the north bank is a junction with the Tahoma Creek Trail, which has suffered flood damage in recent years and is no longer maintained. Turn right (northeast) and once again begin climbing above the stream, sometimes in trees but more often through brushy areas. By now you've probably noticed how the trail on the west side of Mount Rainier is a constant series of tiring ups and downs. This pattern will continue for the next couple of days, and it explains why we recommend saving this most difficult part of the Wonderland Trail for the end of your trip. The current climb reaches an open area beside the rubble and meadows of an old glacial moraine and then makes a final set of switchbacks to the top of Emerald Ridge. From this windswept viewpoint you can look north to the deep trough holding Tahoma Glacier and northeast to towering Mount Rainier. Mountain goats, no doubt enjoying the scenery as much as we are, can often be seen along Emerald Ridge.

The Wonderland Trail turns southwest along the spine of Emerald Ridge, traveling through rocky areas and brilliant green alpine meadows.

TIP: A small pond a little below the trail on your left makes a superb photo spot for capturing Mount Rainier.

The trail now descends rapidly from the alpine zone in a series of steep switchbacks.

WARNING: The tread here is eroded and rocky. Watch your footing.

The steep grade becomes gentler once you reach a bench above the South Puyallup River, along which you ramble downstream to a junction.

> **SIDE TRIP TO "DEVILS PIPE ORGAN":** The South Puyallup River Trail goes straight (west) from this junction, immediately reaching pleasant South Puyallup Camp. It then continues another 0.2 mile to a terrific columnar basalt formation that shouldn't be missed. This feature has no official name but is sometimes referred to as either the Colonnades or the Devils Pipe Organ.
>
> **TIP:** Located in the forests on the north side of Emerald Ridge, this tall rock formation's setting provides very little natural light. A tripod will come in handy if you want to take a photograph in these dark conditions.

Back on the main trail, you go north to cross the South Puyallup River, then turn right (east) and once again go uphill. The ascent this time is an arduous 1,900-foot climb on a south-facing slope. There is a fair amount of shade but no water, and on a hot summer day this section can be exhausting. Numerous irregularly spaced switchbacks break up the climb, as do occasional views. After about 2.3 miles the route reaches more attractive terrain, as it tops the ridge and travels through partial forest and pretty meadows. The climbing doesn't end once you reach the ridge, however, as the trail turns right (east) and ascends along the top of the ridge. Finally, where the trail curves north, it stops climbing and traverses an attractive open slope for about 0.6 mile to Saint Andrews Lake, a small but lovely mountain pool with terrific views of massive Mount Rainier. Ice remains on the water of this lake well into August, and wildflowers carpet the nearby meadows and knolls.

TIP: Off-trail explorations to the east into the upper reaches of Saint Andrews Park are highly rewarding.

From Saint Andrews Lake the trail descends briefly to a little saddle with good views, and then goes along the side of a hill to tiny Aurora Lake in the meadow at Klapatche Park. This alpine jewel has a small designated camp above its northwest shore near a junction with the Klapatche Park Trail. The view looking east over the lake to the dark pinnacle of Tokaloo Rock and up to Mount Rainier is classic. This scenery invites an overnight stay despite the numerous mosquitoes through mid-August and the difficulty of getting a permit for one of the few camps here.

From Klapatche Park the Wonderland Trail descends a wide gully to the northeast and then makes a long series of short switchbacks on a 2,000-foot, toe-jamming descent into the canyon of the North Puyallup River. The moderately steep route down crosses slopes covered with a mix of evergreen forests and deciduous brush. After you reach the welcome waters of a small stream, you switchback and briefly follow the creek downstream. The descent soon picks up again in a series of small switchbacks, finally bottoming out at the end of the closed and mostly overgrown West Side Road (now maintained as a trail). Massive Tokaloo Rock looms over the skyline to the east, and several waterfalls stream down the adjacent cliffs. Now the trail heads north and crosses the North Puyallup River and a small trickling creek before reaching North Puyallup Camp. The sites here are only fair because they have lots of gravel, so tent stakes tend to suffer from abuse. They are also located right beside the trail, so privacy is limited. There is, however, plenty of shade and lots of big trees to provide shelter if it gets windy.

Now your trail sets about regaining the elevation it lost from Klapatche Park. Initially the grade is barely noticeable, as you make a long, almost level crossing of a heavily forested hillside. Once the trail rounds a small ridgecrest, the ascent picks up markedly. You cross a creek and then continue uphill at a steady, tiring grade. After you cross a second creek, the scenery improves because you break out of the trees and enter a large meadow with small scattered trees and lots of bear grass, which in July of favorable years covers the meadow with white blooms. This open area, called Sunset Park, is the result of a large fire in 1930 that burned down the forest that once covered these slopes. The grade of your climb eases as the trail rounds a ridgeline, where an abandoned and hard-to-follow trail heads east up to a high point that once held a lookout and still features stupendous views of Mount Rainier.

The main trail, heading north-northeast, now goes up and down through the attractive meadows and open forests of Sunset Park, rounds a low ridge, and then descends about 200 feet to the ranger cabin at Golden Lakes.

WARNING: The numerous small ponds in this area serve as a nursery for a large population of mosquitoes in July and early August. The bugs here are the worst along the entire circuit.

If you can stand the blood-sucking invertebrates, excellent designated camps are scattered in the trees above a good-size lake west of the ranger cabin.

TIP: Stock up on water at Golden Lakes, as there are few sources for several miles.

From Golden Lakes the trail drops to an insignificant saddle and then goes northwest on a gentle up-and-down route along the side of a ridge. About 1.9 miles from Golden Lakes, the trail reaches a grassy pass and turns sharply right (northeast) into the forests on the north side of the ridge.

TIP: A superb but rarely taken side trip from the pass follows an abandoned jeep track to the west, passes the park boundary, and in 0.5 mile reaches an open knoll that provides excellent views of Mount Rainier.

To complete your trip, follow the Wonderland Trail north as it descends a seemingly endless series of switchbacks and loses 2,100 feet on a route that will test even the strongest knees. Water is scarce and views are nonexistent, but your spirits will be buoyed by the knowledge that this is the final long downhill of the trip. The trail bottoms out in the flatlands beside the glacial waters of the South Mowich River, which you cross on a series of narrow logs. About 0.2 mile past the crossing, you'll reach the short side trail to the wooden shelter at pleasant South Mowich Camp.

TIP: To avoid using the silty river water, you can obtain clearer water from a small stream about 0.1 mile farther north on the Wonderland Trail.

From South Mowich Camp the main trail leads through ancient forest to a log crossing of North Mowich River, another glacial stream, and then begins its final climb to Mowich Lake. You keep right (east) at a junction with the rarely traveled Paul Peak Trail and continue ascending the nicely shaded Wonderland Trail. The climb alternates between switchbacks and uphill traverses, eventually traveling beside the waters of clear Crater Creek. The trail crosses this stream just below a cascading waterfall and climbs a bit more to a junction with the Spray Park Trail. You turn left (north) here and retrace your route from day one for 0.2 mile back to the Mowich Lake trailhead, the end of a long but spectacular trip on the aptly named Wonderland Trail.

VARIATION

If you don't have the time or energy to tackle the entire loop at once, it breaks up nicely into more manageable three- to four-day segments, with trailheads at Mowich Lake, Sunrise, Box Canyon, and Longmire. All of these, however, require dealing with the logistics of car shuttles.

POSSIBLE ITINERARY

	CAMP	MILES	ELEVATION GAIN
Day 1	Cataract Valley Camp	6.7	1,700'
	Side trip to Spray Falls	0.4	100'
	Side trip to Upper Spray Park	2.4	700'
Day 2	Mystic Camp	7.0	3,000'
Day 3	Sunrise Camp	8.7	2,500'
	Side trip to Sunrise Day Lodge	1.8	100'
Day 4	Summerland	9.9	2,500'
Day 5	Nickel Creek	11.3	2,400'
Day 6	Paradise River	10.3	2,500'
	Side trip to Narada Falls	0.2	0'
Day 6	Devils Dream Camp	9.1	2,700'
	Side trip to Longmire	0.4	100'
Day 7	Klapatche Park	10.4	3,850'
	Side trip to Mirror Lake	1.4	150'
	Side trip to "Devils Pipe Organ"	0.4	100'
Day 8	South Mowich Camp	13.7	1,700'
Day 9	Out	4.1	2,300'

BEST SHORTER ALTERNATIVES

The best short samplers of the Wonderland include an overnighter to Indian Bar from Box Canyon, a day hike to Spray Park from Mowich Lake, a day hike to Skyscraper Pass from Sunrise, and an overnighter to Devils Dream with a side trip up to Indian Henry's Hunting Ground from Longmire.

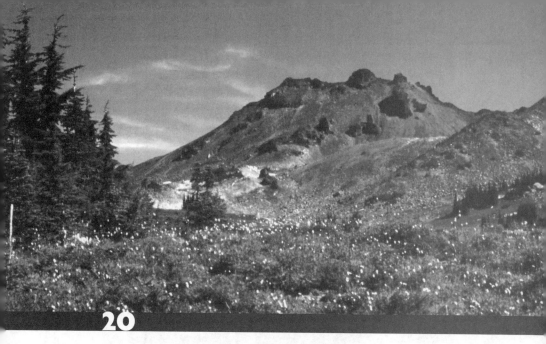

20

GOAT ROCKS CIRCUIT

RATINGS: Scenery 10   **Solitude** 5   **Difficulty** 6

MILES: 37 (39)

ELEVATION GAIN: 6,050' (6,500')

DAYS: 3–5 (4–6)

SHUTTLE MILEAGE: 18

MAPS: USFS *Goat Rocks plus Tatoosh and Glacier View Wildernesses*; Green Trails *Packwood (#302), White Pass (#303),* and *Walupt Lake (#335)*

USUALLY OPEN: July–October

BEST: Mid-July–mid-August

PERMIT: Required. Free and available at the trailhead.

RULES: Maximum group size of 12 people and/or stock; no fires within 0.25 mile of Goat Lake

CONTACT: Gifford Pinchot National Forest, Cowlitz Valley Ranger District, 360-497-1100, fs.usda.gov/main/giffordpinchot

SPECIAL ATTRACTIONS •

Wildflowers, outstanding mountain scenery, wildlife

CHALLENGES •

Dangerously exposed section along the Pacific Crest Trail, some crowded spots

Above: *Old Snowy Mountain over Snowgrass Flat*
photographed by Douglas Lorain

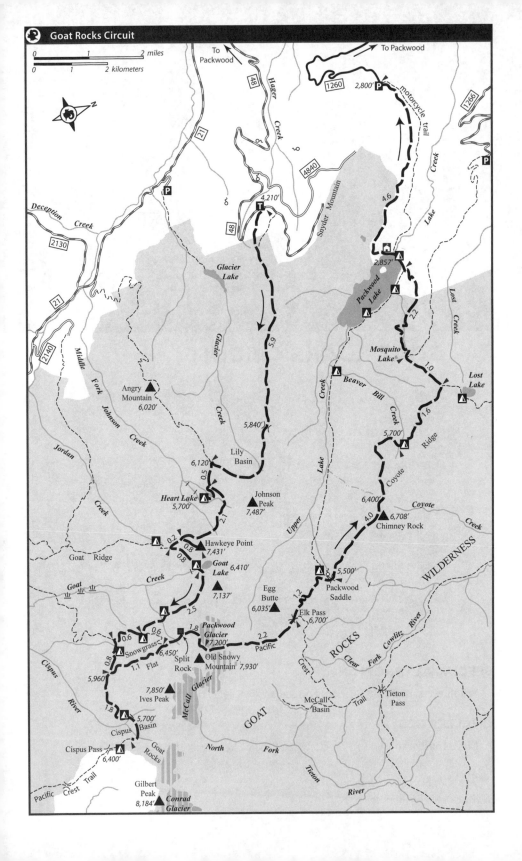

0   1   2 miles
0   1   2 kilometers

To Packwood

To Packwood

1260   2,800'   P

motorcycle trail

1266

P

Deception

Creek

2130

48

Huger

Creek

4840

4.6

Snyder Mountain

27

P

48

4,210'

T

2,857'

Glacier
Lake

Packwood Lake

Lost

Creek

2140

27

Middle

Fork

Johnson

Creek

Glacier

Creek

5.9

Beaver

Bill

Creek

Mosquito
Lake

2.2

Lost
Lake

Jordan

Angry
Mountain
6,020'

5,840'

Lily
Basin

Creek

Upper

Lake

1.0

5,700'

1.6

Coyote

Ridge

6,120'

0.5

Johnson
Peak
7,487'

6,400'

Coyote

4.0

6,708'
Chimney Rock

Coyote

Creek

Heart Lake
5,700'

2.1

Goat   Ridge

0.2

0.8

Hawkeye Point
7,431'

0.8

Goat
Lake   6,410'

7,137'

Egg
Butte
6,035'

.8

5,500'

Packwood
Saddle

WILDERNESS

Goat

2.5

Creek

1.2

Goat

2.5

Elk Pass
6,700'

0.6

1.8

Packwood
Glacier
7,200'

2.2

Pacific

ROCKS

Clear

Fork

Cowlitz

River

0.8

Snowgrass

6,450'

Split
Rock

Old Snowy
Mountain 7,930'

1.1   Flat

5,960'

Cispus

River

7,850'
Ives Peak

McCall Glacier

McCall
Basin

Tieton
Pass

Crest

Trail

1.8

5,700'
Basin

GOAT

North

Fork

Cispus Pass
6,400'

Goat
Rocks

Pacific

Crest

Trail

Gilbert
Peak
8,184'

Conrad
Glacier

Tieton

River

HOW TO GET THERE ••

Drive to Packwood, south of Mount Rainier, on US 12; Packwood lies 71 miles west of Yakima and 75 miles east of Chehalis. To reach the north (ending) trailhead, turn east onto Snyder Road (which becomes Forest Service Road 1260) beside the former Packwood Ranger Station (now vacation rentals). The large, well-marked Packwood Lake Trailhead is at the end of this good road, 5.7 miles from town.

To reach the south (starting) trailhead, from the US 12 intersection with Snyder Road, drive south on US 12 W about 3 miles, and turn left (southeast) on FS 21. Go 1.1 miles, and at a fork, continue straight another mile. Merge onto FS 48. This gravel route, which gets rocky and steep in a couple of spots, climbs in long switchbacks up a hillside of forests and numerous clear-cuts. Stay on FS 48 at each of several junctions to reach the Lily Basin Trailhead, 8.9 miles from the highway.

WARNING: Break-ins are common at this trailhead. The U.S. Forest Service warns people not to leave valuables in their car, especially overnight.

NOTE: You'll need a Northwest Forest Pass to park at these trailheads.

GPS TRAILHEAD COORDINATES:
Southern (Lily Basin): N46° 33.858' W121° 35.994'
Northern (Packwood Lake): N46° 36.504' W121° 37.626'

INTRODUCTION ••

Nestled along the Cascade Divide south of Mount Rainier, Goat Rocks are the spectacularly eroded remains of an ancient volcano. Nature's sculpting by ice and water has left behind a beautiful region of jagged peaks, glaciers, and mountain meadows. The area was named for the mountain goats that live among these crags, but the wilderness is also home to a healthy population of elk, black bears, and all the other wildlife common to the Cascade Range.

The most popular long backpacking trip in the Goat Rocks Wilderness follows the Pacific Crest Trail (PCT) north from Walupt Lake to White Pass. Although this is an exceptional trip, the hike described below includes the most spectacular part of this PCT hike, while adding many miles of view-packed ridges, two sparkling mountain lakes, and some impressive forests. In addition to the improved scenery, this circuit is less crowded and has a shorter car shuttle than the PCT option. For all of these reasons the authors believe this is a superior alternative. The trip is equally scenic in either direction but is described here so you'll have a net elevation loss of 1,400 feet.

DESCRIPTION ••

The path begins by going east, past large trees and through an old fire scar, and passes a junction with a new horse trail at 0.6 mile. It then makes an uneven climb to the top of a wooded ridge. Trees limit the views as the route works uphill along this divide. About 4 miles from the trailhead, you'll reach a large break in the trees, framing a classic view to the north. Large Packwood Lake, with its distinctive island, sits below you in a forested basin, providing a perfect foreground for the distant icy mass of Mount Rainier. Only its relative isolation keeps this perfect setting from being featured in national calendars.

The scenery is consistently better now as the trail alternates among trees, flower-sprinkled meadows, heather, and bouldery hillsides with frequent views. The tour leads east along the ridge, then goes through a little saddle as it gradually gains elevation amid several ups and downs. Where the ridge rises abruptly toward prominent Johnson Peak, the trail veers to the right (south), away from the ridgecrest, and contours across Lily Basin on the west side of the peak. This sloping basin includes several small creeks (the first water of the trip), but it's very rocky, so camping is unattractive.

WARNING: The south side of the basin is prone to washouts. You can usually bypass any problem areas with some careful scrambling, but it might slow you down.

Now the path reenters forest and comes to a junction at the top of a low ridge. You'll want to spend some time here to enjoy the excellent views, especially of hulking Mount Adams, which dominates the rolling landscape to the south. This landmark will be a major feature of all southerly views on this hike, just as Mount Rainier will adorn any vista to the north.

You turn left (east) at the ridgetop junction and drop gradually through trees and meadows to an unsigned junction with the short spur trail to Heart Lake. The attractive lake setting invites an overnight stay at any of the several good camps in the trees near the outlet.

From the Heart Lake turnoff, the trail makes a long climb through large, open meadows around the head of the basin holding the lake.

WARNING: Steep snowfields linger on the north-facing slopes of this basin well into the summer.

At the top of the ridge is a world-class view of the Heart Lake basin, Mount Rainier, and nearby Johnson Peak. Delicate alpine wildflowers like phlox and heather add color and intricate beauty to the scene.

SIDE TRIP TO HAWKEYE POINT: For an even higher grandstand, drop your pack and follow the 0.8-mile spur trail east up an exposed ridge to Hawkeye Point—magnificent!

The trail now descends the south side of the ridge to another junction, where you turn left (east) and contour across an open slope of heather and a veritable sea of wildflowers to the glacial cirque holding Goat Lake. This milky-green-colored alpine lake remains ice-covered for most of the summer, but the setting is tremendous. Fine but fragile campsites can be found near the south shore. Fires are prohibited.

TIP: Pull out your binoculars here to search for mountain goats on the surrounding cliffs.

From Goat Lake your trail goes south across another open slope with only minor ups and downs on its way to famous Snowgrass Flat. This multitiered meadow, carpeted with wildflowers in midsummer, features picturesque scattered trees and bubbling creeks. Wonderful views from this meadow include the nearby crags of Old Snowy Mountain and Ives Peak, as well as distant Mount Adams to the south.

WARNING: This wonderland is justifiably popular with weekend backpackers. Try to schedule your visit for midweek, and avoid damage to the fragile meadows by camping only in designated sites and staying on the trail.

Near the north end of Snowgrass Flat is a trail junction with a confusion of trails, most of which simply dead-end at campsites. The shortest way to continue your trip is to turn left (northeast) on Trail #96 and climb to a junction with the Pacific Crest Trail (PCT). A more interesting option, however, is to continue straight (south) from the junction to reach a lovely meadow, where camping is now prohibited.

Unless the weather is bad, be sure to schedule a late afternoon or evening side trip to spectacular Cispus Basin. To reach it, hike south from the meadow at the lower end of Snowgrass Flat to a junction with Trail #97, then turn left (southeast), pass a creek with good nearby campsites, and climb 0.7 mile to a large cairn marking the junction with the PCT. Here you turn right (southeast) and hike gently downhill another 1.8 miles through Cispus Basin, a sloping parkland situated beneath the crags of Ives Peak. As the PCT rounds this basin, it overlooks waterfalls on the creek, passes through fields of wild-flowers, offers wonderful viewpoints, and provides several vantage points to search for mountain goats. All in all, side trips don't get much more rewarding than this. For more extensive views, continue beyond the basin another mile to windswept Cispus Pass.

TIP: If you'd rather not fight the crowds in Snowgrass Flat, you can camp in Cispus Basin, but only in designated sites.

Back at the PCT junction with the trail from Snowgrass Flat, proceed north on the PCT through beautiful open meadows to a junction with Trail #96. From here continue north on the main trail through a flower-covered and view-packed wonderland to appropriately named Split Rock, a house-size boulder split in two, with trees growing in the gap. The route now makes a gradual but steady climb toward the alpine zone, as the trees disappear and views, especially south to Mount Adams, improve with every step. The PCT follows cairns as it ascends snow-fields, bouldery areas, and small meadows.

WARNING: The next few miles follow the exposed crest of the Goat Rocks, one of the highest elevations reached by the PCT in Washington. The very narrow trail stays well above timberline for several miles, and shelter is nonexistent. Come prepared for the environment, and do not attempt this section in bad weather. More than one hiker has died from hypothermia in this area.

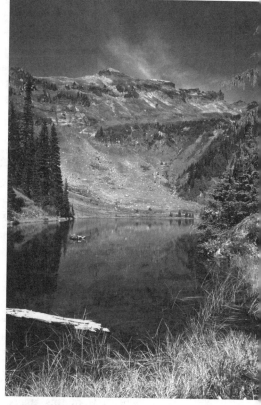

Heart Lake
photographed by Douglas Lorain

The trail tops out on a narrow ridge above Packwood Glacier, where the view down the valley of Upper Lake Creek to towering Mount Rainier is breathtaking. Now you cross the upper reaches of Packwood Glacier (potentially icy on cold mornings or late in the summer), and then traverse some rocky areas below Old Snowy Mountain. Where the trail regains the ridgetop, you'll be able to enjoy vistas to the east, as well as the now-familiar ones to the west and north. In places, the route has been blasted into the side or top of this narrow ridge, and there is limited room for passing.

TIP: Keep a lookout for oncoming horse parties, and find a place to get off on the lower side of the trail well before meeting them.

The trail makes several ups and downs along the ridge but always features great scenery. Near Egg Butte, at the north end of the ridge, early-morning hikers commonly encounter mountain goats, and elk may also be seen in the meadows far below.

TIP: A particularly photogenic view from the ridge above Egg Butte looks northwest to the long expanse of Coyote Ridge, which serves as a foreground for distinctive Mount Rainier.

The trail now drops a bit to Elk Pass and a junction. The PCT turns right (east) here, but your route goes straight (north) and makes a switchbacking descent on the west side of the ridge. As you lose elevation, the terrain becomes much friendlier than it was along the Goat Rocks crest, with lush meadows and trees to provide shelter and shade. The trail drops a little over 1,200 feet from Elk Pass before reaching forested Packwood Saddle and another junction. The fastest route back to civilization follows the Upper Lake Creek Trail past a campsite and spring, then down the valley to the left (west). This trail is only irregularly maintained, however, and has only marginal views. A better and much more scenic alternative goes straight (north) through the saddle and follows Coyote Ridge.

WARNING: Water is scarce along Coyote Ridge.

The rugged and view-packed Coyote Ridge Trail begins with a rapid climb to the open terrain and rock outcrops around Chimney Rock, where you can look across Upper Lake Creek's valley to towering Johnson Peak, all cliffs and snowfields from this angle. The

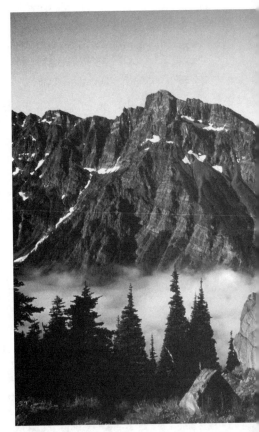

Johnson Peak from Coyote Ridge
photographed by Douglas Lorain

up-and-down route then contours away from the ridgetop, staying on the southwest side of the divide. A rocky promontory about 1 mile from Chimney Rock has a particularly appealing view and makes an ideal lunch or rest stop.

The trail continues its westward course, rounds the shoulder of a bulky high point in the ridge, and then drops to a lovely basin. Nice shade trees and small but reliable Beaver Bill Creek make this basin an inviting campsite. Beyond Beaver Bill Creek, the trail stays mostly in heavy forest, so views are limited, but elk are common and often seen by quiet hikers. Before long the trail comes to a junction.

TIP: From here you can turn right (north) and make a worthwhile 0.6-mile side trip to Lost Lake, a deep pool that features meadows and good camps.

To complete your tour, turn left (west) at the junction south of Lost Lake, and follow a gentle trail through forest and past lush meadows. After 1 mile you turn left (west) at the next junction, drop past tiny but ominously named Mosquito Lake, and then make a long, forested descent to a junction just above the shores of large Packwood Lake.

Your route goes right (west) and follows the path to the lake's outlet stream, where a small resort used to be and where there is still a fine view. Johnson Peak forms a distinctive backdrop for this lake, and a large, forested island adds to the scene. Detracting from the scenery, especially on weekends, are the hundreds of fellow admirers, the result of easy access on a nearly level trail.

TIP: The lake's location, just outside the officially protected wilderness, means the tranquility is often broken by motorcycles. Try to visit on a weekday.

The final part of the trip crosses the lake's dammed outlet stream, passes a historical U.S. Forest Service guard station, and works away from the lake into attractive old-growth forests. Motorcycles can often be heard racing along an old pipeline road to the right (north). The gentle access trail ends at the large Packwood Lake Trailhead, about 4 miles from its namesake.

POSSIBLE ITINERARY

	CAMP	MILES	ELEVATION GAIN
Day 1	Heart Lake	6.6	1,300'
Day 2	Cispus Basin	9.0	2,050'
	Side trip to Hawkeye Point	1.6	450'
Day 3	Beaver Bill Creek	12.1	2,500'
Day 4	Out	9.4	200'

BEST SHORTER ALTERNATIVE

From the Goat Creek Trailhead to the south, a long day hike or one-night backpacking trip to Snowgrass Flat is incredibly rewarding, especially when done as a loop to include Goat Lake.

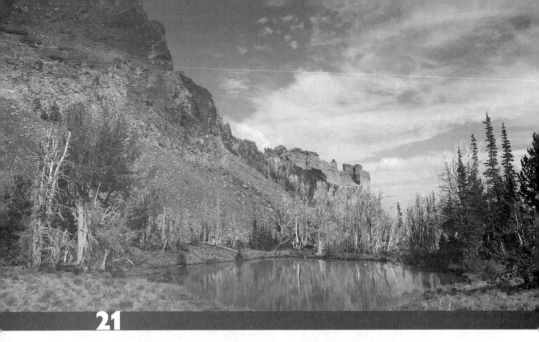

21

MOUNT ADAMS HIGHLINE TRAIL LOOP

RATINGS: Scenery 10   **Solitude** 5   **Difficulty** 9

MILES: 33 (35)

ELEVATION GAIN: 6,700' (7,550')

DAYS: 4–5 (4–6)

SHUTTLE MILEAGE: n/a

MAP: USFS *Mount Adams, Indian Heaven, and Trapper Creek Wildernesses*

USUALLY OPEN: Mid-July–mid-October

BEST: Late July–August

PERMIT: Required (separate permits for the wilderness and the Yakama Indian Reservation). The wilderness permit is free and available at the South Climb Trailhead. Contact the Yakama Nation at the number below or visit yakamanation-nsn.gov/tract-d.php or ynwildlife.org/Recreation.php for current information regarding permits for the reservation.

RULES: Maximum group size of 12 people and/or stock; fires prohibited above the Round-the-Mountain, Pacific Crest, and Highline Trails

CONTACTS: Gifford Pinchot National Forest, Mount Adams Ranger District, 509-395-3400, fs.usda.gov/main/giffordpinchot; Yakama Nation Department of Natural Resources, Forest Development Program, 509-865-5121 ext. 4185, yakamanation-nsn.gov

Above: *Goat Peak over a pond in Avalanche Valley*

photographed by Mark Wetherington

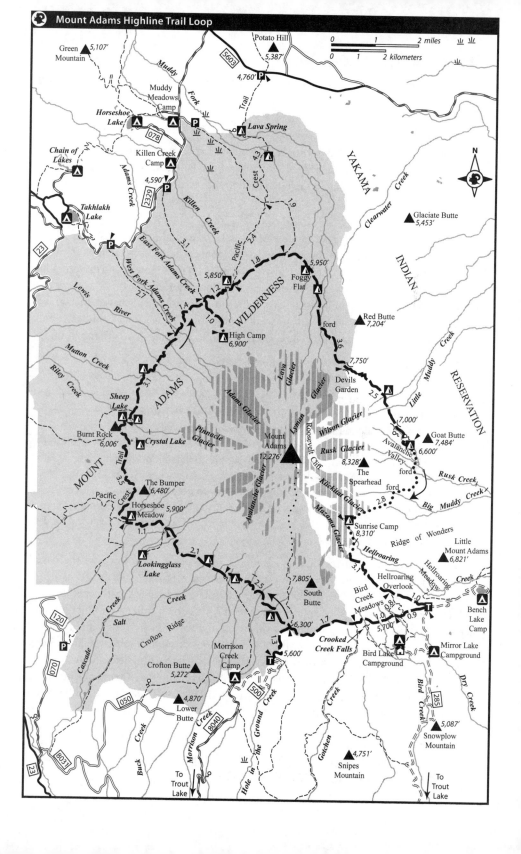

Green Mountain 5,107'

Potato Hill 5,387'

5603

0 1 2 miles
0 1 2 kilometers

4,760' P

Muddy Fork

Muddy Meadows Camp

Horseshoe Lake

078

Lava Spring

YAKAMA

Clearwater Creek

Chain of Lakes

Killen Creek Camp

4,590'

2326

Takhlakh Lake

Adams Creek

4.3

Crest Trail

Glaciate Butte 5,453'

East Fork Adams Creek

West Fork Adams Creek

3.1

2.7

Pacific

2.4

1.9

5,850'

1.2

1.8

Foggy Flat

5,950'

INDIAN

Red Butte 7,204'

Lewis River

1.4

1.0

WILDERNESS

High Camp 6,900'

ford

3.6

7,750'

Little Muddy Creek

RESERVATION

Mutton Creek

ADAMS

Lava Glacier

Lyman Glacier

Devils Garden

7,000'

2.5

Riley Creek

3.1

Sheep Lake

Adams Glacier

Wilson Glacier

Goat Butte 7,484'

Burnt Rock 6,006'

Crystal Lake

Pinnacle Glacier

Mount Adams 12,276'

Roosevelt Cliff

Rusk Glacier

8,328'

Avalanche Valley 6,600'

ford

MOUNT

3.5

Pacific

The Bumper 6,480'

Horseshoe Meadow 5,900'

1.1

Avalanche Glacier

The Spearhead

Klickitat Glacier

ford

2.8

Rusk Creek

Big Muddy Creek

Crest

Lookingglass Lake

2.1

2.5

Mazama Glacier

Sunrise Camp 8,310'

Ridge of Wonders

Little Mount Adams 6,821'

Trail

7,805'

3.1

Hellroaring

Creek

Salt

Creek

South Butte

Bird Creek Meadows

Hellroaring Overlook

Hellroaring Meadow

1.0

120

Crofton Ridge

1.7

6,300'

1.0

0.8

5,700'

0.9

Bench Lake Camp

070

Cascade Creek

P

1.3

5,600'

Crooked Creek Falls

Bird Lake Campground

Mirror Lake Campground

Snowplow Mountain 5,087'

Crofton Butte 5,272'

Morrison Creek Camp

500

Bird Creek

Dry Creek

285

050

Lower Butte 4,870'

8040

Morrison Creek

Hole in the Ground Creek

Gotchen Creek

Snipes Mountain 4,751'

8037

23

Buck Creek

To Trout Lake

To Trout Lake

SPECIAL ATTRACTIONS

Relatively easy trail (for most of the route), terrific mountain scenery, wildflowers, interesting geology

CHALLENGES

Yakama Indian Reservation permit requirements, exposed sections on the north and east sides of the mountain, unbridged crossings of glacial streams, challenging off-trail section for those doing the full loop, rough road to the starting point

HOW TO GET THERE

Start from the picturesque community of Trout Lake, 22 miles north of White Salmon on WA 141. Drive north from town on the paved Mount Adams Recreation Highway for 1.2 miles, then veer right (northeast) at a fork to remain on the highway, and drive another 0.7 mile. If you're starting from the South Climb Trailhead, go left (north) and follow Forest Service Road 80 for 3.7 miles. Then turn right (north) onto initially paved, then gravel, FS 8040, and go 5.4 miles to Morrison Creek Campground. Turn right (southeast) onto FS 500, and climb this rough dirt road another 2.7 miles to Cold Springs Campground.

NOTE: You'll need a Northwest Forest Pass to park at the South Climb Trailhead.

TIP: If you plan to do the full loop around the mountain, it's much easier from a logistical standpoint to begin from Bird Creek Meadows. This way, on the drive in, you can buy the required tribal recreation permit from either the self-issue permit kiosk near Mirror Lake or the Yakama ranger who is usually stationed near Bird Lake. A self-issue permit station is located at the Round-the-Mountain Trailhead for overnight permits if you plan to spend the night on the reservation. If you start the loop at Cold Springs, it's difficult and very inconvenient to go out of your way to get your permit.

Entering the reservation without a permit is considered trespassing. Before setting out for this trip, check with the Yakama Nation regarding current regulations, and respect any closures in place.

If you're starting from Bird Creek Meadows, drive north from town on the paved Mount Adams Recreation Highway for 1.2 miles, then veer right (northeast) at a fork to remain on the highway, and drive another 3.3 miles. Turn right (east) on FS 82, and follow signs to Bird Creek Meadows. Stick with FS 82 for 6 miles to a junction, and keep straight on FS 8290. Slowly pick your way along this narrow, rough dirt route for 4.1 miles to a junction beside tiny Mirror Lake. There is usually a self-issue kiosk here, or you can obtain a Yakama Indian Reservation permit by turning left and visiting the ranger station at Bird Lake. Once you have a permit, go back to the Mirror Lake junction, and drive north another 1.1 miles. Head northwest on the trail, and climb 0.6 mile to the Round-the-Mountain Trailhead.

GPS TRAILHEAD COORDINATES:
South Climb (Cold Springs): N46° 08.154' W121° 29.856'
Bird Creek Meadows: N46° 09.272' W121° 25.584'

INTRODUCTION ••

Of the five major volcanic peaks in the Washington Cascades, only Mount Baker lacks any sort of around-the-mountain trail. The remaining four all have very scenic routes that showcase lots of wildflowers, terrific mountain scenery, and great views. The journey around Mount Adams includes the same attractions as the others but also has some significant differences. First of all, the trail here is less strenuous, generally managing to avoid the deep canyons and high ridges found on the other trips. Second, the weather on Mount Adams is usually better because it's located farther east. Finally, longer road access over sometimes-rough gravel and dirt roads ensures that Mount Adams is somewhat less crowded, so while you won't exactly be lonesome, you should enjoy more solitude.

Note for loop hikers: Almost any backpacker can enjoy this trip as a fun out-and-back by turning around at either Foggy Flat or Devils Garden and returning the way you came. Some hikers, however, will be interested in doing the entire, rugged circuit all the way around the peak.

The feasibility of doing the full loop depends on three main factors: First is whether the Yakama Nation, which owns the east side of the mountain, allows nontribal members to use its lands and/or to camp overnight. Large parts of the Yakama Indian Reservation have been closed in recent years due to safety concerns and recovery efforts from large forest fires. Although some hikers go through anyway, that is trespassing, illegal, and not recommended. Call ahead for the latest status on land closures.

The second factor is how experienced and comfortable you are with off-trail travel. Some of the trails, especially on the Yakama Indian Reservation, are sketchy and rough. Even more important, the section from Avalanche Valley to Sunrise Camp is entirely off trail. This off-trail portion requires at least one (and sometimes several) potentially difficult creek crossing, some tricky navigation issues, snow travel, and negotiating large boulder fields. By the proper route, it is certainly feasible for athletic and experienced hikers, but novices should not consider it.

WARNING: Before setting out on this trip, confirm with the Yakama Nation if camping is allowed on the reservation.

Finally, consider the time of year and the weather. The annual window of opportunity for the off-trail section is relatively short—typically from about mid-August to mid- or late September. Heavy snowmelt earlier in the summer makes the creek crossings too difficult for safety, and the cold temperatures, possible snow, and constant wind in autumn make things decidedly uncomfortable at best (and dangerous at worst) when traveling through miles of exposed above-timberline terrain. Even the daily weather matters because you definitely don't want to face a ford of Big Muddy Creek or, to a lesser extent, some of the other glacial streams on a hot afternoon, when the creeks are roaring with meltwater from the glaciers just upstream. All that said, if you can safely and legally do it, the full loop, especially the rugged portion on the east side, is lots of fun and wildly scenic. It's just not for everybody.

This adventure has two logical starting points, and which one is better depends on your preferences. The first option is Bird Creek Meadows in the Yakama Indian Reservation.

This entry allows you to immediately savor the spectacular scenery and famous wildflower gardens of Bird Creek Meadows. On the downside, it requires a longer drive on poorer roads, and you must buy a use permit from the Yakama Nation, regardless of whether you plan to complete the full loop. The second starting point is Cold Springs Campground, where the standard Northwest Forest Pass is acceptable and the road access is marginally better, but you will miss Bird Creek Meadows. To get the best of both worlds, some hikers who don't plan to do the full loop start at Cold Springs, then make a side trip to Bird Creek Meadows. (Loop hikers will pass through Bird Creek Meadows on their final day.) Another consideration: The Cold Springs Trailhead is the starting point for the popular southside climbing route of Mount Adams, so the small campground and trailhead here are often crowded, especially on summer weekends. Competing for a parking spot with early-arriving climbers can be difficult. We advise starting at Bird Creek Meadows (check on road conditions; the road was notoriously bad for many years but was rebuilt in 2019) and paying the few extra dollars for a Yakama permit, even if you don't plan to complete the full loop. The beauty is well worth the price, and it's still a cheap vacation.

DESCRIPTION

If you begin at Bird Creek Meadows, start by hiking west from the Round-the-Mountain Trailhead just below the picnic area. The scenery starts off with a bang amid acres of colorful wildflowers and terrific views to the hulking, rounded summit of Mount Adams. After just 0.1 mile is a junction. The trail to the right (northwest) climbs to Hellroaring Overlook and Sunrise Camp. If you make the full loop around the mountain, you will return that way.

The main Round-the-Mountain Trail goes west from the Hellroaring Overlook turnoff, exploring more of the glories of Bird Creek Meadows on a gentle path that crosses several little creeks on picturesque wooden logs and bridges. The Yakama Nation manages this area exclusively for day use, so overnight camping is prohibited except at the designated car camps at Bird, Bench, and Mirror Lakes, all well below the trail.

TIP: While early to mid-August is the peak wildflower time, you can also enjoy lovely fall colors in early to mid-October, when there are many fewer people. At that time, the meadows are golden brown and the huckleberry bushes have turned bright red.

Over the next 0.9 mile you pass three different junctions with trails that explore the meadows. At each junction you keep straight (west), staying on the Round-the Mountain Trail as it makes a long, rolling ascent through a delightful subalpine terrain of meadows, small creeks, and forests of mountain hemlocks and subalpine firs. At 1.6 miles you come to another junction.

TIP: It's well worth your time here to make a 0.2-mile one-way downhill side trip on the trail to the left (south) to a viewpoint just below beautiful Crooked Creek Falls.

The Round-the-Mountain Trail continues straight 0.3 mile to a junction with Snipes Mountain Trail and the boundary between the Yakama Indian Reservation and the Mount Adams Wilderness area. Keep straight (west) and continue the intermittent uphill trek as you cross meadows, areas of lava, and some burn areas for 2.3 miles to the four-way junction with the South Climb Trail. To reach the Cold Springs (South Climb) trailhead, the alternate starting point, you would turn left (south) here and travel 1.3 miles down a rocky old jeep road (now used as a trail).

This junction is also the takeoff point for those interested in climbing Mount Adams. The long, tiring, but not technically difficult climb follows a trail north a little over 1 mile, and then goes up rocky ridges and long snowfields to the summit glaciers. The view from the top is outstanding.

TIP: An ice ax and raingear come in handy, especially for sliding down snowfields on the return.

NOTE: A Cascade Volcano Pass is required for all climbers traveling above 7,000 feet on Mount Adams. These are available from the Mount Adams Ranger Station in Trout Lake (bring exact change: cash or check). In 2019 a weekday pass cost $10, a weekend pass cost $15, and an annual pass was $30.

From the Cold Springs junction, the Round-the-Mountain Trail leads west, making a gently rolling traverse through sections of burned forest. It then goes over a small ridge to a nice view of Mount Adams. The terrain is generally open, with some mountain hemlocks adding patches of shade and variety. You cross intermittent Morrison Creek (adequate camps nearby) and continue the easy up-and-down hike to the west. On clear days there are fine views looking south to Mount Hood in the distance in Oregon. Now you cross some old lava flows and sometimes-dry creekbeds to a campsite a little before the junction with the Shorthorn Trail. Keep straight (northwest) and soon reach Salt Creek, where there are more possible camps.

The main trail goes northwest, continuing with its amazingly gentle grade. Unlike the trails around other major Pacific Northwest peaks, the one encircling Mount Adams avoids significant climbs and descents. The easy walking makes this trip ideal for hikers who want to explore a glacier-clad volcano but aren't up to the challenge of Mount Rainier's Wonderland Trail or the rugged trips around Glacier Peak and Mount St. Helens.

Although the trail is fairly level, the surrounding terrain is not because much of the south side's landscape consists of jumbled rock and sand, the result of a massive landslide almost a century ago. The trail eventually reenters gentler alpine terrain and then crosses two branches of aptly named Cascade Creek just before reaching a junction.

TIP: A good side trip drops fairly steeply down the trail to the left (south) on the way to tiny Lookingglass Lake (0.9 mile). The pool features pleasant camps and partially obstructed views of Mount Adams.

The main trail continues west for 1.1 miles, passing through another patch of burned forest, to the welcome expanse of Horseshoe Meadow, a large, flat meadow covered with tiny wildflowers and featuring an excellent view of Mount Adams. The best photos are from the southwest side of the meadow. The tiny creek that crosses Horseshoe Meadow sometimes runs dry by late summer, but if water is available, excellent camps are just beyond the creek crossing.

WARNING: Horse parties often use this camp.

TIP: For privacy and reliable water, walk cross-country up the meadow, follow the right branch of the "creek," and scramble uphill to a lovely little pumice meadow, which offers nice views and good camps.

At the west end of Horseshoe Meadow, you turn right (northwest) at a junction with the Pacific Crest Trail (PCT) and gain a bit of elevation along a small ridge. Then the trail makes an up-and-down transit of numerous small ridges and gullies as it takes a circuitous course to the north. Ridges block views of nearby Mount Adams, but there are nice views to the west of distant Mount St. Helens. You round a ridge and then, about 2.8 miles from starting on the PCT, begin to lose elevation along the side of a second ridge.

TIP: Just before beginning this descent, a terrific cross-country side trip goes steeply east up a grassy gully for 0.2 mile. It then climbs to the left into a rocky area with scattered trees holding a small tarn called Crystal Lake. The lake is so small that it can be difficult to find, but if you succeed, there are good camps here and a terrific view across the water to bulky Mount Adams.

The reader may have noticed that the adjectives used to describe Mount Adams often include *hulking, bulky,* or *massive.* This peak cannot boast of the delicate, pointed beauty of other Cascade summits, as from every angle, the mountain looks like it needs to go on a diet. In its own way, however, Mount Adams is every bit as spectacular as its daintier neighbors.

From its location below unseen Crystal Lake, the PCT loses elevation, crosses a small saddle, and then descends to tiny Sheep Lake, which has a small but decent (although not terribly private) campsite at its northeast end. Beyond this lake, you continue north as the trail contours across a partly forested slope, crosses milky Riley Creek (very nice camps along an unofficial footpath that heads upstream just after the crossing), and then comes to a junction with the little-used Riley Camp Trail going left (west). Keep straight

Falls on Killen Creek
photographed by Douglas Lorain

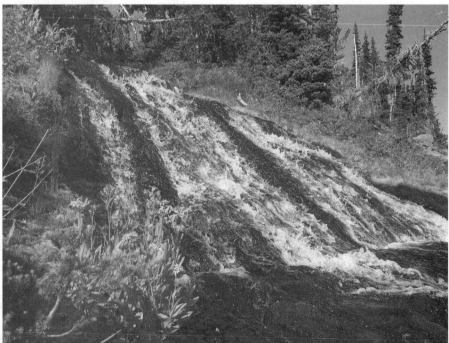

(north) on the PCT and soon come to Mutton Creek beside a very recent-looking lava flow and a nice campsite. From here the trail gradually gains elevation as it crosses this rugged landscape of jagged lava.

Past the jumbled lava, the trail reenters gentler terrain and soon reaches the rock-hop crossing of not-quite-clear Lewis River. The gentle trail through this area features some superb views of Mount Rainier and the Tatoosh Range to the north. You keep straight (northeast) at a junction with the Divide Trail, and immediately thereafter reach the crossing of West Fork Adams Creek. This muddy, glacial stream can be forded, but if you prefer to keep your feet dry, you can usually find a small log across the creek just upstream from the official trail crossing. Nervous hikers may prefer to scoot across the log with the aid of a larger contact point than just their feet.

Continuing your hike north on the PCT, a short stretch of mostly level walking takes you to the junction with the Killen Creek Trail.

HIGH CAMP SIDE TRIP: A signed trail goes right here, climbing steeply over rocky terrain for 1 mile to High Camp in the beautiful alpine country to the southeast. If you have the time, it's well spent on this side trip and in exploring the alpine benches near the camp. The entire area is spectacularly scenic, especially the terrific views of Mount Adams. Camping at this exposed location is amazing, *if* the weather permits, in part because the sunrises and sunsets are breathtaking.

From the Killen Creek junction, your loop route goes straight (northeast) on the PCT. In 0.7 mile the path drops a bit to reach a lovely little meadow with a seasonal pond and a great view of Mount Adams. At the far end of this meadow, the trail crosses Killen Creek on a bridge just above a sloping waterfall, and then makes a short switchback down to a beautiful little basin. Nearby ponds, a cascading waterfall, and wonderful views of Mount Adams combine to make this a choice location. Other hikers seem to agree with this assessment, as this is a very popular campsite, especially on summer weekends. About 200 yards beyond this basin is a junction with the Highline Trail, where you turn right (northeast).

The pleasant Highline Trail leads you through attractive, primarily open forests as it quickly passes two small ponds and makes an irregular climb to the northeast. The climb tops out on a wide ridge with good views and then loses about 250 feet to a junction. The Highline Trail continues east, makes a series of steep little ups and downs (more ups than downs), and comes to a lush meadow called Foggy Flat. A clear stream flows through this green oasis, with excellent camps in the nearby trees and Mount Adams picturesquely crowning the scene. As always, please do not camp on the fragile meadow vegetation.

TIP: Stock up on water here because the sources for the next several miles are either undependable or muddy with glacial silt.

Foggy Flat is an inviting base camp for those who do not plan to complete the full loop but still want to visit Avalanche Valley, arguably the highlight of this trip, via a long day hike. A day hike seems like a logical plan since you will have to return by the same route. The authors recommend, however, that if camping is currently allowed on Yakama land, you carry your heavy pack all the way to Avalanche Valley. The place is just too spectacular to appreciate in the hour or two you would have on a day hike. In addition, the early-morning view of Mount Adams over Avalanche Valley is a memory that will last a lifetime.

However large a pack you're carrying, the trail soon climbs above the forest just past Foggy Flat and enters a rugged area of boulders and glacial outwash. At the edge of this wasteland, an acceptable campsite lies near a small, reasonably clear creek.

From here the trail features lots of small ups and downs, but *up* is dominant. Views north to distant Mount Rainier and the Goat Rocks become more impressive as you climb, helping to compensate for the sweat. Only a few weather-stunted mountain hemlocks and whitebark pines survive in this inhospitable landscape, where even grass is rare. The only animals are a few marmots and pikas, ravens flying overhead, and an occasional herd of mountain goats. The sometimes-faint path climbs steeply beside boisterous and glacial Muddy Fork and then drops briefly to cross the creek. A snowbridge may provide reasonably safe passage across this torrent for most of the summer, but you should probe carefully with an ice ax or a walking stick to avoid thin spots.

WARNING: If the snowbridge has collapsed, the crossing may be dangerous or even impossible on a warm afternoon with lots of snowmelt from upstream.

After crossing the creek, look for huge rock cairns on the far side and follow these as the trail resumes climbing through this above-timberline moonscape.

WARNING: This area is very exposed and often windy. Avoid it in bad weather.

You climb moderately steeply through more boulder fields and lava and then reach a small flat area covered with volcanic cinders. Here you will enjoy fine views of Red Butte, a prominent cinder cone about 1 mile to the northeast, and the distant icy summit of Mount Rainier. Towering above this entire scene, of course, is the enormous mass of Mount Adams and large Lyman Glacier. The trail finally tops out at about 7,750 feet on an exposed ridge called Devils Garden. Winds are almost constant here, so you may have to take cover behind one of the large rock cairns to rest and enjoy the view.

The route now turns east and reenters the Yakama Indian Reservation. Beyond this point, the trail exists only by virtue of hiker's boots, as the Yakamas do not maintain this remote route. The Yakama Nation requires a permit for using this area, which you can obtain from the ranger at Bird Lake before you start. The few camps in this area are not specifically designated for use by nontribal members, but the Yakamas have traditionally allowed backpackers to use them. To ensure that the tribe isn't forced to impose restrictions on public use in the future, it's particularly important that you never build campfires and that you treat the land with special care. It is of paramount importance that you confirm with the Yakama Nation that camping is allowed.

The scenic tour goes east to a small drop-off, descends steeply into a little basin, and then turns south. The rolling alpine terrain here is varied and attractive with boulders, meadows, small creeks, and rocky ridges.

WARNING 1: Water sources in this sandy, volcanic soil sometimes dry up by late summer.

WARNING 2: The trail is easy to lose in this open terrain. If you're not sure, go back to the last obvious tread and look for one of the small cairns hikers have put up to aid in navigation.

You gradually descend and cross a couple of usually flowing creeks (adequate camps) to a ford of silty Little Muddy Creek. From there you climb a bit to a low saddle northwest of prominent Goat Butte. South of this saddle, the trail descends past some springs to two small but incredibly scenic ponds amid the glorious expanse of Avalanche Valley. A large, gushing spring feeds a good-size creek of extremely cold water at the head of the meadows, and colorful wildflowers carpet the entire area. The craggy edge of Goat Butte forms a beautiful backdrop along the meadow's eastern edge. It will be hard to notice any of these features, however, as your attention is turned to the jaw-dropping view of Mount Adams to the west. Cliffs and 4,000-foot-high ramparts support streaking waterfalls that pour out of Rusk and Klickitat Glaciers, shimmering in the sun. Higher still rises Roosevelt Cliff, then more glaciers, and finally the rounded summit of the great volcano. The scene is one of the best these authors have ever enjoyed. A few wildly scenic campsites are in the area, but please treat this fragile area lightly.

TIP: Bring binoculars to search the cliffs for mountain goats.

After arriving at Avalanche Valley . . . well, first of all, enjoy! This is, after all, one of the most spectacular backcountry locations in Washington State. Next, you need to carefully consider your options. As previously discussed, you can always turn around and happily return the way you came. For all but experienced off-trail hikers, in fact, that is exactly what you should do.

Hikers with the necessary skills and ambition, however, might want to do the full loop around the mountain. If you are a member of that rugged cadre, and you are here during the late summer window of opportunity, then all you need to complete this circuit is a bit of determination and knowledge of the proper route. The first is up to you. For the second, read on.

Although there is no route between Avalanche Valley and Sunrise Camp that could be described as easy, taking the proper route will make your life dramatically easier and the trip more reasonable. First, do not follow the route shown on the Green Trails map of Mount Adams. This takes you much too high on the mountain, forcing you to deal with some dangerously steep slopes with loose rocks, as well as a very difficult crossing of a rock glacier at the base of Klickitat Glacier. Only contemplate this tough route if you are really concerned about how high the meltwaters are filling Big Muddy Creek and you have the necessary skills and equipment required for glacier travel. The much better route is to take the low road, so to speak, through the valleys well below Klickitat Glacier.

Begin by descending on sketchy trail through the lower end of Avalanche Valley. After a little less than 0.2 mile, leave the trail and continue downhill and south through rolling forests and meadowlands until you reach the eroded canyon of Rusk Creek, now about 350 feet lower in elevation than the ponds in Avalanche Valley. Search around a bit until you find a reasonably safe route down to Rusk Creek, then cross this glacial stream.

TIP: Try to time this crossing for early morning before the meltwaters get too high. Even then, you should expect wet feet on a not-too-difficult ford, although if you really search around, you may find a place to rock-hop it.

Once across Rusk Creek, scramble up the steep opposite bank, then hike through open forests and across sloping hillsides, going around the base of a ridge while remaining near the 6,250-foot contour. This takes you into the next scenic canyon, which holds Big

Muddy Creek. This glacial stream tumbles through a boulder-strewn landscape with awe-inspiring views up to nearby Mount Adams and the icy Klickitat Glacier that feeds the creek. Hiking up the canyon is relatively straightforward and not overly difficult, except for the fact that somewhere along the way, you'll have to cross the creek. The best plan is to hike upstream until you locate a reasonable spot and to make the crossing as early in the day as possible. You can expect a short (maybe 10–12 feet), knee- to thigh-deep crossing through cold, swift, and very silty water. Use trekking poles for added balance and have wading shoes with good traction. It isn't a simple cakewalk, but under the right conditions, experienced hikers should be fine.

Once across Big Muddy Creek, you complete the long climb up the valley amid boulders to the bottom of a large snowfield that abuts the south side of sprawling Klickitat Glacier. You will need to climb this snowfield to reach Sunrise Camp, which is located at the low point of the ridge at the top of the snowfield just to the right of a large rocky abutment. The snowfield is long and requires about a 1,000-foot climb, but it's not terribly steep. Unless it is a cold and icy morning, you can often carefully climb the snowfield without the aid of an ice ax or crampons. The views as you ascend—both of tall and icy Mount Adams and down the valley you just climbed to pyramid-shaped Goat Butte—are superb. Mountain goats are often seen in this area.

At the top of the snowfield, you cross a small area of boulders. Immediately on the other side, you should see the stark and flat sandy expanse of Sunrise Camp, with its numerous user-constructed rock walls to help keep tents from blowing away in the wind. The location, near a meltwater creek, is wildly scenic, with very up close looks at Mazama Glacier and distant views looking south to pointed Mount Hood in Oregon.

Finding the faint route down from Sunrise Camp is tricky. Fortunately, if the weather is clear, it's a simple matter to look south and down to your next destination, a large muddy lake at the foot of Mazama Glacier. The lake usually has icebergs floating in it throughout

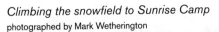

Climbing the snowfield to Sunrise Camp
photographed by Mark Wetherington

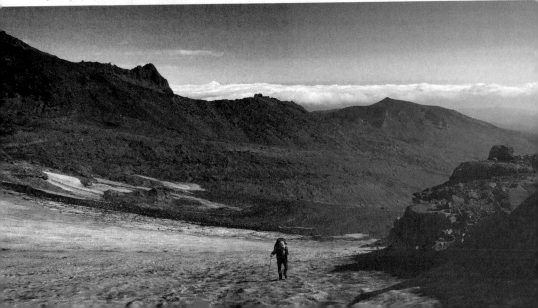

the summer. Even without the rocky and hard-to-find semi-official trail, making your way down to the lake is relatively simple and straightforward. It involves some boulder-hopping, descending areas of loose scree, and negotiating a couple of steep spots, but navigation is simple. After a fairly quick 1.3 miles, you'll reach the lake. Hikers have built a couple of rock walls here to protect tents, but you should only camp here in an emergency, as the Yakama Nation does not consider this to be a legal campsite.

Things get easier now; after a careful examination, you'll find a faint official trail (look for cairns and orange paint marks on rocks as guides) just below and southeast of the lake. This route leads you across a scree slope to the top of a side ridge. From here you follow the ridgetop downhill to the southeast for about 80 yards, then switchback down to the left (east) side of the relatively flat meadowlands below. From here you follow an initially faint tread that goes south along a minor view-packed ridgeline with scattered conifers. Expect awesome views of Mount Adams, Little Mount Adams to the east, and a tall water-fall on the creek that flows down from near Sunrise Camp. The large, green expanse below Little Mount Adams is Hellroaring Meadow.

At an obvious viewpoint location known as Hellroaring Overlook, about 3.1 miles down from Sunrise Camp, or 1.8 miles from the meltwater lake, is a possibly unsigned junction. If you started at Bird Creek Meadows, you veer left (southeast), sticking with the ridge, and descend through open forest for 1 mile to the Round-the-Mountain Trailhead.

If your destination is the Cold Springs trailhead, then bear right (south) at the junction beside Hellroaring Overlook, descend through flower-covered meadowlands for 0.3 mile, and then go right (southwest) at a second junction. After another 0.5 mile, you reach a junction with Round-the-Mountain Trail #9, where you turn right (west) and proceed as described at the beginning of this hike.

VARIATIONS

As discussed previously, you can skip the off-trail portion of this loop and make this an out-and-back hike by turning around at either Devils Garden or Avalanche Valley. With a long car shuttle, you could also turn this into a point-to-point trip by finishing your hike at either the Muddy Meadows Trailhead or the Pacific Crest Trailhead on Forest Service Road 5603 near Potato Hill.

POSSIBLE ITINERARY

	CAMP	MILES	ELEVATION GAIN
Day 1	Horseshoe Meadow	9.3	1,100'
Day 2	Killen Creek Meadows	9.2	900'
	Side trip to High Camp	2.0	850'
Day 3	Avalanche Valley	7.9	2,400'
Day 4	Out	6.9	2,300'

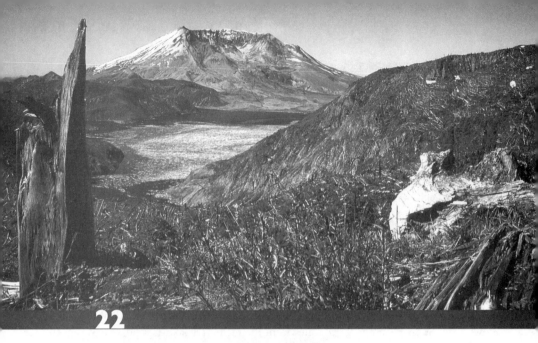

22

MOUNT MARGARET
BACKCOUNTRY LOOP

RATINGS: Scenery 9   **Solitude** 3   **Difficulty** 9/7

MILES: 28/30 (29/31)

ELEVATION GAIN: 6,300'/7,450' (6,900'/8,050')

DAYS: 3–5 (3–5)

SHUTTLE MILEAGE: n/a

MAP: Green Trails *Mount St. Helens National Volcanic Monument (#332S)*

USUALLY OPEN: Mid-June–October

BEST: Late June–July

PERMIT: Required. Permits must be reserved in advance by visiting recreation .gov or by calling 877-444-6777. A $6 nonrefundable reservation fee applies.

RULES: Maximum group size of 4 people; camping allowed only at one of the eight designated campsites; livestock, dogs, and fires strictly prohibited; access prohibited to the areas around Boot Lake and St. Helens Lake, and on all lands south of the Boundary Trail; all off-trail travel, even for short distances, prohibited; backpackers strongly encouraged to use bear canisters (hanging food from trees is not an option given the small size of the regrowing forest)

CONTACT: Mount St. Helens National Volcanic Monument, 360-449-7800, fs.usda.gov/main/giffordpinchot

Above: *Mount St. Helens from Norway Pass*
photographed by Douglas Lorain

SPECIAL ATTRACTIONS ····································

Amazing and unique geology and volcanic scenery, botanical interest as plants regrow in the devastated area, great views

CHALLENGES ··································

Very limited shade; frequent washouts; lack of water, even at designated camps, especially by late summer (call ahead about conditions); extremely rugged and possibly dangerous route if you take the Mount Whittier Trail; potential for volcanic activity closing trails; difficulty in getting permits

HOW TO GET THERE ····································

Take I-5 to Exit 49, and head east on WA 504. Go 42.7 miles, and veer right (southwest) to continue on WA 504. Proceed 9 miles to the huge road-end parking lot for the Johnston Ridge Observatory.

NOTE: You'll need a Northwest Forest Pass to park at this trailhead.

GPS TRAILHEAD COORDINATES: N46° 16.602' W122° 13.008'

INTRODUCTION ····································

While the Loowit Trail around Mount St. Helens (see Trip 23) offers a better up close and personal look at the volcano, if you really want to get a larger scale overview of the mountain and the destruction wrought by the 1980 eruption, you have to step back a few miles. That is precisely the opportunity afforded by the wonderfully scenic trails in the popular Mount Margaret Backcountry north of the mountain. Here, the views across the still log-choked waters of Spirit Lake to the volcano's crater and steaming dome are like nothing else in North America, making this trip a must-do for any Washington backpacker. But the loop exploring this remarkable region offers much more than just volcanic views. You will visit several beautiful lakes, follow view-packed ridgelines, marvel at a number of impressive rock formations, and possibly see herds of elk browsing in the meadows. It's a fun experience, albeit one that is best enjoyed during cooler weather (to avoid the relentless sun on the shadeless, open slopes) and one that requires jumping through hoops to get a reserved permit well in advance of your trip.

DESCRIPTION ····································

The paved hiker-only trail begins near a large signboard at the northeast end of the parking lot. The surrounding area was completely devastated in the big eruption of May 1980, but vegetation is returning, with an increasing abundance of willows and Sitka alders. Pacific silver firs seem to be the dominant evergreens so far, although none have grown to more than 25 feet or so. Wildflowers taking advantage of the abundant sunshine include lupine, yarrow, pearly everlasting, wild strawberry, fireweed, and cliff penstemon.

As interesting and attractive as the flowers, grasses, and shrubs are, however, the real star of the show is Mount St. Helens, which dominates the view to the south. You can

continued on page 216

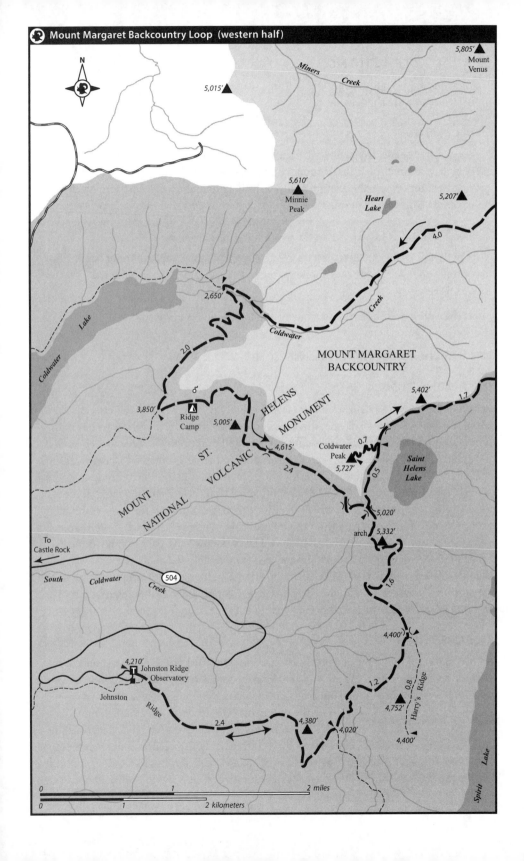

N

5,805' ▲
Mount
Venus

Miners   Creek

5,015' ▲

5,610'
▲
Minnie
Peak

Heart
Lake

5,207' ▲

4.0

Creek

2,650'

Coldwater

MOUNT MARGARET
BACKCOUNTRY

2.0

5,402' ▲   1.7

HELENS

3,850'   ♂
          △
         Ridge
         Camp   5,005' ▲

MONUMENT

Coldwater
Peak   0.7

4,615'

ST.

5,727'

0.5

Saint
Helens
Lake

2.4

VOLCANIC

5,020'

arch   5,332'

MOUNT

NATIONAL

1.6

To
Castle Rock

South   Coldwater   Creek

504

4,400'

4,210'
  ⊤ Johnston Ridge
  ■ Observatory

Johnston

1.2   0.8

Harry's Ridge

4,752' ▲

Ridge

2.4   4,380'
              ▲   4,020'

4,400'

Spirit
Lake

0   1   2 miles

0   1   2 kilometers

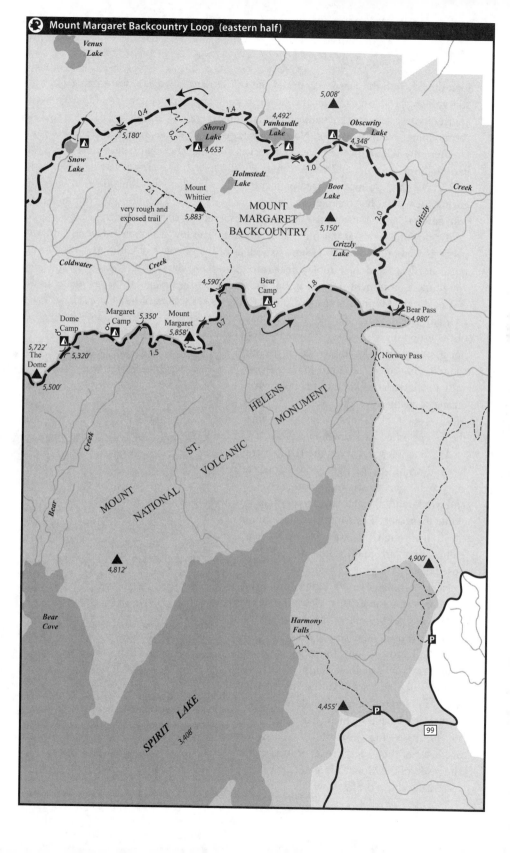

continued from page 213

look directly into the massive crater of the volcano and often see steam rising from the still-growing lava dome inside. The view is particularly impressive as you look across the enormous devastated area of wildly eroded mudflows and volcanic debris between you and the mountain. No other view in North America is remotely like the scene in front of you.

After only 100 yards, the paved trail makes a turn to the right (southwest) on its way back to the observatory and visitor center. For this hike, however, you veer left (southeast) on a gravel- and pumice-covered path that takes you gradually downhill. Although the environment looks harsh and unwelcoming to wildlife, elk are actually quite common here, with herds as large as 40 animals commonly observed, especially early in the morning.

The downhill ends at 0.8 mile, after which you follow a rolling ridgeline with stupendous views of Mount St. Helens, as well as of the pinnacle of Coldwater Peak to the north-northeast and the jumbled peaks around Mount Margaret to the northeast. When you round a prominent ridge near 2 miles, you gain your first good views looking to the east of distant Mount Adams and down to the closer waters of large Spirit Lake. Even after all these decades, the lake still has many logs floating in it. These logs are the result

of the eruption, when a superheated wall of hot gas and ash killed the trees on the surrounding hillsides. The explosion also began with a massive landslide into the lake, which created a giant wave that washed up those hillsides and took the dead trees with it when the water sloshed back down into the lake.

At a junction at 2.4 miles, the Truman Trail heads downhill to the right (south), but you go straight (northeast) on the Boundary Trail and wind uphill through an area particularly prone to erosion. Posts mark the location of the trail through this wasteland filled with gullies. The surrounding hillsides are composed of very colorful soils and rocks.

Near 3.6 miles, Harry's Ridge Trail, a 0.8-mile one-way route to a viewpoint above Spirit Lake, goes right (south). The main trail goes left (north) and steadily ascends long switchbacks to the top of a ridge, where on clear days you can look south to Oregon's Mount Hood and north to the rugged Goat Rocks and Mount Rainier. The deep waters of Saint Helens Lake—which, like Spirit Lake, still has many logs in it—fill the basin just northeast of this ridge. The contorted ridges and peaks of the Mount Margaret area can be seen rising above the lake's waters.

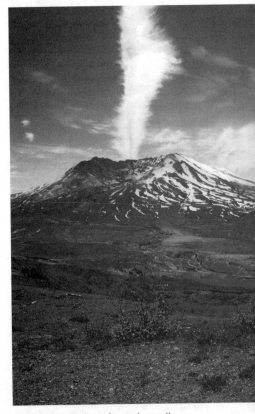

Mount St. Helens from the trail on Johnston Ridge
photographed by Douglas Lorain

The narrow and rugged trail now descends a pair of switchbacks, passes through a small rock arch, and then goes up and down to a junction and a saddle on the south flank of Coldwater Peak. If you skip the dangerously airy Mount Whittier/Whittier Ridge Trail later in the loop, you will return via the Coldwater Trail, which goes left (northwest) here.

Keep straight (north) on the Boundary Trail, which makes its way across the steep slopes of Coldwater Peak well above Saint Helens Lake on your right. After 0.5 mile you reach a junction.

> **SIDE TRIP TO COLDWATER PEAK:** Turn left (west) and begin a rather steep ascent of the northeast ridge of Coldwater Peak. The path makes numerous short switchbacks, and, as always in this area, there is no shade, so you'll be fully exposed to the sun's heat. The rewards, however, are numerous and superb. The rock here is often a very attractive reddish color, the wildflowers are abundant, and the views, especially looking far to the north to Mount Rainier, are excellent. After 0.7 mile you reach the summit, where you'll have dramatic vistas over parts of Spirit Lake to Mount St. Helens and looking east to Mount Adams. Be sure not to disturb the scientific equipment at the summit.

The Boundary Trail goes straight (north-northeast) at the Coldwater Peak junction, passes through a saddle, and then curves east across a scenic slope north of Saint Helens Lake. High on the ridge to your left, you can see a cluster of very impressive and jagged rock formations, while the lower slopes near the trail are carpeted with early-July wildflowers, especially lupine.

An extended climb gains 500 feet and takes you to a high point below the summit of a rocky peak called The Dome. Then you descend to a signed turnoff to Dome Camp at 7.4 miles. This view-packed camp sits high on a ridge northeast of The Dome and has three designated sites for overnight visitors. A really tiny spring near the outhouse and lower campsite is the only source of water, and this spring often runs dry later in the summer. If you are scheduled to stay at this site, ask the rangers about the availability of water or carry everything you will need.

The wildly scenic Boundary Trail continues east from Dome Camp, going uphill along the ridge and connecting The Dome with Mount Margaret. The views looking south across the log-choked waters of Spirit Lake to the massive crater of Mount St. Helens are breathtaking. About 0.5 mile from Dome Camp, you come to the short spur trail that goes left to Margaret Camp. Another small but somewhat more reliable spring provides water for the campers at this very scenic location.

The next mile of up-and-down hiking offers amazing scenery as you go through little saddles and loop around high points along the ridge. This is followed by a pair of long-legged uphill switchbacks that takes you high on the slopes of ruggedly scenic Mount Margaret to a junction at 8.9 miles. The short spur trail to the left (west) leads to the summit of Mount Margaret and outstanding panoramas.

The Boundary Trail goes straight (north) at the Mount Margaret junction and makes a rolling descent for 0.7 mile past a rock outcrop to a junction in a saddle. The Mount Whittier/Whittier Ridge Trail goes left (north) here and includes a sign warning hikers about the dangerous exposure along this rough trail. Take this warning seriously because this could be the most exposed, difficult, and, in a few places, even potentially dangerous official trail you will ever hike. But the decision on whether to hike it will come later in the trip, so bear right (east), staying on the Boundary Trail, and contour around the head of a small stream feeding into Spirit Lake. After a little over 0.4 mile, you pass a short spur trail that goes left (north) and leads to scenic Bear Camp. This attractive site gets its water from a usually reliable (check first) spring feeding a creek that flows down to Grizzly Lake.

An extended mostly moderate descent over open, view-packed slopes takes you down to Bear Pass and a junction. Wildflowers are abundant here in early to midsummer, with the more common varieties including yarrow, paintbrush, lupine, pearly everlasting, and fireweed. The blossoms add excellent color to outstanding photographs of southwest views across the log-strewn waters of Spirit Lake to the gaping crater of Mount St. Helens. This will be your last view of the volcano for the next several miles. As has been true in many places along this trip, the trail here is covered with dirt mixed with fine-grain ash and pumice deposited here in the massive eruption of 1980. Other evidence of the eruption comes in the form of thousands of downed logs scattered all about the hillsides.

The Boundary Trail veers right (east) at this junction, but for this loop you turn left (northeast) and descend at a moderately steep grade on a narrow and sometimes dangerously eroded trail. This circuitous path takes you across a steep hillside, over a pair of little ridges, and through an area with lots of massive deadfall before reaching Grizzly Lake about 0.8 mile from Bear Pass. This beautiful and quite deep lake fills a steep-walled cirque that, after being swept clear of nearly all life in the eruption of 1980, is now choked with regrowing shrubs, young willows and evergreens, and alpine wildflowers such as pink heather and partridge foot. The outlet to the lake is still choked with logs from trees killed in the volcanic fury of 1980.

After crossing the outlet to Grizzly Lake, you make a mile-long rolling traverse across a hillside to Obscurity Lake. This hourglass-shaped pool, backed by a small rocky butte above its northwest shore, has a designated camping area near the inlet creek at the lake's west end. Anglers can try their luck here and match wits with the resident brook trout.

The loop trail climbs steadily away from Obscurity Lake, taking you through a narrow pass before descending to deep Panhandle Lake. A downhill spur trail goes right (east) to reach the designated campsites near a small inlet creek.

Now comes some of the Mount Margaret country's best scenery, as you steeply ascend a ridge west of Panhandle Lake. This ridgeline offers amazing views looking down into the deep cirque holding sapphire-blue Shovel Lake. Mount Whittier's snow-streaked cliffs offer a dramatic backdrop, while at your feet, colorful cliff penstemon blossoms provide a wonderful foreground for photographs. The higher you go on this ridge, the better the distant views become, with nice sight lines to Mounts Adams and Rainier, as well as to the forested depths of the nearby Green River Valley. Herds of elk spend their summers feeding in the meadows in this area, so keep an eye out for these large mammals.

At a ridgetop junction, look for a spur trail that goes left (south) and descends rather steeply for 0.5 mile to the designated campsites at the west end of Shovel Lake.

The loop trail goes straight (west) at this junction, contouring along for a little over 0.4 mile to reach a wide and often windy pass and a junction with the north end of the Mount Whittier/Whittier Ridge Trail.

Here you face a choice. The more scenic (actually, make that *much* more scenic) and shorter route turns left (south) on the Mount Whittier/Whittier Ridge Trail. Before you commit yourself to that course, however, be prepared for a very tough and perhaps even somewhat dangerous undertaking. This trail is steep and frequently washed out or obliterated by rockslides that offer no reasonable possibility for detours. It's also so narrow in places that a hiker carrying a heavy external frame pack with a sleeping mat attached probably can't make it through (use a narrower internal frame pack, if you have one). If you have the slightest fear of heights, then forget it because the exposure is pretty extreme at times. And if any snow or ice is still on the trail, then forget it too because this route is scary enough without the possibility of slipping on ice. Navigation is sometimes very difficult, as the trail is poorly marked and often obscured by washouts. I simply cannot stress enough that what you just read must be taken seriously. We are all familiar with guidebooks that give you a pro forma warning about a trail that, when you hike it, turns out to be not nearly as bad as it was made out to be. This is *NOT* such a warning. Unless you are a very confident scrambler with no fear of heights, then *do not take this route.* On the positive side, however, the views (assuming you can tear your eyes off the frightening narrowness of the tread at your feet) are amazing and extend over thousands of square miles of rugged and scenic terrain.

If you take this 2.1-mile route, the previous description pretty much covers the highlights. The general course of the trail steeply ascends to the top of, and then follows, a jagged ridgeline, with scary drop-offs on either side, until you finally descend to the Boundary Trail. At a minimum, you will have to use your hands for stability and safety at several locations, and you may have to take off your pack at times just to make it through particularly narrow bits. It's a real adventure, but it's lots of fun if you are up for the challenge. Once back on the Boundary Trail, go west and retrace your route 9.6 miles back to the Johnston Ridge Observatory. Fit hikers can make the trip back in one day, but it might be more fun (and it's certainly easier on your body) to spend another night at either Margaret or Dome Camp along the way.

Hikers who lack the necessary scrambling skills for the Mount Whittier/Whittier Ridge Trail, or anyone who understandably values safety over scenery, should go straight (west) at the junction in the saddle west of Shovel Lake. Descend through partial forest for 0.4

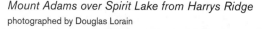

Mount Adams over Spirit Lake from Harrys Ridge
photographed by Douglas Lorain

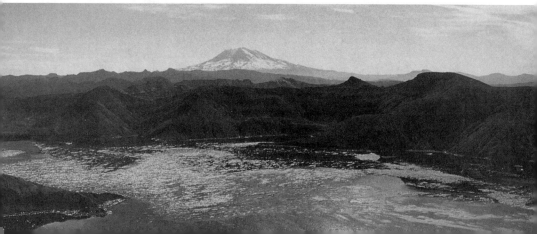

mile to the spur trail that accesses the designated camps at the northeast end of small Snow Lake. More downhill hiking, actually quite a bit more, takes you through partial forest until you finally reach the waters of Coldwater Creek and reenter the devastated area, now regrowing with forest. You follow the north bank of the creek about 1.7 miles (well past where the old Green Trails maps indicate a junction) before finally reaching a junction in the wide and nearly level valley above Coldwater Lake.

You turn left (southeast) here, soon cross a wooden bridge over cascading Coldwater Creek, and climb a series of long-legged switchbacks on a relatively steep and brushy slope. As you ascend, there are increasingly fine views of Minnie Peak to the northeast and the huge expanse of Coldwater Lake, a 3.5-mile-long body of water that did not even exist before mudflows from the 1980 eruption dammed the flow of Coldwater Creek. After the switchbacks, a gentler ascent over mostly open slopes leads to a junction, from which you'll enjoy particularly outstanding views down the entire length of Coldwater Lake, with waving grasses and regrowing trees in the foreground.

To complete the loop, go left (east) at the junction and climb to a broad ridgecrest, where you'll find Ridge Camp. In early summer a small spring about 0.2 mile north of this camp offers water, but this trickle dries up later in the year. Still climbing, the narrow and rocky path comes to a ridgecrest, where you turn south and cross the very steep east face of an unnamed butte. Shortly after this traverse, you walk through a saddle, then make a moderately graded climb across the southwest side of Coldwater Peak back to the junction with the Boundary Trail above Saint Helens Lake. Turn right (south) here and follow the Boundary Trail 5.2 miles back the way you came to the Johnston Ridge Observatory.

VARIATION

With a very long car shuttle, you can make this into a fun one-way trip by skipping the lakes northeast of Mount Margaret and ending your route at the Norway Pass Trailhead on Forest Service Road 26 east of Bear Pass.

POSSIBLE ITINERARY

	CAMP	MILES	ELEVATION GAIN
Day 1	Dome Camp	7.4	2,100'
	Side trip to Coldwater Peak	1.4	600'
Day 2	Panhandle Lake	7	1,250'
	via Mount Whittier:		
Day 3	Out	13.5	2,950'
	via Coldwater Creek:		
Day 3	Ridge Camp	8.1	2,100'
Day 4	Out	7.3	2,000'

BEST SHORTER ALTERNATIVE

A one-night trip to either Dome or Margaret Camp gives you some of the best views of Spirit Lake and Mount St. Helens, although it misses the lovely lake country northeast of Mount Margaret.

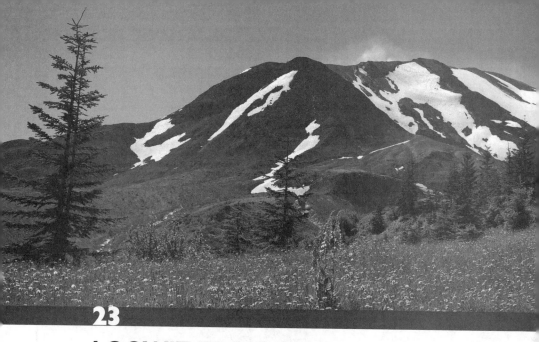

LOOWIT TRAIL LOOP

RATINGS: Scenery 9 **Solitude** 4 **Difficulty** 9
MILES: 34 (35)
ELEVATION GAIN: 4,700' (4,900')
DAYS: 3 (3)
SHUTTLE MILEAGE: n/a
MAP: USFS *Mount St. Helens National Volcanic Monument & Administrative Area* (although mileages are missing)
USUALLY OPEN: Late June–late October
BEST: Late June–mid-July
PERMIT: None required
RULES: Off-trail travel prohibited in the restricted area north of the mountain; climbing permit required for travel on the mountain above 4,800 feet (which is always above the described trail)
CONTACT: Mount St. Helens National Volcanic Monument, 360-449-7800, fs.usda.gov/main/giffordpinchot

SPECIAL ATTRACTIONS ●

Unique volcanic scenery, unobstructed views

Above: *View of Mount St Helens from near Studebaker Ridge*
photographed by Mark Wetherington

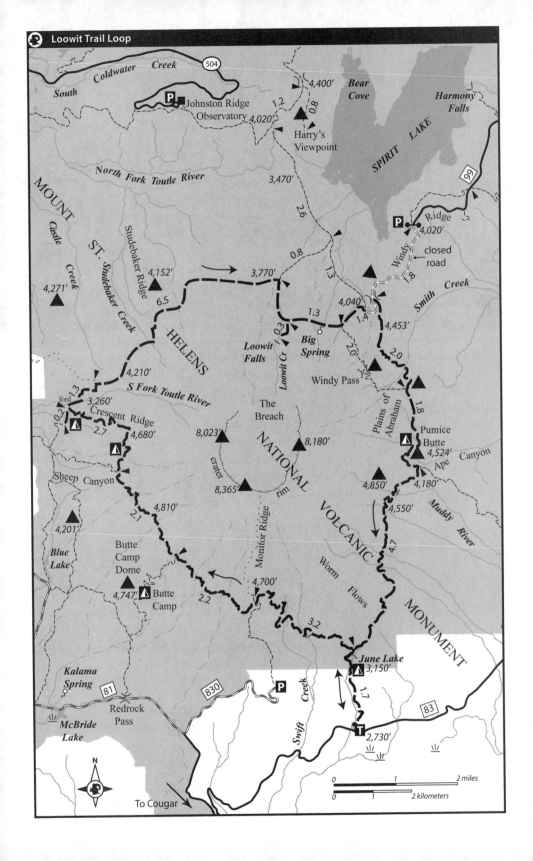

Coldwater Creek 504

South

Bear Cove

Harmony Falls

Johnston Ridge Observatory 4,020'

4,400'

1.2

0.8

Harry's Viewpoint

SPIRIT LAKE

99

North Fork Toutle River

3,470'

2.6

Windy Ridge 4,020'

closed road

MOUNT

Castle Creek

4,271'

ST. Studebaker Ridge

Studebaker Creek

4,152'

6.5

HELENS

3,770'

0.8

1.3

1.3

4,040'

1.4

4,453'

1.8

Windy

Smith Creek

Loowit Falls

Loowit Cr

0.3

Big Spring

1.3

2.0

2.0

Windy Pass

4,210'

S Fork Toutle River

ford 3,260'

0.2

1.3

Crescent Ridge

2.7

4,680'

The Breach

8,023'

NATIONAL

8,180'

crater

8,365'

rim

Plains of Abraham

Pumice Butte 4,524'

1.8

Ape Canyon

Sheep Canyon

2.1

4,810'

4,201'

Blue Lake

Butte Camp Dome

4,747'

Butte Camp

2.2

Monitor Ridge

4,700'

4,850'

4,180'

4,550'

Muddy River

4.7

VOLCANIC

Worm Flows

3.2

MONUMENT

June Lake 3,150'

Kalama Spring

81

830

Swift Creek

83

Redrock Pass

1.7

McBride Lake

T 2,730'

N

To Cougar

0   1   2 miles

0   1   2 kilometers

CHALLENGES

Very rough trail in places, limited water and camping choices, long stretches with almost no shade, noisy sightseeing helicopters

NOTE: Intermittent eruptions have closed many of the trails, especially on the north side of the mountain. Call ahead and/or check the website to determine the current status.

HOW TO GET THERE

Take I-5 to Exit 21, then drive east on WA 503 for 31.4 miles past Cougar. The road becomes Forest Service Road 90. Continue 3.4 miles, and turn left (northwest) onto FS 83. Follow this road 6.8 miles to a signed turnoff for June Lake o the left (north). The trailhead is approximately 0.25 mile from the pavement.

NOTE: You'll need a Northwest Forest Pass to park at this trailhead.

GPS TRAILHEAD COORDINATES: N46° 08.238' W122° 09.414'

INTRODUCTION

Mount St. Helens was once the prettiest mountain in the Pacific Northwest. The mountain's almost perfect conical shape, glistening white glaciers, and deep-green surrounding forests made it strikingly attractive. That all changed, of course, one Sunday morning in May 1980, when this volcano put on a demonstration of violence that will be remembered for generations to come. The devastation left by that eruption is still amazing to behold, even though trees, flowers, and shrubs are slowly replacing the wasteland of brown and gray. The mountain and its surroundings can no longer be called pretty, but the barren landscape is fascinating to observe.

NOTE: From a logistics standpoint, the Loowit Trail around Mount St. Helens is easier than the Mount Margaret Loop (see Trip 22) because you are not restricted to designated camps and no reservations are required. In all other respects, however, this loop is more difficult, due to rugged lava flows, lots of ups and downs, and limited camping choices.

DESCRIPTION

From the June Lake Trailhead, you hike north on the well-used trail for 1.4 miles as it gently climbs uphill and reaches popular June Lake. The lake was formed about 500 years ago when a lava flow blocked a creek and left behind this shallow pool. Willows crowd the shore, and until late summer, a tall waterfall drops off a forested cliff almost directly into the lake. Adequate campsites are available for backpackers who got a late start.

TIP: This is a popular day hike. Visit on a weekday for more privacy.

Continue 0.3 mile from the lake up the forested hillside to reach the Loowit Trail junction and the start of the loop, where you turn left (northwest). Attempt to find comfort in the fact that you are not delaying the inevitable, and that your legs are fresh, because you now face the most strenuous uphill of the entire loop. The trail soon reaches a rough lava flow, which you steeply ascend by following survey stakes. You then cross Swift Creek near a waterfall and enter old-growth forest. The circuitous route wanders up through forests and avalanche chutes, where many trees have been toppled by snowslides. After gaining about 1,400 feet from June Lake, you abruptly reach a level section of trail and contour across meadows and wooded slopes to a junction with the Ptarmigan Trail, which is the heavily used climber's route up the south side of the peak. The less-traveled Loowit Trail heads southwest, crosses the Ptarmigan Trail, and goes up and down in rocky lava flows and ravines before reaching some attractive alpine meadows and flower fields.

WARNING: By midsummer, water is scarce in this area.

The sometimes-faint Loowit Trail continues its rugged course of rocks, meadows, and lava fields on an undulating route to the northwest. Watch for posts in the lava to help you follow the proper course. Views to the southwest of Goat Mountain, Goat Marsh Lake, and distant Mount Hood are superb. About 2.2 miles from the last junction, you meet the Butte Camp Trail. Very attractive Butte Camp is an ideal campsite, but it's a rather dis-

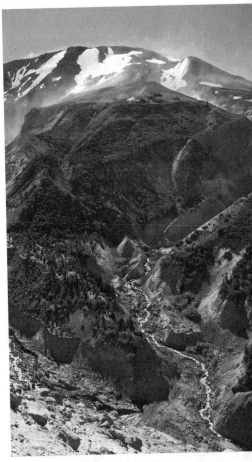

tant 1.3 miles away and fully 800 feet down. By going straight (northwest) and sticking with the Loowit Trail, you are compensated with lots of colorful heather and good views of Butte Camp Dome, Mount St. Helens, and Mount Hood. You should also keep an eye out for elk here.

The Loowit Trail continues to circle the mountain close to timberline, but the terrain is now much less rough and more pleasant to hike. Good views and wildflowers abound. Your route wanders along, crossing several gullies that sometimes have water (and some- times have washouts) and traversing pleasant forested areas. Shortly before reaching a junc- tion with the Sheep Canyon Trail, you must cross a troublesome gully with very loose soils that is difficult to scramble through but not generally too dangerous. Beyond this gully, your route goes straight (north) and continues up and down over open slopes.

TIP: About 0.5 mile from Sheep Canyon, you will find water and adequate campsites at a couple of small ponds below the trail.

Once you reach Crescent Ridge, the scen- ery quickly changes. Having now completely circled the south side of the volcano, you enter the eruption area, where the forests turn to charred snags and views extend north into

View of South Fork Toutle River gorge
photographed by Mark Wetherington

the devastated area. The trail alternates between snags and living forest as it makes a long, often steep downhill along the ridge. Numerous switchbacks help to save your knees on this 1,400-foot descent.

The downhill ends just as you're curving into the wasteland of the South Fork Toutle River Canyon. At a marked junction with the Toutle Trail near the edge of the gorge, be sure to turn left (south) and hike about 0.2 mile to a nice campsite beside a clear creek with shade from old-growth trees. This is an excellent spot for the first night's camp, although less enchanting campsites can be eked out closer to the river.

The Loowit Trail turns right (northeast) at the junction, traverses a rocky hillside, and comes to a crossing of muddy South Fork Toutle River.

TIP: In the afternoon on hot days, this unbridged crossing can be an adventure. It's much better to camp at the place described previously and cross in the morning.

Once on the north bank, you scramble up the unstable soils of mudflow material and relocate the path. You should be able to see it going diagonally up the ridge to the north. As you switchback up this narrow trail, the views of Mount St. Helens rapidly improve and soon become quite impressive. Just after you top out on the ridge, there is a junction with a lightly used trail that goes left (west) toward Castle Lake.

The main loop trail goes right (northeast) and gently climbs near the top of the ridge, where you'll enjoy excellent views into the South Fork's gorge and up to the mountain. You turn north away from the canyon and once again hike through the barren wasteland of the devastated area. The often-strenuous hiking is completely exposed to both sun and wind. As you hike you'll cross lots of rocky areas, mudflows, and creeks that may or may not have water. The route is sometimes faint, so watch where you're going. Drop down to cross the mudflow of Studebaker Creek, and then climb a bit to go over Studebaker Ridge. The crater is higher in elevation than you are, but you will begin to see its inner walls as you continue going east.

NOTE: The area for the next few miles is prone to landslides. This has led to extended closures in recent years and frequent reroutings of the trail. Call ahead to see if the trail is currently open to hikers and if it can be reasonably followed. Out of necessity, the following is only a general description, as the terrain and the exact route change from year to year.

The trail curves around the slopes above a flat basin, then drops down from Studebaker Ridge to a large, rocky, flat plain below the crater. With no trees or anything else to get in the way, views are unrestricted across the devastated area to Spirit Lake, the peaks around Mount Margaret, and Mount St. Helens. The trail follows cairns and posts across the wasteland for about 1.5 miles, crosses Loowit Creek, and comes to a junction. You go right (south) and, after a 0.7-mile ascent, come to a junction with the Loowit Falls Trail.

LOOWIT FALLS SIDE TRIP: Don't miss the popular 0.6-mile round-trip from here to an overlook of the impressive 250-foot-tall waterfall in a dark gorge.

The main trail is now well defined and more heavily traveled by day hikers from Windy Ridge, as it goes up and down to the east and crosses several clear little springs and creeklets that have attracted a host of lush riparian plants. About 1.3 miles from the Loowit Falls turnoff is a signed junction with Trail #216E. Turn left (northeast), leaving the Loowit Trail proper and avoiding the often-sketchy climb to and descent from Windy Pass, and descend this path for 0.8 mile to a junction with the Truman Trail on a closed road.

Hike east on the road to reach the Abraham Trail junction, and then turn right (south) on the view-packed Abraham Trail, which ascends a narrow, north-south ridge, sometimes with the help of stairs. Penstemon, paintbrush, and other wildflowers provide color to superb photos of the mountain from this ridge. The path leaves the ridgecrest and goes up and down across a rugged area of gullies with a surprisingly good display of wildflowers in June and July. Once you round a hill, the ash-gray volcano comes prominently back into view, and you descend to a crossing of often-dry Smith Creek.

From here you begin to cross the spectacular Plains of Abraham. This nearly level, rocky wasteland of mudflow and pyroclastic flow material has almost no vegetation but features a smashing up close view of the east side of Mount St. Helens. You are so close, in fact, that even the widest-angle camera lens has difficulty capturing the scene in one frame. You soon reconnect with the Windy Pass Trail, where you go straight (south), following cairns and rocks that line either side of the path to help you navigate. Work your way around the west side of a knoll, and cross a sometimes-trickling creek near the south end of the Plains. Since you have now left the restricted area, you may camp here. There is little shade, but you will find plenty of flat ground, as well as water in early summer. Tucked in the stands of new-growth trees are some nice sites for tents, and the view east to distant Mount Adams is remarkable. The trail now goes around the west side of small Pumice Butte, crosses another trickling creek, and enters an area just barely touched by the eruption. The snags, trees, and smaller plants here are right on the edge of the eruption impact line, and the contrast with the wasteland to the north is striking.

June Lake
photographed by Mark Wetherington

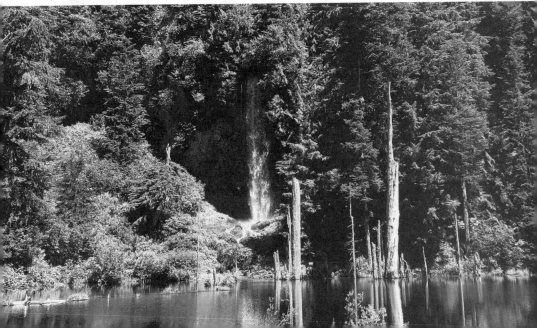

Leaving the Plains of Abraham, you travel downhill briefly and come to a junction with the Ape Canyon Trail.

SIDE TRIP TO APE CANYON VIEWPOINT: Be sure to make a short 0.1-mile detour down this trail to view the amazing slotlike gorge of Ape Canyon.

The Loowit Trail turns right (south) at the junction and almost immediately begins to display its ruggedly difficult character. Much of the next several miles travel over either rocky terrain or extremely rough lava flows, where your navigation abilities are occasionally tested (look for cairns and posts marking the route), and your conditioning is constantly on trial. Views of the mountain are not as spectacular on this side of the peak, but they are still frequent and attractive. Also, water and shade, while still at a premium, are much more common than on the north side of the mountain.

Beyond the Ape Canyon Trail, the path first climbs over rocks and meadows to a crossing of Muddy River in a ravine with a waterfall and snowbanks that remain well into summer. From here you climb a bit more to a crossing of the meltwater stream from snowfields above. The terrain is very broken and subject to landslides, so watch your step. You now generally lose elevation as you work your way to two small creeks with acceptable water and nice views of the volcano. You could make a poor emergency camp in this area, but shade is limited. The scattered trees here, mostly mountain hemlock or true fir, were safe from the eruption's impact. Soon after the creeks, you round a steep hillside and begin crossing the rugged lava of the Worm Flows. Both your legs and your boot soles take a beating as you make your way down through the rough rocks. Eventually, you enter denser stands of trees and hear a creek in a wooded ravine on the left shortly before the junction with the June Lake Trail. To complete your hike, simply go left (south) and retrace your steps back to the trailhead, well satisfied with your experience in this grand volcanic landscape.

POSSIBLE ITINERARY

	CAMP	MILES	ELEVATION GAIN
Day 1	South Fork Toutle River Camp (including 0.2-mile detour to campsite)	12.1	2,400'
Day 2	Pumice Butte	15.0	1,300'
	Side trip to Loowit Falls	0.6	150'
Day 3	Out	6.6	1,000'
	Side trip to Ape Canyon Viewpoint	0.2	50'

BEST SHORTER ALTERNATIVE

An excellent day hike sampler of the volcanic wasteland on the north side of the mountain starts from the Windy Ridge Trailhead to the northeast to explore either Loowit Falls or Plains of Abraham.

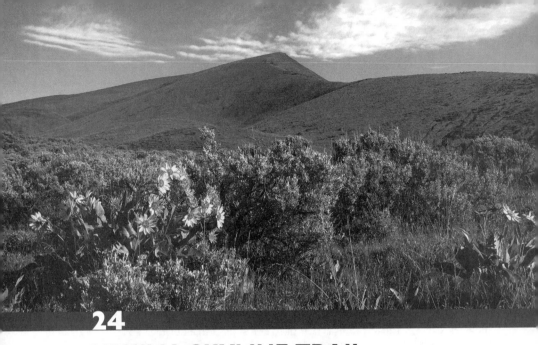

24

YAKIMA SKYLINE TRAIL

RATINGS: Scenery 6   **Solitude** 3   **Difficulty** 4
MILES: 27 (27)
ELEVATION GAIN: 6,800' (7,000')
DAYS: 2–3 (2–3)
SHUTTLE MILEAGE: n/a
MAPS: Washington Department of Natural Resources *Wenas Green Dot Map*.
    This map is very detailed and useful but not topographic. Four USGS topo-
    graphic maps are needed to cover this area: *Pomona, Selah, The Cotton-
    woods,* and *Wymer.* It may be easier to print a contour map off the internet at
    a site such as Caltopo.
USUALLY OPEN: Year-round, though infrequent rain and snow can make road
    conditions difficult
BEST: April–early June
PERMIT: None
RULES: No fires allowed April 15–October 15
CONTACT: Washington Department of Fish and Wildlife, 509-697-4503,
    wdfw.wa.gov/places-to-go/wildlife-areas/wenas-wildlife-area

SPECIAL ATTRACTIONS ·

Wildflowers, birds and other wildlife, high desert scenery, expansive views

Above: *Looking up to Umtanum Ridge from near the Roza site*
photographed by Douglas Lorain

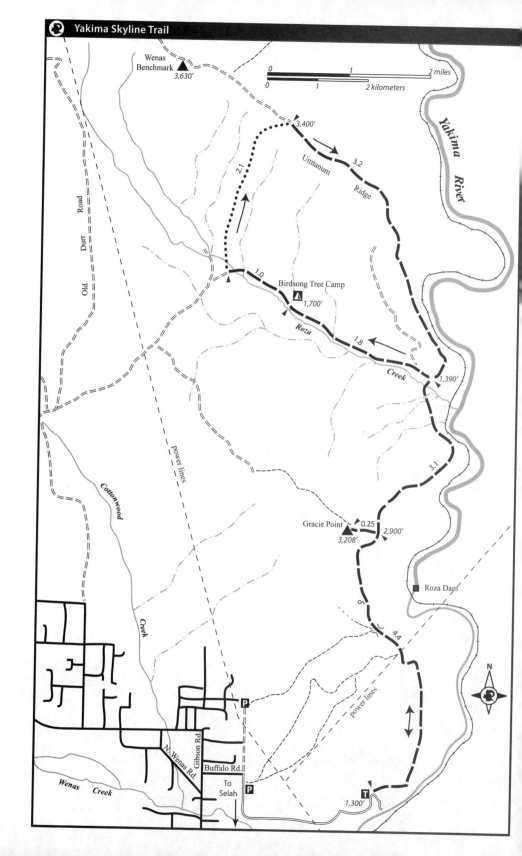

Wenas
Benchmark
3,630'

0   1   2 miles
0   1   2 kilometers

3,400'

Umtanum
Ridge

3.2

Yakima River

2.1

1.0

Birdsong Tree Camp
1,700'

Roza

1.8

Creek

1,390'

Old
Durr
Road

power lines

Cottonwood
Creek

3.1

Gracie Point   0.25
3,208'   2,900'

Roza Dam

.8

4.4

N. Wenas Rd.
Gibson Rd.

P

Buffalo Rd.
P

To Selah

Wenas   Creek

power lines

T
1,300'

N

CHALLENGES

Heat; lack of shade; lack of water; rattlesnakes; traffic and train noise; phone towers and roads often interrupt the natural views; roads form part of the route

HOW TO GET THERE

Take I-82 to Exit 26 for Selah. Head north on WA 821, and in 0.3 mile turn left (west) onto WA 823 (also known as Harrison Road). Follow Harrison Road about 2 miles, and then turn sharply right (north) onto North Wenas Road. Drive approximately 3 miles, and turn right (north) onto Gibson Road at a junction, then make a right (east) onto Buffalo Road in 0.3 mile. The pavement ends 1 mile after you turn on Buffalo Road, at which point you make a right (south), and follow the road 1.8 miles to a large but primitive parking area, passing through a gate and cattle guard along the way. The road is rough but suitable for most passenger cars unless it is muddy. From the parking area, you follow the road downhill (north) about 200 feet to where the trail leaves the road and begins its ascent to the rim of the Yakima Canyon. A few parking spots are available at the bottom of the hill, but the steep and rocky descent and limited parking make this an effort that's more trouble than it's worth.

NOTE: You'll need a Discover Pass to use this trailhead.

GPS TRAILHEAD COORDINATES: N46° 42.763' W120° 28.560'

INTRODUCTION

Although decidedly lacking in wilderness character, this trip provides backpackers with a fantastic opportunity to experience eastern Washington's desert landscape. Wildflowers bloom and mild temperatures prevail early in the season, when most mountain passes are

Mule deer on the Yakima Skyline Trail
photographed by Mark Wetherington

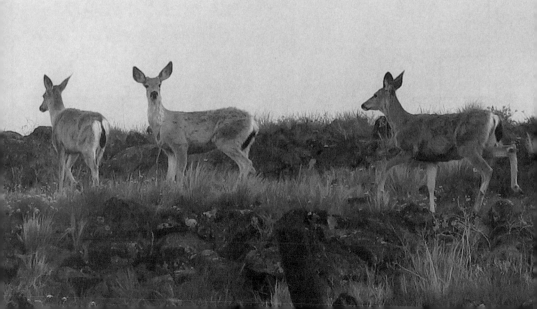

still under several feet of snow, making this a terrific conditioning hike to start off your backpacking season. Fine views of Mounts Adams and Rainier are available from many places along the Yakima Skyline Trail, and the panorama from Gracie Point is particularly stunning. Roza Creek offers riparian charm, and a campsite at the Birdsong Tree is well suited as a base camp for multiple possible day trips.

DESCRIPTION

The Yakima Skyline Trail begins as a distinct singletrack path through the sagebrush that winds its way east then north toward the rim of the Yakima River Canyon. The views, which feel expansive even from the trailhead, improve greatly as the trail climbs higher above the Yakima River. In spring, balsamroot and lupine make the scenery at your feet nearly as excellent as the peeks over your shoulder toward the distant peaks. The sagebrush-steppe landscape seems to lack variety, but it's surprisingly enchanting once you allow yourself to be immersed in the theme of arid beauty. The smells of sage and blooming wildflowers, the steady breezes, and the nearly endless views and vast sky make this hike as much a sensory experience as a physical one. Weathered fence posts flanking the trail serve as reminders of the area's ranching history and also allow hikers something to fixate on while hiking uphill.

WARNING: Rattlesnakes are common in this area, so be vigilant.

After 2 miles of steady climbing, you reach a hitching post and breathtaking (if you have any breath to spare after the constant climb) views into the Yakima River Canyon. This is a popular turnaround point for day hikers and a pleasant place to take a break. Continuing along, you briefly veer away from the rim of the canyon as the trail heads toward a saddle, unfortunately going under a power line on its way. The saddle provides an excellent vantage point for enjoying the natural beauty and appreciating the sheer magnitude of the canyon, as well as of the Roza Dam and less exciting components of transportation infrastructure, such as a railroad, several local roads, and distant highways. A distinct doubletrack path leaves the saddle to the southwest (it connects with an alternate trailhead), and a fainter trail exits the saddle in a northwesterly direction, becoming increasingly indistinct in short order; but you want to continue on the most distinct trail that is closest to the canyon rim.

From the saddle the Yakima Skyline Trail makes a brief descent to a cluster of trees, which shields a small spring that has been piped into a modest tank. On a warm day, this location would perhaps be more preferable for an extended break than the shadeless saddle or hitching post. Although the tank is becoming overgrown and filled with algae, the cold, clear water can easily be procured for filtering or other treatment to replenish your water supply.

WARNING: This is the last water source before Roza Creek, but it might not be dependable in dry years. Pack enough water to reach Roza Creek.

The trail quickly regains the elevation it lost to reach the spring and remains on a fairly steady contour for the next few miles. The views remain consistent as well, with the rugged canyon and mellow river being your constant companions. At 4.4 miles you reach a large cairn and a falling-down fence post, where a faint boot path intersects the main trail.

GRACIE POINT SIDE TRIP: The boot path to the left (west) follows fence posts for 0.25 mile and gains 200 feet of elevation to reach Gracie Point, a broad summit with views of the area that are the textbook definition of panoramic. This point provides hikers with top-of-the-world views without any chance of vertigo. This side trip is well worth the effort and should be considered an almost mandatory detour.

From the junction with the path to Gracie Point, the main trail begins a steady descent to Roza Creek. The small valley created by Roza Creek and backed by massive Umtanum Ridge gradually becomes the main focal point. The trail threads its way among sagebrush, crosses two small creekbeds (the only way you would get wet as you cross these creeks is if you spilled your water bottle), and passes through an old fence line before reaching the banks of tiny but lively Roza Creek. After crossing the creek, which should present no challenge except in catastrophic flooding events, continue straight until you reach an old road and use this to continue your journey upstream (northwest).

TIP: There is plenty of room to camp near where the trail crosses Roza Creek, but the nearby BNSF Railway, as well as lights from distant houses and roads, will likely compel you to head upstream and choose a more remote campsite.

Abundant grasses, trees, and the sloping hillsides that hem in Roza Creek create a remarkable contrast to the initial miles of this hike. While the sagebrush is still a constant, the high lonesome views have been replaced with comforting creekside scenery. Views up broad gullies toward the ridgetops still allow you to stretch your eyes. Scattered rock outcrops add a quintessential desert element to this section.

The level ground and charm of the Birdsong Tree campsite, 1.8 miles from the Roza Creek crossing, makes an ideal destination for your first night and can serve as an excellent base camp. Several large trees—with the stately locust known as the Birdsong Tree being the centerpiece—provide welcome shade and help anchor the site. Water can be procured from Roza Creek, which, despite its limited size, is loud enough early in the season to provide a subtle soundtrack on quiet nights, while chirps from the area's avian occupants provide healthy competition. While not a stunning alpine camp with a lake in the foreground and

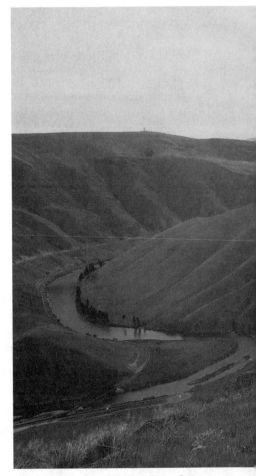

Looking down into Yakima River Canyon
photographed by Mark Wetherington

a glaciated peak reaching for the sky, the Birdsong Tree campsite is delightful in its own way. Watching impossibly soft desert light settle across sagebrush hillsides is a sublime way to wind down your evening and something every backpacker should experience.

From here, you can either retrace your steps, if you have only one night to spare, or you can use the site as a base camp and explore to your heart's content. An abundance of seldom-used roads spiderweb this area, providing ambitious hikers with all-day hikes that loop back to the campsite. However, the real beauty (not to mention the solitude and unspoiled scenery) lies off the trails and roads.

> **UMTANUM RIDGE DAY HIKE:** For the most highly recommended day hike from camp, continue along Roza Creek nearly 1 mile until the old road crosses the creek. At this point, you can choose your own adventure. The best plan is to leave the road and follow the creek and game trails upcanyon until you find an appealing slope and work your way north toward Umtanum Ridge. The hillsides aren't terribly steep, and there are no box canyons or concerns of reaching a dead end or obstacle. As far as off-trail hiking goes, it's actually pretty relaxing. This unscripted adventure, with occasional game trails providing some assistance in making forward progress, is an excellent opportunity to spot wildlife—elk and deer, as well as bighorn sheep, exist in healthy populations—and to enjoy the floral highlights of the hillsides. The open views, simple navigation, and relatively forgiving terrain make the elevation gain (approximately 1,600 feet over about 2 miles from Roza Creek to Umtanum Ridge) an easygoing affair that shouldn't pose a challenge to most hikers.

The number of miles to the singletrack section of the Yakima Skyline Trail, which takes you back to Roza Creek, will vary depending on where you reach the ridge and the old road that follows its crest. Most hikers, unless they choose to follow Roza Creek nearly to its headwaters, will find themselves walking anywhere from 2 to 3 miles on this dusty dirt road, which offers easy travel and views of the Stuart Mountain Range to the northwest on clear days. At the end of the ridge, a rough road drops off to the right, a sign straight ahead notes a motor vehicle closure, and an appealing singletrack trail heads to the left, veering southeast. Take the singletrack and follow it as it descends, steeply at times, back to Roza Creek. From here, you can head back upstream to your base camp at the Birdsong Tree for another night of desert sights and sounds, before hiking back out the way you came.

POSSIBLE ITINERARY

	CAMP	MILES	ELEVATION GAIN
Day 1	Birdsong Tree	9.3	2,600'
	Side trip to Gracie Point	0.5	200'
Day 2	Birdsong Tree		
	Day hike loop on Umtanum Ridge	8.1	2,000'
Day 3	Out	9.3	2,200'

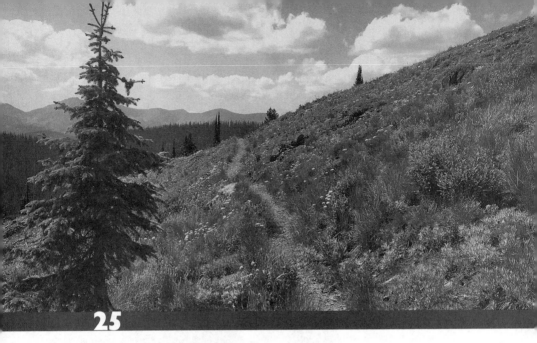

25

SALMO-PRIEST LOOP

RATINGS: Scenery 7   **Solitude** 8   **Difficulty** 5
MILES: 37 (38.5)
ELEVATION GAIN: 5,800' (6,300')
DAYS: 3–4 (3–4)
SHUTTLE MILEAGE: n/a
MAP: USFS *Salmo-Priest Wilderness*
USUALLY OPEN: July–October
BEST: July
PERMIT: None
RULES: Maximum group size of 12 people and/or stock
CONTACT: Colville National Forest, Sullivan Lake Ranger District, 509-446-7500, fs.usda.gov/colville

SPECIAL ATTRACTIONS ••

Unusual wildlife, solitude, fine views

CHALLENGES ••

Grizzly bears—use extreme bear precautions; limited water and campsites along ridge trail

Above: *Shedroof Divide Trail*
photographed by Mark Wetherington

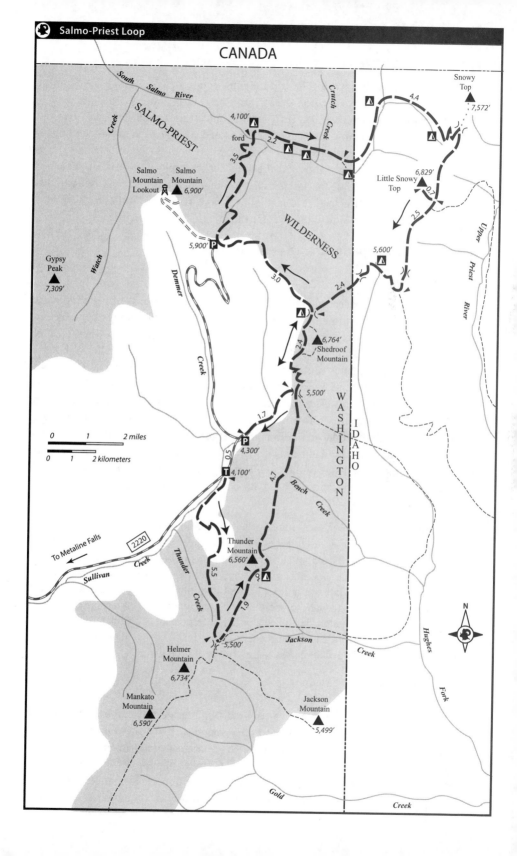

CANADA

South Salmo River

Crutch Creek

Snowy Top
7,572'

4.4

SALMO-PRIEST

4,100'

ford

2.2

3.5

Creek

Salmo
Mountain
Lookout

Salmo
Mountain
6,900'

WILDERNESS

6,829'

Little Snowy
Top

0.7

2.5

Gypsy
Peak

7,309'

5,900'

5,600'

Watch

3.0

2.4

Demmer

Upper Priest River

6,764'
Shedroof
Mountain

2.4

Creek

5,500'

1.7

WASHINGTON

IDAHO

4,300'

0.5

4,100'

4.7

Bench Creek

To Metaline Falls

2220

Sullivan

Creek

Thunder Creek

Thunder
Mountain
6,560'

0.4

5.5

1.9

N

5,500'

Jackson

Creek

Hughes

Helmer
Mountain
6,734'

Fork

Mankato
Mountain

6,590'

Jackson
Mountain
5,499'

Gold

Creek

0   1   2 miles

0   1   2 kilometers

HOW TO GET THERE •

Start from the small town of Tiger, at the intersection of WA 20 and WA 31 in the northeastern corner of Washington. Head north on WA 31, and go 16 miles, passing through the town of Metaline Falls. Turn right (southeast) onto Sullivan Lake Road, and drive 4.9 miles to a junction with Forest Service Road 22, signed SALMO MOUNTAIN 21 MILES. To reach the Sullivan Lake Ranger Station, where you can get information, maps, and bear canisters, go straight and drive 0.4 mile. For the trailheads, turn left (east) here and follow good gravel FS 22 for 5.3 miles to a prominent junction. Stay left (east), now on FS 2220, and follow this road as it parallels Sullivan Creek for 6.7 miles to the marked turnoff on the right (east) side of the road for the small Thunder Creek Trailhead.

GPS TRAILHEAD COORDINATES: N48° 54.018' W117° 04.908'

INTRODUCTION •

The Salmo-Priest Wilderness, in the extreme northeast corner of Washington, protects a remarkable region. The mountains here, an offshoot of the Selkirk Range, combine several attributes that set them apart from all other mountains in the state. Their location is ideally suited to receiving precipitation, making this the wettest area in Washington east of the Cascade Mountains. As a result, the forests here contain species more commonly associated with the wetter west slope of the Cascades than the normally drier east slope. Hikers familiar with western Washington's rainforests will feel right at home. Also at home here is an unusual assortment of rare wildlife, including lynx, wolverines, grizzly bears, and mountain caribou. In addition, the ridges and peaks here are more rugged and heavily eroded than those in neighboring ranges, so the landscape is more dramatic than is normal for the east side of the state. This trip visits all the major highlights of this wilderness and will delight backpackers with both wonderful scenery and a surprising degree of solitude.

> **WARNING:** This is grizzly bear country. You are more likely to see them here than anywhere else in the state. Accordingly, the following precautions are in order: Avoid hiking alone or at night, avoid areas with recent signs of bears, take special care to avoid spilling food or garbage near your camp, make plenty of noise while you hike, and hang all food and garbage at least 15 feet from the ground and 500 feet away from your camp. You may want to use the bear canisters that are available from the Sullivan Lake Ranger Station. If you see a grizzly bear, consider yourself fortunate that you saw one of these rare and magnificent creatures in the wild, and report the sighting to the U.S. Forest Service—it likes to keep track of such things.

DESCRIPTION •

The Thunder Creek Trail begins as an old roadbed that steadily climbs south through pleasant forest. Sullivan Creek provides a nice soundtrack at times, but the views are limited. Although you hike up the Thunder Creek drainage later in the hike, the trail never gets too close to its namesake stream. After 2 miles of fairly monotonous but easy hiking, the roadbed turns to singletrack, and the forest noticeably changes character— more charming, more inviting, and more scenic. Your footpath continues steadily gaining elevation, and the forest soon becomes downright awesome. Old-growth cedars and hemlocks inspire wonder and provide shade, making this section of trail exceptionally enjoyable. As you gain more elevation during the final push to a small saddle and trail junction, you leave this primeval forest behind, but it serves as a nice prelude to the wonderful scenery you will pass through later along the South Salmo River.

At the ridgetop junction you head left (north) on the Shedroof Divide Trail. Shortly after, you will also pass a junction for a trail heading east and dropping down into Jackson Creek. Continue on through thick forest, with occasional eastward views, for 1.9 miles to a small spring and a campsite of matching proportions a few hundred feet later. This is the only reasonable water source and campsite for a considerable distance, and it makes an excellent destination for the first night's camp. Walk a few hundred feet past the campsite to a decent opening in the forest to enjoy a panorama with dinner. While Thunder Mountain is a tempting objective for those with summit fever, the long-abandoned trail leading up is difficult to follow, so it's probably better to delay gratification until you reach the slightly more distinct trail up Shedroof Mountain or, even better, the easily followed trail to Little Snowy Top later in the trip.

After about 1.5 miles of hiking from the campsite near Thunder Mountain, you enter an area of forest recovering from a recent burn. The trail is in reasonably good shape, but the scenery leaves a bit to be desired, and the area will be prone to deadfall for years to come, as the blackened trees succumb to gravity and the forces of nature. You eventually leave the burn and drop to a small saddle that has a signed four-way junction. A primitive trail heads east to Hughes Fork in Idaho, while the Shedroof Cutoff Trail leads southwest back toward FS 2220. You will be taking the Shedroof Cutoff Trail on your return.

For now continue straight (north) and begin to climb steeply up brushy switchbacks to the crest of the ridge. After the ascent, a mile or so of easy hiking delivers you to a faint junction with a rugged footpath that climbs to the top of Shedroof Mountain. The view from the former lookout site (the lookout is gone, but, oddly, the outhouse is still there)

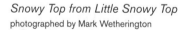

Snowy Top from Little Snowy Top
photographed by Mark Wetherington

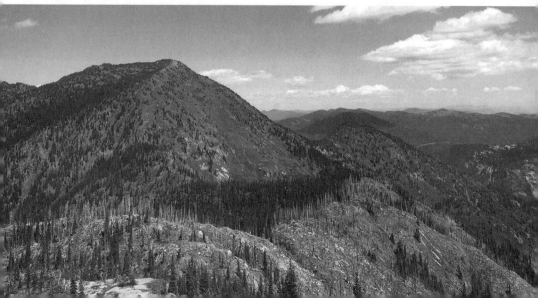

is excellent, but the trail conditions make the reward-to-effort ratio a bit skewed, especially since the phenomenal and more easily attained vantage point from Little Snowy Top remains on the agenda.

Bypassing the excursion to Shedroof Mountain, you continue north and descend down the flank of the mountain to an inviting saddle and the junction with the Salmo Divide Trail. An unreliable spring (it was barely a trickle on a recent summer visit) provides water a few hundred yards to the east on the Shedroof Divide Trail, and a small spot for tents near the junction is a notable amenity to hikers who don't mind a potentially dry camp and have brought sufficient water from elsewhere. You head left (northwest) on the Salmo Divide Trail as it undulates through the forest and passes through open areas that allow for great views of Crowell Ridge and Gypsy Peak to the west. At 7,309 feet, Gypsy Peak has the distinction of being the highest point in eastern Washington.

After 2 miles, you exit the wilderness and your trek continues on an old road. The views are pleasant enough, and the old road allows for a quick pace as you descend to the trailhead for the Salmo Basin Trail, which is the next leg of your odyssey.

The Salmo Basin Trail begins off the access road about 50 yards west of the north trailhead parking area and immediately drops into the trees. The forest here is typical of the ridgetops in these mountains, with subalpine fir dominating and a good number of Engelmann spruce mixed in for variety. The well-graded trail drops steadily but moderately, making occasional switchbacks and crossing several small creeks in the first mile. Views are limited, but the forest is interesting as it slowly changes from high-elevation species to lower-elevation conifers like western hemlock and western red cedar. The undergrowth follows a similar pattern, going from huckleberry bushes to a verdant lushness of mosses, ferns, thimbleberry plants, western yews, and small forest wildflowers like queen-cup.

Your path descends a hillside in dark forest, with a creek well below you on the left, and then switchbacks and drops to a rock-hop crossing of the creek. A boardwalk has been placed over the worst boggy areas near the creek to reduce mud and erosion. From the crossing, you descend above the west bank of the creek. The magnificent trees, especially the cedars, increase in size as you go. Near the bottom of the canyon, you make a few lazy switchbacks, then arrive at the South Salmo River in the cool depths of this beautiful forest. Excellent campsites are on the north side of this bridgeless crossing.

Fording the river is feasible but not terribly inviting, as the water is cold and often at least knee-deep even in midsummer. Fortunately, there is usually a log across the water upstream from the trail. On the north shore the trail climbs a bit from the spacious camping area and soon meets an abandoned trail that goes downstream. Your route turns right (east) and begins the long, forested climb to the river's headwaters. The well-engineered route sometimes gains elevation and is sometimes level, but it rarely wastes previous uphill effort by losing elevation. Although views are nonexistent, the thick forest canopy nicely shades the path, and you are constantly accompanied by the sounds of birds and the murmur of the rushing river.

About 1 mile beyond the river crossing, you'll go over a boardwalk and pass a very good riverside campsite, followed by another just 0.3 mile farther upstream. The trail now crosses cascading Crutch Creek on a broken-down log bridge and continues climbing through lush forests well above the river to a signed fork. To the right a 0.3-mile trail drops southeast to the South Salmo River at the old Salmo Cabin, where there is a good camp.

Your trail bears left (east) and follows the canyon as it curves north. Not long after the junction, you leave the wilderness and enter Idaho. A wilderness sign directed at visitors traveling in the other direction marks the state boundary. The climb out of this canyon is more gradual than the descent was, so you may not notice the change in the forest around you, as first the cedars disappear and then the hemlocks, replaced with Engelmann spruces, firs, and a few western white pines.

You'll pass a good camp on a bench about 150 yards before you come to a crossing of the South Salmo River. The ford is a bit tricky, so try looking upstream, where a usually dry crossing is available on shaky logs. The climb is steeper now as you steadily ascend through forests that gradually become more open. You hop across another tributary creek, the last stream of any consequence on this trip, as the climb continues unabated. For a while, you follow a splashing creek, and then gradually climb through the stream's large upper basin, which has several open areas, numerous small creeks, and possible camps. Here you will obtain your first good views of the surrounding ridges.

TIP: Get water at one of the small creeks in this basin because, once you reach the ridge, there will be none for several miles.

Now you switchback fairly steeply out of the basin, obtaining ever-improving views back down the Salmo River Canyon to the sharp pinnacles of peaks in British Columbia's Stagleap Provincial Park.

WARNING: This sheltered slope is often covered with snowfields into July, and the trail is easy to lose.

You'll reach the ridge at a small saddle on the side of hulking Snowy Top. Really ambitious hikers can make the rugged scramble to the top of this 7,572-foot landmark.

WARNING: Even though there is limited water along the ridge, mosquitoes are abundant in late June and July.

Your trail turns sharply right (south) at the ridgeline and goes up and down along the top of this scenic divide. The trail then cuts across the view-packed eastern slopes of Little Snowy Top and comes to a fork.

LITTLE SNOWY TOP SIDE TRIP: To the right (northwest), the mandatory 0.7-mile side trip climbs steeply to Little Snowy Top. The views from here, including the peaks and valleys of two states and one Canadian province, are superb. Plan on spending at least an hour at the summit to soak in the views. Unfortunately, the lookout cabin that sat atop this prominence for over 80 years is no more. It burned completely in 2016, likely from careless use of its wood stove by visitors.

Back at the Little Snowy Top junction, the main trail continues south 0.2 mile to a junction with an unmaintained trail to Upper Priest River. Your route goes straight (south), continuing its extended tour across the mostly open eastern side of the ridge. Eventually, you cross a small saddle and briefly travel on the western slopes before returning to the east. The trail now gradually loses elevation until it comes to a ridgetop junction. Your trail turns back to the right (northwest). It descends nine short switchbacks to a nice camp beside a pleasant little creek that usually flows for most of the summer. From this inviting spot, the trail loses a bit more elevation to a narrow saddle, and then sets about regaining the lost altitude.

Partway up this sometimes-steep path, you pass a Salmo-Priest Wilderness sign, indicating your return to the state of Washington. You now climb past more good views and return to the prominent junction with the Salmo Divide Trail in a wide saddle.

Retrace your steps to the south along this section of trail for 2.4 miles as it skirts Shedroof Mountain and comes to the Shedroof Cutoff junction. Take a right (southwest) on the Shedroof Cutoff Trail as it descends and parallels a small stream through dense forest. It reaches FS 2220 after 1.7 miles. To return to your vehicle and close this loop, hike downhill along FS 2220 for 0.5 mile to the Thunder Creek Trailhead.

POSSIBLE ITINERARY

	CAMP	MILES	ELEVATION GAIN
Day 1	Spring near Thunder Mountain	7.4	2,000'
Day 2	South Salmo River ford	13.6	1,000'
Day 3	Campsite southwest of Little Snowy Top	10.1	2,000'
	Side trip to Little Snowy Top	1.4	500'
Day 4	Out (including 0.5-mile road walk)	6.0	800'

BEST SHORTER ALTERNATIVE ●

For a shorter trip, start from the Salmo Basin Trailhead below Salmo Mountain (about 6.5 miles of driving beyond the Thunder Creek Trailhead), and hike the 19-mile loop beginning from the parking area there.

TIP: Before you start hiking, an excellent side trip goes up a rough dirt road from the saddle west of this trailhead to the commanding viewpoint at Salmo Mountain Lookout.

South Salmo River
photographed by Mark Wetherington

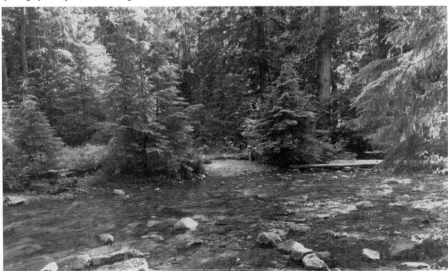

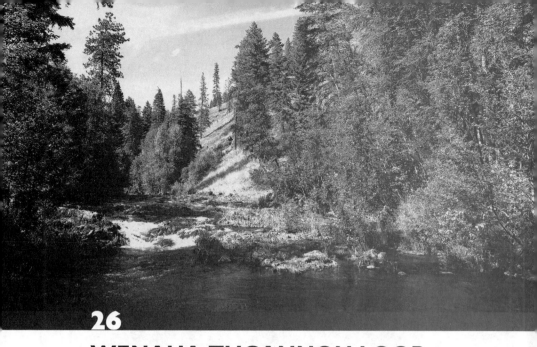

26

WENAHA-TUCANNON LOOP

RATINGS: Scenery 7   **Solitude** 8   **Difficulty** 8
MILES: 46 (64)
ELEVATION GAIN: 8,450' (10,300')
DAYS: 4–7 (6–7)
SHUTTLE MILEAGE: n/a
MAP: USFS *Wenaha-Tucannon Wilderness*
USUALLY OPEN: Late May–November
BEST: Early to mid-June
PERMIT: None
RULES: No camping within 75 feet of water
CONTACT: Umatilla National Forest, Pomeroy Ranger District, 509-843-1891, fs.usda.gov/main/umatilla

SPECIAL ATTRACTIONS

Wildlife, solitude, canyon scenery

CHALLENGES

Rattlesnakes (in lower canyons), limited water sources, some steep sections, large recent burn areas, indistinct and minimally maintained trails

Above: *Crooked Creek*
photographed by Mark Wetherington

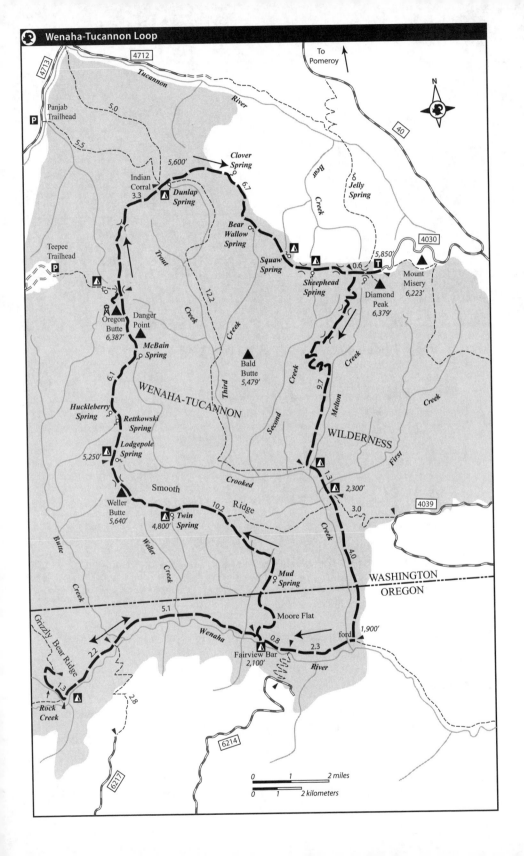

HOW TO GET THERE ··

From Pomeroy, drive south on WA 128 E. After 7.6 miles, continue straight (south) onto Mountain Road. Go 7.3 miles, and continue straight (south) onto Forest Service Road 40. Follow this gravel road 15.7 miles as it climbs into the forests and open ridges of the Blue Mountains.

> **TIP:** Be sure to stop at Sunset Point along the way, about 12.5 miles after joining FS 40, to enjoy a fine view of the rugged Tucannon River Canyon.

Near the top of a low pass, you turn right (west) onto FS 4030 (also known as Diamond Creek Road), and follow it 5 miles to the road end.

> **WARNING:** As the road rounds the north side of Mount Misery, it changes from gravel to rough dirt. You may prefer to walk the final 2.5 miles.

> **NOTE:** You'll need a Northwest Forest Pass to park at this trailhead.

GPS TRAILHEAD COORDINATES: N46° 07.152' W117° 32.190'

INTRODUCTION ··

With so much nearby mountain splendor to keep them occupied, most Washington backpackers know little or nothing about the Wenaha-Tucannon Wilderness. They may have noticed it on maps, tucked away in the state's southeast corner, or perhaps heard stories about the region's elk or canyon scenery, but relatively few have bothered to explore this land. Those who do learn that Washington has more to offer than rugged mountains and scenic beaches. Here you'll discover a land of forested plateaus and ridges, with terrific views down into impressively deep canyons. Along the canyon bottoms, you can camp beside joyous streams and savor views back up to the canyon rims, which are unlike anything found elsewhere in the state. Elk are abundant in this ideal habitat, and they are joined by bighorn sheep, black bears, mountain lions, and many other species not often seen in the more densely forested Cascade and Olympic Mountains.

The mountains here, a northern extension of Oregon's Blue Mountains, enjoy better weather than the soggier ranges to the west. As a result, these trails open sooner and are less prone to endless days of overcast conditions and rain. This dry climate carries a significant drawback, however, as water can be hard to find. Ridge trails often go for miles between springs, and even these water sources may diminish to nothing more than muddy trickles by late summer. You should carry 2 quarts or more of water and refill at every opportunity.

> **WARNING:** In late fall, hunters arrive looking for all those elk. Backpackers must be sure to advertise themselves with bright red or orange clothing.

DESCRIPTION ··

From the end of the road, the trail makes a brief climb west through thick forests on the north side of Diamond Peak. You soon come to a junction with the Tucannon River Trail and a short unsigned path to the top of Diamond Peak. Keep straight (west) at this intersection and descend 0.2 mile to another junction.

Turn left (south) here, following signs for Crooked Creek, and hike out to an open ridge with fine views of the nearby ridges and canyons. The trail leaves the ridge and switchbacks to the right as it begins a long descent into the Melton Creek drainage. The steep route follows the west side of a ridge, and then goes through a saddle with excellent views of deep canyons on both sides. You switchback down the south slope, hit another saddle, and steeply descend still more switchbacks, as the trail makes its way down rocky, open slopes with good views.

NOTE: The authors recommend doing this loop clockwise to avoid climbing this long, dry, sun-exposed slope.

Eventually, your aching knees get a break, as the trail bottoms out just above Melton Creek.

The trail stays on the slope above Melton Creek and takes a roller-coaster course to the south. The path includes several good viewpoints of the canyon and surrounding ridges, with picturesque ponderosa pines adding to the scenery. As you near the bottom of the canyon, a small arch just to the right of the trail offers an item of geological interest.

WARNING: Rattlesnakes inhabit these lower canyon environments. Watch your step, and check carefully before sitting down to rest.

Just as the narrow canyon of Melton Creek ends, you'll come to a pleasant campsite and a junction with the Crooked Creek Trail.

Crooked Creek is one of the largest streams in the wilderness, draining a very scenic 2,000-foot-deep canyon. Anglers might want to try their luck in these waters, as the creek supports a healthy population of trout. Your route goes left (southeast). The trail crosses Melton Creek and continues downstream through partial forest and open areas above Crooked Creek. About 0.7 mile from Melton Creek, the trail makes a relatively easy ford of First Creek. In an open area just upstream from the crossing are a cabin and a camping area.

WARNING: This area is popular with horses and cattle, so the camps are often dusty and "aromatic."

Continue south on the Crooked Creek Trail. The path wanders downstream through an attractive mix of vegetation. Ponderosa pine is the dominant tree, although some Douglas and grand firs are also present. Near the stream are willows and other riparian shrubs, while a smattering of wildflowers brightens the open areas away from the water.

WARNING: Less welcome than the flowers are the occasional sprigs of poison ivy, which you may encounter along any of the lower canyon trails. Learn to identify and avoid it.

In addition to the pleasant stream and vegetation, there are continuous neck-craning views up to the steep-walled rim of the canyon.

About 0.6 mile from First Creek is a junction with Trail #3133, a popular horse access to this area. You keep straight (south) and hike downstream through partial forest and open rocky areas with good views. Keep an eye out for ospreys and eagles overhead, various reptiles underfoot (especially in the sunny areas), and mammals like deer, coyote, and porcupine. As you near the Oregon state line, marked by a sign on a tree, you enter forest recovering from an intense burn in 2015 and continue south to a junction with the popular Wenaha River Trail.

Your route turns right (west) at this junction and crosses a muddy area of riparian vegetation to Crooked Creek. There is no bridge over Crooked Creek. The Umatilla National Forest plans to replace the bridge at some point, but until a new structure is built, you will need to ford or cross using downed trees. At normal water levels, this will not be a hazardous or challenging proposition. For the next few miles you follow the Wenaha River's spectacular canyon along a well-maintained path that generally stays on the hillsides as it travels through an area recovering from a catastrophic burn. Views of the river and the flanking canyon walls are frequent, and, apart from all the blackened snags, the hiking is very pleasant on this gently graded up-and-down trail. You pass a junction with the Hoodoo Trail that goes left (south). Continue upstream another 0.8 mile to a large river-level flat called Fairview Bar, which used to be a delightful place to camp. However, as it recovers from a forest fire, it is overgrown with vegetation, and the abundance of hazard trees makes it an undesirable, not to mention unsafe, place to camp. A small and somewhat more appealing campsite is located approximately 0.25 mile before reaching Fairview Bar.

GRIZZLY BEAR RIDGE SIDE TRIP: A long but excellent day hike from Fairview Bar follows the Wenaha River Trail upstream for 7.3 scenic miles to Rock Creek. At that point you turn right (north) and climb the Grizzly Bear Ridge Trail for 1.3 miles to a ridgetop switchback with a spectacular view of the Wenaha River Canyon. This side trip features some of the canyon's best scenery and gives you the opportunity to fully appreciate the many joys of this wilderness stream.

WARNING: Large sections of the trail along the river and up to Grizzly Bear Ridge are still recovering from an intense wildfire. The junction with the Grizzly Bear Ridge Trail, located just before you cross Rock Creek, may be indistinct. You should also expect to encounter significant downfall along this side trip for the next few years.

NOTE: Hikers who don't want to go all the way to Grizzly Bear Ridge can turn back at any time, amply rewarded by fine canyon scenery.

From Fairview Bar your loop route follows an unsigned trail that goes north from the burned trees at the north end of the meadow. The beginning of this trail is indistinct, but, once located, the route is easy to follow as it traverses the open slopes. The route is steep at times as you climb in irregular traverses and switchbacks through partial forest, and then break out onto steep, grassy slopes covered with wildflowers in May and early June. Look for Lomatium, clarkia, buckwheat, gilia, paintbrush, and a host of other colorful blossoms. The trail climbs steadily through this scenic area, but with all the rest stops needed to look at flowers and take pictures of the canyon, it's easy not to notice the climb.

Eventually, you'll reach the top of the canyon's steepest slopes, but the trail continues to gradually gain elevation as it enters forest recovering from an intense burn in 2015 along the edge of Moore Flat.

WARNING: The trail is extremely difficult to follow in this area. Be prepared to rely on maps and a compass or GPS to stay on course.

Continue climbing through recovering forest, and come to a small creek on the left. You bear left (west) here, cross the creek, and climb mostly in trees but with occasional open areas. Several unmarked routes take off in various directions to points used by hunters and livestock ranchers. Stick with the main trail. Your route crosses another small creek, and then works up to the top of Smooth Ridge, where there is a poorly marked junction with the Packer Trail and partly obstructed views of the Crooked Creek Valley to the north.

Your route goes west along this forested ridge and then comes to a large meadow, where there is a hunter's camp with water from Twin Spring, which has a convenient trough made from a tree trunk. Evidence of the intensity of the burn diminishes noticeably as you approach Twin Spring, and as you continue to Weller Butte, you finally reenter unburned forest. The main trail goes left (downhill) around the camp before regaining the lost elevation back up to Smooth Ridge, which gets narrower as the path continues to climb. At the top of Weller Butte there are good if somewhat obstructed views of the deep canyons on both sides. The forests at these higher elevations are composed of Douglas firs, western larches, lodgepole pines, and subalpine firs.

NOTE: Although there are ups and downs yet to come, the hardest climbing of the trip is now over. From Fairview Bar you have gained a total of about 3,600 feet.

From Weller Butte your trail steeply loses elevation on the rocky north slope of the peak, reaches a saddle, and then once again climbs up the ridge. At the top you come to a gentler ridgetop and turn north. After another 0.3 mile you'll come to the edge of an irregularly shaped open area (the vegetation is too sparse to call it a meadow), with good camps in the nearby trees. Lodgepole Spring, a vital source of water, is located a bit below the trail on the right.

NOTE: It can be easy to lose the main trail around Lodgepole Spring, as it braids and leads to various hunting camps or meadows for grazing. The main trail remains in the woods and stays below the open areas as it leaves Lodgepole Spring.

TIP: Elk are common here, as they are throughout the Wenaha-Tucannon Wilderness. An evening or morning stroll through the open areas above the trail is a good way to see these impressive animals.

From Lodgepole Spring you continue north along a relatively gentle ridgetop. You pass the uninviting trickle of Rettkowski Spring and shortly thereafter Huckleberry Spring, both less appealing than Lodgepole Spring for camping. Now you return to the wide ridgeline and make a series of gentle ups and downs. About 1.4 miles north of Huckleberry Spring, the trail leaves the ridge and drops briefly into the trees to the right at a signed junction with the short trail to McBain Spring.

WARNING: Early in the year, the route here may be lost in snow and downed trees. Navigate carefully.

After leaving the wide ridge, you continue north past an outcrop called Danger Point and hike along a narrow ridgeline with excellent views. Upper Crooked Creek Canyon drops off to the east; to the west are the rugged upper reaches of East Fork Butte Creek, and straight ahead is Oregon Butte, the highest point in the wilderness.

As the ridge rises to Oregon Butte, the trail cuts across the east side of a very scenic hillside with wildflowers, rocky viewpoints, and scattered trees. The path then gains some elevation to a saddle north of Oregon Butte, where there is a trail junction.

OREGON BUTTE SIDE TRIP: Don't miss the short side trip to the fire lookout atop Oregon Butte. Lookouts are always fun to visit for their interesting history, architecture, and views, but the one atop Oregon Butte—with a 360-degree panorama of the rugged canyons, forests, and ridges of the Wenaha-Tucannon country—is especially worthwhile. At 6,387 feet, Oregon Butte is the high point of this trip, in more ways than one.

TIP: Thirsty hikers will want to make a short side trip to Oregon Butte Spring. To reach it, hike west from the junction north of Oregon Butte, and go 0.2 mile on Trail #3143. You can camp at the spring or on nearby ridges, from which you will enjoy spectacular sunsets.

Back on the main trail, you descend through forests, following the ridgeline to the north. You reach a narrow saddle and then go up and down another mile through rather monotonous forests with only occasional views through the trees. The trail finally reaches a wider ridgetop, turns northeast, and begins to emerge from the forest into large meadows.

TIP: Look for elk and black bear in this area, especially in the mornings and evenings.

The trail climbs a bit and enters a large, gently rolling ridgetop meadow, where several unsigned paths intersect your route. An especially confusing path goes southeast out a wide ridge, but the proper route travels north for 0.4 mile to a signed junction near Indian Corral.

NOTE: This sign was tied to a tree on a recent summer hike and is easy to miss.

Here you turn right (northeast) and go through an attractive mix of open areas and trees for 0.2 mile to another junction. To reach the welcome clear waters and good camps at bubbling Dunlap Spring, turn right (east) at this junction and descend 0.1 mile through forest.

TIP: If you spend the night here, be sure to return to the open meadows near the trail junction around dusk. You'll have a good chance of seeing elk, deer, owls, and other wildlife.

To complete your tour, return to the trail junction above Dunlap Spring and hike northeast. The route alternates between open ridges, rocky areas, and high forests as it loops first east then south. In the sloping meadows around Clover Spring are some fine views to the southwest of Oregon Butte. Most of the hiking is fairly gentle, with only short steep sections. Unmarked routes branch off to small springs and unnamed ridges, but the main path is fairly obvious. Past Bear Wallow Spring, about 3 miles from Dunlap Spring, the view-packed trail skirts the edge of some cliffs above the headwaters of Third Creek. Although it has several small ups and downs, the trail generally gains elevation as it continues southeast. At Squaw Spring, in the trees on your left, you'll find water and a good campsite.

Beyond Squaw Spring you alternate between low hills and saddles, as the trail turns more directly east, passes a superb clifftop viewpoint above the canyon of Second Creek to the south, and then drops to a saddle with a good campsite above trickling Sheephead Spring. Just beyond here, more clifftop viewpoints provide occasional glimpses to the south.

WARNING: This section of trail is at elevations over 6,000 feet, so there are occasional snow patches here through mid-June. If snow hides the tread, stick with an easterly course and you should be fine.

The many open areas along this section of trail support lots of colorful wildflowers in June and early July.

The final part of your hike drops to a saddle before returning to the junction near Diamond Peak that you passed on day one. From here you head east to your vehicle by making the short hike back out the way you came in.

VARIATION

Although the trails are almost completely melted out by early June, lingering snow on the road to the Mount Misery Trailhead often makes it inaccessible until as late as mid-June. If you'd like to hike this before the road opens up, or would prefer to avoid driving the rough section of road near the trailhead, this loop can also be accessed via the Panjab Trailhead off Forest Service Road 4713 on the northwest border of the wilderness. Hike the Panjab Trail approximately 5.5 miles east (with 2,500 feet of elevation gain) to Indian Corral and then proceed to hike this loop as described.

POSSIBLE ITINERARY

	CAMP	MILES	ELEVATION GAIN
Day 1	Melton Creek	10.3	200'
Day 2	Fairview Bar	8.4	300'
Day 3	Fairview Bar		
	Day hike to Grizzly Bear Ridge view	17.2	1,600'
Day 4	Lodgepole Spring	10.2	5,300'
Day 5	Dunlap Spring	10.0	1,450'
	Side trip to Oregon Butte	0.5	250'
Day 6	Out	7.2	1,200'

BEST SHORTER ALTERNATIVES

The best day hike sampler here is the short ramble to Oregon Butte from the Teepee trailhead to the west. For a fun short overnight option, try a loop trip in the northwest part of the wilderness that goes up the Tucannon River to Jelly Spring and Diamond Peak and then turns west along the scenic ridge to Dunlap Spring before exiting to the northwest from near Indian Corral.

OTHER BACKPACKING OPTIONS

Though this book includes what the authors consider to be the best long backpacking trips in Washington, there are many other options for the adventurous hiker. With some creativity and a good set of topographic maps, a backpacker could spend a lifetime exploring the mountains, forests, and shorelines of this state.

What follows is an overview of some additional recommended trips, with just enough description to whet the appetite. As these are only general suggestions without detailed descriptions, no permit information or maps are provided for these hikes.

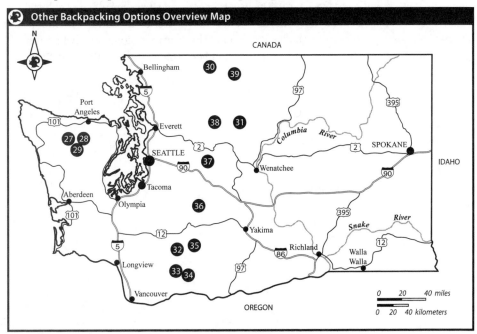

Other Backpacking Options Overview Map

27

BAILEY RANGE TRAVERSE

RATINGS: Scenery 10   **Solitude** 6   **Difficulty** 10

MILES: 40–60

DAYS: 6–10

MAPS: Custom Correct *Elwha Valley* and *Seven Lakes Basin–Hoh*

USUALLY OPEN: Late July–September

BEST: August

SPECIAL ATTRACTIONS

Amazing mountain scenery, wildlife

CHALLENGES

Many miles of off-trail travel over very rugged terrain, route-finding difficulties, unpredictable (and often just plain lousy) weather

GPS TRAILHEAD COORDINATES: N47° 57.297' W123° 50.092'

S trictly for very experienced hikers who are comfortable with tough off-trail travel, this rugged outing in the central Olympic Mountains features some of the greatest scenery in North America (no exaggeration)—assuming, that is, that the weather is good and you are willing to work for it. The usual itinerary starts at the Sol Duc Trailhead (see Trip 3); you hike up to High Divide, then follow the trailless divide south from Mount Carrie. You can exit either from Dodwell-Rixon Pass by returning along the Elwha River or, for a shorter alternative, leave the ridge at Mount Ferry and cut over to the Long Ridge Trail at Dodger Point.

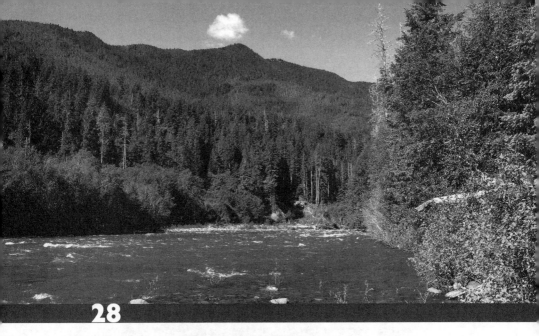

28
ELWHA–QUINAULT
CROSS-OLYMPICS TRAVERSE

RATINGS: Scenery 5   **Solitude** 4   **Difficulty** 4
MILES: 45
DAYS: 3–5
MAPS: Custom Correct *Elwha Valley* and *Quinault–Colonel Bob*
USUALLY OPEN: Late June–October
BEST: July/mid-October

SPECIAL ATTRACTIONS

Beautiful rivers, waterfalls, historical interest

CHALLENGES

Limited mountain views, sometimes crowded, long car shuttle

GPS TRAILHEAD COORDINATES: Elwha (start): N47º 58.075' W123º 34.950'
North Quinault (end): N47º 34.549' W123º 38.884'

This is a popular north-south route across the Olympic Mountains. It starts on the Elwha River near Port Angeles and ends at the North Fork Quinault River Trailhead above Lake Quinault. Most of the path follows lovely streams that cascade

Above: *Elwha River below Humes Ranch*
photographed by Douglas Lorain

through the heavy forests of these viewless canyons. Only near Low Divide do you get a quick glimpse of the peaks.

TIP: Don't miss a side trip from just north of Low Divide into the alpine wonderland of Martins Park.

Probably the biggest attraction of this trip is that it follows the historic route of the Press Expedition of 1889–1890. It took this intrepid group more than six months to explore the interior of the Olympic Mountains—one of the last wild areas in the Lower 48 states to be surveyed. You, however, can now comfortably complete the trip in about four days.

29

NORTH QUINAULT–SKYLINE TRAIL LOOP

RATINGS: Scenery 8   **Solitude** 7   **Difficulty** 10
MILES: 42
DAYS: 3–6
MAP: Custom Correct *Quinault–Colonel Bob*
USUALLY OPEN: Mid-July–October
BEST: August

SPECIAL ATTRACTIONS

Wildlife, solitude, excellent views

CHALLENGES

Very rough and sketchy trail along ridge; black bears are common—use a bear canister

GPS TRAILHEAD COORDINATES: N47º 34.549' W123º 38.884'

This rugged loop explores the southwestern Olympic Mountains by following the North Quinault River Trail to Low Divide and returning along the rarely used Skyline Trail. The varied scenery includes a beautiful river, lush forests, and a long ridge with outstanding views. Wildlife is abundant, with good opportunities to observe both elk and black bears. Much of the route along the Skyline Trail, however, is so faint and rugged that it requires an extraordinary amount of both physical and mental energy to follow. The trip is only recommended for very fit backpackers who are experienced at route finding. Anyone else would probably find this hike too difficult to enjoy.

30

BEAVER LOOP

RATINGS: Scenery 7   **Solitude** 5   **Difficulty** 6
MILES: 30+
DAYS: 3–5
MAP: Trails Illustrated *North Cascades National Park (#223)*
USUALLY OPEN: Late July–October
BEST: August–September

SPECIAL ATTRACTIONS

Beautiful old-growth forests

CHALLENGES

Boat transportation complexities and expense

GPS TRAILHEAD COORDINATES: Ross Lake Resort: N48° 43.665' W121° 03.760'

Big trees, especially cedars, are the star attraction of this loop in the northeastern part of North Cascades National Park. Mountain views are limited, but for a few miles around Beaver Pass, there are some fine vistas of the mountains and glaciers of Luna Cirque.

To reach the north trailhead you must take the Ross Lake shuttle boat to Little Beaver Creek. Follow Little Beaver Trail up this forested canyon, then turn south on Big Beaver Trail and climb over Beaver Pass. From here you follow Big Beaver Creek down through huge forests and past meadows and marshes back to Ross Lake.

To return to civilization you can either arrange for the boat to pick you up or follow a pleasant shoreline trail and cross the dam. To reserve a boat trip, call the Ross Lake Resort water taxi service at 206-486-3751. For a free but required backcountry camping permit, contact the Marblemount Ranger Station at 360-854-7245.

31

NORTH FORK ENTIAT RIVER LOOP

RATINGS: Scenery 7   **Solitude** 7   **Difficulty** 6
MILES: 25+
DAYS: 2–5
MAP: Green Trails *Lucerne (#114)*
USUALLY OPEN: Late June–October
BEST: Very late September–early October

SPECIAL ATTRACTIONS

Excellent views, larch trees in full autumn glory

CHALLENGES

Steep and poorly defined trail in some places

GPS TRAILHEAD COORDINATES: N48º 00.673' W120º 34.327'

High meadows, high lakes, and even higher ridges sporting terrific fall colors and fine scenery highlight this outing that visits North Fork Entiat River, gorgeous Fern Lake, Grouse Pass, and Pyramid Mountain. That last destination features an almost scary view that looks seemingly straight down almost 7,000 feet to Lake Chelan.

32

JUNIPER AND LANGILLE RIDGES

RATINGS: Scenery 8   **Solitude** 6   **Difficulty** 6
MILES: 29
DAYS: 3–4
MAP: Green Trails *McCoy Peak (#333)*
USUALLY OPEN: Late July–October
BEST: August–September

SPECIAL ATTRACTIONS

Great ridgetop views, interesting rock formations

CHALLENGES

Rugged trails, motorcycles allowed on trails

GPS TRAILHEAD COORDINATES: Juniper (start): N46° 23.802' W121° 45.918'
Langille (end): N46° 22.903' W121° 49.836'

These two adjacent ridges at the headwaters of the Cispus River south of Randle feature high and ruggedly scenic trails. They can be combined into a fun horseshoe
loop with a reasonable car shuttle. Expect endless views, photogenic rock outcrops, and wildflower-filled meadows. Sadly, the trails are often badly eroded by motor-
ized wheels.

33

INDIAN HEAVEN COUNTRY

RATINGS: Scenery 7   Solitude 5   Difficulty 3
MILES: Varies
DAYS: Varies
MAP: USFS *Mount Adams, Indian Heaven, and Trapper Creek Wildernesses*
USUALLY OPEN: July–late October
BEST: Early–mid-October

SPECIAL ATTRACTIONS

Gentle terrain (good family hiking), lots of lakes and meadows, great fall colors,
huckleberries

CHALLENGES

Clouds of mosquitoes in July, many of the best older trails are no longer shown on maps

GPS TRAILHEAD COORDINATES: East Crater (suggested): N45° 58.866' W121° 45.492'

The Indian Heaven Wilderness is a compact area in the Gifford Pinchot National
Forest west of Trout Lake. The wilderness lacks high peaks but makes up for it with
countless scenic lakes and absolutely gorgeous meadows. The landscape is especially attractive in early October, when the golden-colored meadows, red vine maples,
and orange huckleberry bushes put on one of the best fall-color displays in the state. The
wilderness's small size limits the opportunities for long-distance backpackers, but this is a
wonderful area to spend time with the kids exploring from a base camp. There are a number of possible options, but one excellent base camp is at centrally located Junction Lake.

THE PACIFIC CREST TRAIL

The primary selection criterion for the hikes included in this book was outstanding scenery, with additional consideration given to "special" features like fall colors and unique geology. With more places to see in Washington than you could possibly visit in a lifetime, the authors see no sense in wasting your time on less than the best. Other hikers, however, have different and no less worthy goals. Many backpackers, for example, have an ambition to hike the entire Washington section of the Pacific Crest Trail (PCT). Although several parts of the PCT have been included in the featured trips section, they are there only because the authors felt they were among the best trails in the state. No effort was made to include the PCT (or any other trail) just for the sake of its name recognition.

For the benefit of backpackers who are doing the PCT in segments (the usual plan), the following is a quick overview of the most logical one- to two-week trips.

TIP: No extended trip on the Washington section of the PCT would be complete without a copy of *Pacific Crest Trail: Oregon and Washington* (Wilderness Press). This unique guidebook provides a wealth of detailed and very useful information on campsites, dangers, and wildlife, and it provides a complete description of every mile along the trail. Anyone hiking the PCT for more than a few days will find this to be an invaluable resource.

34

COLUMBIA RIVER TO MOUNT ADAMS

MILES: 82
BEST: Mid-October

GPS TRAILHEAD COORDINATES: North Bonneville (start): N45º 39.024' W121º 55.967'
FS 23 (end): N46º 10.236' W121º 37.668'

Most of this section is rather dull, as it travels through viewless forests and often near roads. The best features of the hike are ripe huckleberries in late August and fall colors in October.

35

MOUNT ADAMS TO WHITE PASS

MILES: 65
BEST: Late July

GPS TRAILHEAD COORDINATES: FS 23 (start): N46º 10.236' W121º 37.668'
End: N46º 38.698' W121º 22.953'

This is a fabulously scenic section through two very attractive wilderness areas—Mount Adams and Goat Rocks. Beware of some dangerously exposed sections in the Goat Rocks Wilderness (see description for Trip 20).

36

WHITE PASS TO SNOQUALMIE PASS

MILES: 99
BEST: Late July/early October

GPS TRAILHEAD COORDINATES: Start: N46º 38.698' W121º 22.953'
End: N47º 25.668' W121º 24.810'

The southern part of this segment is quite pleasant, with lots of lakes and flowers, and occasional views of Mount Rainier. North of the Norse Peak Wilderness, however, the scenery becomes relatively dull with lots of clear-cuts. In addition, the lake country north of White Pass is infested with mosquitoes in July. Most hikers will enjoy the southern part of this section, especially during fall-color time, but the rest is a bit of a slog.

37

SNOQUALMIE PASS TO STEVENS PASS

MILES: 83 (without side trips)
BEST: Very late July–August

GPS TRAILHEAD COORDINATES: Start: N47° 25.668' W121° 24.810'
End: N47° 44.772' W121° 05.160'

This spectacular trail section is fully described in Trip 17.

38

STEVENS PASS TO RAINY PASS

MILES: 117
BEST: August

GPS TRAILHEAD COORDINATES: Start: N47° 44.772' W121° 05.160'
Bridge Creek (end): N48° 30.300' W120° 43.146'

This very long but wildly scenic section initially goes through relatively gentle terrain in the Henry M. Jackson Wilderness. North of that preserve, you'll tour the rugged and spectacular Glacier Peak Wilderness before dropping into the canyons of the Stehekin River and Bridge Creek. There is no road access and the route is rather long, so your pack will be quite heavy at the beginning.

39

RAINY PASS TO CANADA

MILES: 69
BEST: Early August/late September

GPS TRAILHEAD COORDINATES: Bridge Creek (start): N48° 30.300' W120° 43.146'
Manning Park (end): N49° 03.589' W120° 45.665'

This is arguably the finest section of the PCT in Washington because of its great wildflower displays, its expansive views, and the reasonable chance of solitude. There are two outstanding times to make the trip. The first is late July and early August, when the ridgetop meadows are bursting with colorful wildflowers. A less-well-known time to visit is in very late September, when the alpine larches splash the hillsides with gold.

INDEX

C

D

ABOUT THE AUTHORS

Douglas Lorain's family moved to the Pacific Northwest in 1969, and he has been hitting the trails of his home region ever since. With the good fortune to grow up in an outdoor-oriented family, he has vivid memories of countless camping, hiking, bird-watching, and other trips in every hidden corner of this spectacular area. He calculates that, over the years, he has logged well over 32,000 trail miles in this part of the continent, and despite a history that includes developing a nasty case of giardia, being bitten by a rattlesnake, being shot at by a hunter, getting stuck in quicksand, being charged by grizzly bears (twice!), and donating countless gallons of blood to "invertebrate vampires," he happily sees no end in sight.

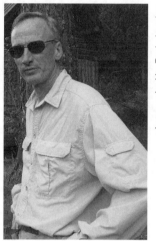

photographed by Becky Lovejoy

Doug is a photographer and recipient of the prestigious National Outdoor Book Award. His books cover only the best trips from the thousands of hikes and backpacking trips he has taken throughout Washington, Oregon, Idaho, and beyond. His photographs have been featured in numerous magazines, calendars, and books, and his other guidebook titles include *Afoot & Afield: Portland/Vancouver, Backpacking Idaho, Backpacking Oregon, Backpacking Wyoming, One Best Hike: Mount Rainier's Wonderland Trail, 100 Classic Hikes in Oregon, 100 Classic Hikes: Montana,* and *Top Trails: Olympic National Park & Vicinity.*

After spending decades exploring the trails of the Pacific Northwest, he now lives in Hamilton, Montana, with his wife, Becky Lovejoy, and their yellow Labrador retriever, Seabrook.

continued on page 268

Mark Wetherington began backpacking in 2007 while a student at the University of Kentucky and obsessively explored the trails and landforms of the Southeast before moving to Montana in 2014. Since arriving in Big Sky Country, he has spent as much time as possible exploring the wilderness areas and other public lands of Montana, Washington, and Idaho via boots, snowshoes, and cross-country skis. Seeking the next "best place to wake up"—from alpine lakes to hot springs to abandoned fire lookouts—serves as his main inspiration for backpacking.

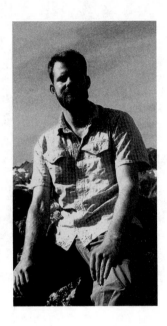

Mark has worked in outdoor retail and libraries, as a freelance writer, and as a visitor services information assistant for the U.S. Forest Service in Kentucky's Red River Gorge. He has been lucky enough to find a career working in public libraries and lives in Hamilton, Montana.